Health Benefits of Mediterranean Diet

Health Benefits of Mediterranean Diet

Special Issue Editors

Giuseppe Grosso
Daniela Martini

MDPI • Basel • Beijing • Wuhan • Barcelona • Belgrade

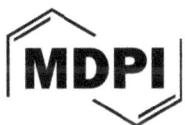

Special Issue Editors
Giuseppe Grosso
University of Catania
Italy

Daniela Martini
University of Parma
Italy

Editorial Office
MDPI
St. Alban-Anlage 66
4052 Basel, Switzerland

This is a reprint of articles from the Special Issue published online in the open access journal *Nutrients* (ISSN 2072-6643) from 2018 to 2019 (available at: https://www.mdpi.com/journal/nutrients/special_issues/Mediterranean_Diet_Benefits)

For citation purposes, cite each article independently as indicated on the article page online and as indicated below:

LastName, A.A.; LastName, B.B.; LastName, C.C. Article Title. *Journal Name* **Year**, *Article Number*, Page Range.

ISBN 978-3-03921-493-8 (Pbk)
ISBN 978-3-03921-494-5 (PDF)

© 2019 by the authors. Articles in this book are Open Access and distributed under the Creative Commons Attribution (CC BY) license, which allows users to download, copy and build upon published articles, as long as the author and publisher are properly credited, which ensures maximum dissemination and a wider impact of our publications.
The book as a whole is distributed by MDPI under the terms and conditions of the Creative Commons license CC BY-NC-ND.

Contents

About the Special Issue Editors vii

Daniela Martini
Health Benefits of Mediterranean Diet
Reprinted from: *Nutrients* **2019**, *11*, 1802, doi:10.3390/nu11081802 1

Elena S. George, Teagan Kucianski, Hannah L. Mayr, George Moschonis, Audrey C. Tierney and Catherine Itsiopoulos
A Mediterranean Diet Model in Australia: Strategies for Translating the Traditional Mediterranean Diet into a Multicultural Setting
Reprinted from: *Nutrients* **2018**, *10*, 465, doi:10.3390/nu10040465 5

Félix Zurita-Ortega, Silvia San Román-Mata, Ramón Chacón-Cuberos, Manuel Castro-Sánchez and José Joaquín Muros
Adherence to the Mediterranean Diet Is Associated with Physical Activity, Self-Concept and Sociodemographic Factors in University Student
Reprinted from: *Nutrients* **2018**, *10*, 966, doi:10.3390/nu10080966 25

Marilena Vitale, Maria Masulli, Ilaria Calabrese, Angela Albarosa Rivellese, Enzo Bonora, Stefano Signorini, Gabriele Perriello, Sebastiano Squatrito, Raffaella Buzzetti, Giovanni Sartore, Anna Carla Babini, Giovanna Gregori, Carla Giordano, Gennaro Clemente, Sara Grioni, Pasquale Dolce, Gabriele Riccardi, Olga Vaccaro and on behalf of the TOSCA.IT Study Group
Impact of a Mediterranean Dietary Pattern and Its Components on Cardiovascular Risk Factors, Glucose Control, and Body Weight in People with Type 2 Diabetes: A Real-Life Study
Reprinted from: *Nutrients* **2018**, *10*, 1067, doi:10.3390/nu10081067 36

Francesca Archero, Roberta Ricotti, Arianna Solito, Deborah Carrera, Federica Civello, Rosina Di Bella, Simonetta Bellone and Flavia Prodam
Adherence to the Mediterranean Diet among School Children and Adolescents Living in Northern Italy and Unhealthy Food Behaviors Associated to Overweight
Reprinted from: *Nutrients* **2018**, *10*, 1322, doi:10.3390/nu10091322 48

José Joaquín Muros and Mikel Zabala
Differences in Mediterranean Diet Adherence between Cyclists and Triathletes in a Sample of Spanish Athletes
Reprinted from: *Nutrients* **2018**, *10*, 1480, doi:10.3390/nu10101480 61

Sara Castro-Barquero, Rosa M. Lamuela-Raventós, Mónica Doménech and Ramon Estruch
Relationship between Mediterranean Dietary Polyphenol Intake and Obesity
Reprinted from: *Nutrients* **2018**, *10*, 1523, doi:10.3390/nu10101523 72

Harriet Kretowicz, Vanora Hundley and Fotini Tsofliou
Exploring the Perceived Barriers to Following a Mediterranean Style Diet in Childbearing Age: A Qualitative Study
Reprinted from: *Nutrients* **2018**, *10*, 1694, doi:10.3390/nu10111694 85

Kenia M. B. Carvalho, Débora B. Ronca, Nathalie Michels, Inge Huybrechts,
Magdalena Cuenca-Garcia, Ascensión Marcos, Dénes Molnár, Jean Dallongeville,
Yannis Manios, Beatriz D. Schaan, Luis Moreno, Stefaan de Henauw and Livia A. Carvalho
Does the Mediterranean Diet Protect against Stress-Induced Inflammatory Activation in
European Adolescents? The HELENA Study
Reprinted from: *Nutrients* 2018, *10*, 1770, doi:10.3390/nu10111770 100

Ramón Chacón-Cuberos, Georgian Badicu, Félix Zurita-Ortega and Manuel Castro-Sánchez
Mediterranean Diet and Motivation in Sport: A Comparative Study Between University
Students from Spain and Romania
Reprinted from: *Nutrients* 2019, *11*, 30, doi:10.3390/nu11010030 109

Qi Jin, Alicen Black, Stefanos N. Kales, Dhiraj Vattem, Miguel Ruiz-Canela and Mercedes
Sotos-Prieto
Metabolomics and Microbiomes as Potential Tools to Evaluate the Effects of the
Mediterranean Diet
Reprinted from: *Nutrients* 2019, *11*, 207, doi:10.3390/nu11010207 123

Cristian Del Bo', Mirko Marino, Daniela Martini, Massimiliano Tucci,
Salvatore Ciappellano, Patrizia Riso and Marisa Porrini
Overview of Human Intervention Studies Evaluating the Impact of the Mediterranean Diet on
Markers of DNA Damage
Reprinted from: *Nutrients* 2019, *11*, 391, doi:10.3390/nu11020391 150

Justyna Godos, Raffaele Ferri, Filippo Caraci, Filomena Irene Ilaria Cosentino,
Sabrina Castellano, Fabio Galvano and Giuseppe Grosso
Adherence to the Mediterranean Diet is Associated with Better Sleep Quality in Italian Adults
Reprinted from: *Nutrients* 2019, *11*, 976, doi:10.3390/nu11050976 163

Justyna Godos, Sabrina Castellano and Marina Marranzano
Adherence to a Mediterranean Dietary Pattern Is Associated with Higher Quality of Life in a
Cohort of Italian Adults
Reprinted from: *Nutrients* 2019, *11*, 981, doi:10.3390/nu11050981 178

Carlotta Biagi, Mattia Di Nunzio, Alessandra Bordoni, Davide Gori and Marcello Lanari
Effect of Adherence to Mediterranean Diet during Pregnancy on Children's Health:
A Systematic Review
Reprinted from: *Nutrients* 2019, *11*, 997, doi:10.3390/nu11050997 190

Annunziata D'Alessandro, Luisa Lampignano and Giovanni De Pergola
Mediterranean Diet Pyramid: A Proposal for Italian People. A Systematic Review of
Prospective Studies to Derive Serving Sizes
Reprinted from: *Nutrients* 2019, *11*, 1296, doi:10.3390/nu11061296 215

Santa D'Innocenzo, Carlotta Biagi and Marcello Lanari
Obesity and the Mediterranean Diet: A Review of Evidence of the Role and Sustainability of the
Mediterranean Diet
Reprinted from: *Nutrients* 2019, *11*, 1306, doi:10.3390/nu11061306 242

About the Special Issue Editors

Giuseppe Grosso's research focuses on evidence-based nutrition, a field emerging from the application of the Health Technology Assessment to food and nutrition. His main interests include the impact of dietary and lifestyle habits on common non-communicable diseases. In doing his research, he has written over 100 papers on the effects of dietary patterns (i.e., the Mediterranean diet) and specific antioxidant-rich foods (i.e., coffee, tea), as well as individual antioxidants (i.e., polyphenols, n-3 PUFA) on cardiovascular and metabolic diseases, cancer, and depression. Collaborating with several research institutions, Dr. Grosso has conducted his research on cohorts of individuals in both Mediterranean and non-Mediterranean countries. He is interested in the synthesis of evidence aimed to generate policy-oriented research in the area of public health nutrition. Dr. Grosso's research also aims to measure planetary health, including the potential impact of nutrition at a global level. Dr. Giuseppe Grosso is also a medical doctor who graduated cum laude. He holds a specialization in public health and a Ph.D. in neuropharmacology. He is currently working as an Assistant Professor of Human Nutrition at the Department of Biomedical and Biotechnological Sciences, School of Medicine, University of Catania, Italy.

Daniela Martini is a Post-Doctoral Research Fellow at the Human Nutrition Unit of the University of Parma. She has attained a PhD in Food Science and Nutrition. Her expertise includes the following: The analysis of antioxidant compounds in foods, the evaluation of the role of bioactive-rich foods in the modulation of markers of oxidative stress in in vivo models, and food legislation (e.g., food labeling, nutrition and health claims)

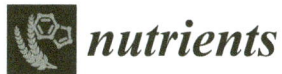

Editorial

Health Benefits of Mediterranean Diet

Daniela Martini *

Human Nutrition Unit, Department of Veterinary Science, University of Parma, 43125 Parma, Italy

Received: 1 August 2019; Accepted: 2 August 2019; Published: 5 August 2019

Growing evidence shows that a dietary pattern inspired by Mediterranean Diet (MD) principles is associated with numerous health benefits [1,2]. A Mediterranean-type diet has been demonstrated to exert a preventive effect toward cardiovascular diseases, in both Mediterranean and non-Mediterranean populations [1,3]. These properties may in part depend on the positive action on the cardiometabolic risk [4,5], by decreasing the risk of diabetes and metabolic-related conditions [6–8]. There is also evidence of a potential role of the Mediterranean diet in preventing certain cancers [9]. Finally, a new field of research has showed that a higher adherence to the Mediterranean diet is associated with a lower risk of mental disorders, including cognitive decline and depression [10–12]. Overall, a better understanding of the key elements of this dietary pattern, the underlying mechanisms, and targets, are needed to corroborate current evidence and provide insights on new and potential outcomes.

The Special Issue "Health Benefits of Mediterranean Diet" was devoted to collect original research and reviews of literature concerning the Mediterranean diet and various health outcomes. New information has been added in this field by means of 16 articles, with nine original papers, six reviews/meta-analysis and one opinion.

A widely considered aspect was the evaluation of the adherence to the MD in different target populations. An Italian study found a poor adherence in 16.7% of a group of 669 subjects (6–16 years) attending five schools from the North Italy, with poor adherence more frequent in primary than in secondary schools [13].

Among two other studies from Spanish groups of research, the first investigated the relationship between adherence to MD, physical activity, self-concept (i.e., the collection of beliefs about oneself), and other sociodemographic factors in a group of Spanish university students. Results showed that MD adherence, measured by means of the Mediterranean Diet Quality Index (KIDMED), was associated with academic and physical self-concept [14].

In the second one, Muros and Zabala investigated the adherence to MD in two groups of cyclists and triathletes, finding a large proportion of the surveyed athletic population not meeting the MD guidelines, with particularly low adherence amongst men and cyclists [15].

The adherence to the MD was also investigated by the group of Chacon-Cuberos who evaluated the relationships between adherence to the MD and motivational climate in sport on a sample of university students from Spain and Romania [16]. Results showed a higher adherence in students from Spain compared to Romanians and observed that ego-oriented climates (measured as unequal recognition, member rivalry and punishment for mistakes) are linked to a better adherence to the MD, especially due to the importance of following a proper diet in sport contexts.

Besides measuring the adherence to MD in different contexts, it is also interesting to identify the perceived barriers to follow the MD, which might lead to low MD adherence. In this scenario, Kretowicz and colleagues considered women of childbearing age and identified five barriers and enablers (Mediterranean diet features, perceived benefits, existing dietary behavior and knowledge, practical factors, and information source) that should be considered in the design and development of an intervention to effectively promote and encourage adherence to the MD [17].

As already mentioned, a high adherence to the MD has been extensively associated with a number of health outcomes, and several manuscripts of this Special Issue explored this association. Firstly, two observational studies by Godos and colleagues [18,19] showed a linear association between the overall quality of life and adherence to the MD score in a cohort of over 2000 Italian adults. Authors also evaluate whether subjects found a better sleep quality by following MD, either toward direct effect on health or indirect effects through improvement of weight status.

The role of MD on body weight and other outcomes has been also investigated by an Italian group who observed that a high MD score was associated with lower values of plasma lipids and glycated hemoglobin, blood pressure and body mass index in people with type-2 diabetes [20], thus supporting the MD as a suitable model also in these subjects. The association between MD and obesity has been also considered and discussed in other two reviews included in this Special issue.

Firstly, Castro-Barquero et al. reviewed the evidence on the relationship between the polyphenol intake in the frame of the MD (e.g., from extra-virgin olive oil, nuts and legumes) and obesity [21]. Findings evidenced that, despite the intake of some specific polyphenols has been associated with body weight improvements, there is no strong evidence of an association between polyphenols intake and lowering of body adiposity.

A second review was proposed by D'Innocenzo and coworkers who highlighted the importance of public policy measures to make a healthy diet easily accessible and affordable. [22] This advice has been deepen as for general population as for target groups (e.g., children and adolescents), in order to tackle obesity epidemic by considering that "Diet as not just a food model, but also as the most appropriate regime for disease prevention, a sort of complete lifestyle plan for the pursuit of healthcare sustainability".

The adherence to the MD has been also associated to inflammation in an investigation performed within the HELENA study [23]. Results evidenced a counteracting effect of stress on inflammatory biomarkers with high MD adherence, with stress being a significant independent negative predictor of a healthy dietary pattern.

Lastly, the study by Del Bo' and colleagues systematically reviewed the human intervention studies evaluating the impact of Mediterranean diet on markers of DNA damage, reporting a reduction in the levels of 8-hydroxy-2′–deoxyguanosine and a modulation of DNA repair gene expression and telomere length [24].

The Special Issue also included other aspects relating to the MD, such as serving size and translation of the MD to other diets. Firstly, D'Alessandro and coworkers performed a systematic review of dose-response meta-analyses of prospective studies, which evaluated the association between the intake of food groups belonging to a variant of the Modern Mediterranean Diet Pyramid and the risk of CVD [25]. Among the different aspects worth to be studied, the serving sizes of the foods seems to have a key role in order to obtain a protective or a not detrimental effect toward selected diseases. This supports the idea that a throughout definition of MD must consider not only the types of food but also their amounts and frequency of consumption. Being the efficacy and feasibility of MD for the management of chronic diseases not been extensively evaluated in non-Mediterranean settings, the paper by George and coworkers [26] increased knowledge about potential strategies for translating the traditional MD into a non-Mediterranean setting.

A different shade of evidence has been added by the work of Biagi et al., a systematic review investigating the effect of the MD during pregnancy on birth outcome [27]. Despite authors concluded that data were insufficient and further randomized control trials are needed to draw clear conclusions, growing evidence seem to suggest a beneficial effect of the Mediterranean diet during pregnancy on children's health.

One of the main challenges when trying to investigate the role of the MD on health is related to the accurate assessment of exposure to this dietary pattern. In this framework, the manuscript by Jin et al. focused on metabolomics and gut microbiota role for evaluating the MD effects by summarizing the current evidence from observational and clinical trials [28].

Overall, the studies included in the Special issue provide new insights on the protective effect of MD on health, although many authors reported the need of performing further investigations to confirm these effects.

Conflicts of Interest: The authors declare no conflict of interest.

References

1. Galbete, C.; Schwingshackl, L.; Schwedhelm, C.; Boeing, H.; Schulze, M.B. Evaluating Mediterranean diet and risk of chronic disease in cohort studies: An umbrella review of meta-analyses. *Eur. J. Epidemiol.* **2018**, *33*, 909–931. [CrossRef] [PubMed]
2. D'Alessandro, A.; De Pergola, G. The Mediterranean Diet: Its definition and evaluation of a priori dietary indexes in primary cardiovascular prevention. *Int. J. Food Sci. Nutr.* **2018**, *69*, 647–659. [CrossRef] [PubMed]
3. Dinu, M.; Pagliai, G.; Casini, A.; Sofi, F. Mediterranean diet and multiple health outcomes: An umbrella review of meta-analyses of observational studies and randomised trials. *Eur. J. Clin. Nutr.* **2018**, *72*, 30–43. [CrossRef] [PubMed]
4. Grosso, G.; Marventano, S.; Yang, J.; Micek, A.; Pajak, A.; Scalfi, L.; Galvano, F.; Kales, S.N. A comprehensive meta-analysis on evidence of Mediterranean diet and cardiovascular disease: Are individual components equal? *Crit. Rev. Food Sci. Nutr.* **2017**, *57*, 3218–3232. [CrossRef] [PubMed]
5. Rosato, V.; Temple, N.J.; La Vecchia, C.; Castellan, G.; Tavani, A.; Guercio, V. Mediterranean diet and cardiovascular disease: A systematic review and meta-analysis of observational studies. *Eur. J. Nutr.* **2019**, *58*, 173–191. [CrossRef] [PubMed]
6. Becerra-Tomás, N.; Blanco Mejía, S.; Viguiliouk, E.; Khan, T.; Kendall, C.W.C.; Kahleova, H.; Rahelić, D.; Sievenpiper, J.L.; Salas-Salvadó, J. Mediterranean diet, cardiovascular disease and mortality in diabetes: A systematic review and meta-analysis of prospective cohort studies and randomized clinical trials. *Crit. Rev. Food Sci. Nutr.* **2019**, 1–21. [CrossRef] [PubMed]
7. Godos, J.; Federico, A.; Dallio, M.; Scazzina, F. Mediterranean diet and nonalcoholic fatty liver disease: Molecular mechanisms of protection. *Int. J. Food Sci. Nutr.* **2017**, *68*, 18–27. [CrossRef] [PubMed]
8. Godos, J.; Zappalà, G.; Bernardini, S.; Giambini, I.; Bes-Rastrollo, M.; Martinez-Gonzalez, M. Adherence to the Mediterranean diet is inversely associated with metabolic syndrome occurrence: A meta-analysis of observational studies. *Int. J. Food Sci. Nutr.* **2017**, *68*, 138–148. [CrossRef]
9. Schwingshackl, L.; Hoffmann, G. Adherence to Mediterranean diet and risk of cancer: An updated systematic review and meta-analysis of observational studies. *Cancer Med.* **2015**, *4*, 1933–1947. [CrossRef]
10. Aridi, Y.; Walker, J.; Wright, O. The Association between the Mediterranean Dietary Pattern and Cognitive Health: A Systematic Review. *Nutrients* **2017**, *9*, 674. [CrossRef]
11. Shafiei, F.; Salari-Moghaddam, A.; Larijani, B.; Esmaillzadeh, A. Adherence to the Mediterranean diet and risk of depression: A systematic review and updated meta-analysis of observational studies. *Nutr. Rev.* **2019**, *77*, 230–239. [CrossRef] [PubMed]
12. Pagliai, G.; Sofi, F.; Vannetti, F.; Caiani, S.; Pasquini, G.; Molino Lova, R.; Cecchi, F.; Sorbi, S.; Macchi, C. Mediterranean Diet, Food Consumption and Risk of Late-Life Depression: The Mugello Study. *J. Nutr. Health Aging* **2018**, *22*, 569–574. [CrossRef] [PubMed]
13. Archero, F.; Ricotti, R.; Solito, A.; Carrera, D.; Civello, F.; Di Bella, R.; Bellone, S.; Prodam, F. Adherence to the Mediterranean Diet among School Children and Adolescents Living in Northern Italy and Unhealthy Food Behaviors Associated to Overweight. *Nutrients* **2018**, *10*, 1322. [CrossRef] [PubMed]
14. Zurita-Ortega, F.; San Román-Mata, S.; Chacón-Cuberos, R.; Castro-Sánchez, M.; Muros, J. Adherence to the Mediterranean Diet Is Associated with Physical Activity, Self-Concept and Sociodemographic Factors in University Student. *Nutrients* **2018**, *10*, 966. [CrossRef] [PubMed]
15. Muros, J.; Zabala, M. Differences in Mediterranean Diet Adherence between Cyclists and Triathletes in a Sample of Spanish Athletes. *Nutrients* **2018**, *10*, 1480. [CrossRef] [PubMed]
16. Chacón-Cuberos, R.; Badicu, G.; Zurita-Ortega, F.; Castro-Sánchez, M. Mediterranean Diet and Motivation in Sport: A Comparative Study BETWEEN University Students from Spain and Romania. *Nutrients* **2018**, *11*, 30. [CrossRef] [PubMed]

17. Kretowicz, H.; Hundley, V.; Tsofliou, F. Exploring the Perceived Barriers to Following a Mediterranean Style Diet in Childbearing Age: A Qualitative Study. *Nutrients* **2018**, *10*, 1694. [CrossRef]
18. Godos, J.; Castellano, S.; Marranzano, M. Adherence to a Mediterranean Dietary Pattern Is Associated with Higher Quality of Life in a Cohort of Italian Adults. *Nutrients* **2019**, *11*, 981. [CrossRef] [PubMed]
19. Godos, J.; Ferri, R.; Caraci, F.; Cosentino, F.I.I.; Castellano, S.; Galvano, F.; Grosso, G. Adherence to the Mediterranean Diet is Associated with Better Sleep Quality in Italian Adults. *Nutrients* **2019**, *11*, 976. [CrossRef]
20. Vitale, M.; Masulli, M.; Calabrese, I.; Rivellese, A.; Bonora, E.; Signorini, S.; Perriello, G.; Squatrito, S.; Buzzetti, R.; Sartore, G.; et al. Impact of a Mediterranean Dietary Pattern and Its Components on Cardiovascular Risk Factors, Glucose Control, and Body Weight in People with Type 2 Diabetes: A Real-Life Study. *Nutrients* **2018**, *10*, 1067. [CrossRef]
21. Castro-Barquero, S.; Lamuela-Raventós, R.; Doménech, M.; Estruch, R. Relationship between Mediterranean Dietary Polyphenol Intake and Obesity. *Nutrients* **2018**, *10*, 1523. [CrossRef] [PubMed]
22. D'Innocenzo, S.; Biagi, C.; Lanari, M. Obesity and the Mediterranean Diet: A Review of Evidence of the Role and Sustainability of the Mediterranean Diet. *Nutrients* **2019**, *11*, 1306. [CrossRef] [PubMed]
23. Carvalho, K.; Ronca, D.; Michels, N.; Huybrechts, I.; Cuenca-Garcia, M.; Marcos, A.; Molnár, D.; Dallongeville, J.; Manios, Y.; Schaan, B.; et al. Does the Mediterranean Diet Protect against Stress-Induced Inflammatory Activation in European Adolescents? The HELENA Study. *Nutrients* **2018**, *10*, 1770. [CrossRef] [PubMed]
24. Del Bo', C.; Marino, M.; Martini, D.; Tucci, M.; Ciappellano, S.; Riso, P.; Porrini, M. Overview of Human Intervention Studies Evaluating the Impact of the Mediterranean Diet on Markers of DNA Damage. *Nutrients* **2019**, *11*, 391. [CrossRef] [PubMed]
25. D'Alessandro, A.; Lampignano, L.; De Pergola, G. Mediterranean Diet Pyramid: A Proposal for Italian People. A Systematic Review of Prospective Studies to Derive Serving Sizes. *Nutrients* **2019**, *11*, 1296. [CrossRef] [PubMed]
26. George, E.S.; Kucianski, T.; Mayr, H.L.; Moschonis, G.; Tierney, A.C.; Itsiopoulos, C. A Mediterranean Diet Model in Australia: Strategies for Translating the Traditional Mediterranean Diet into a Multicultural Setting. *Nutrients* **2018**, *10*, 465. [CrossRef]
27. Biagi, C.; Di Nunzio, M.; Bordoni, A.; Gori, D.; Lanari, M. Effect of Adherence to Mediterranean Diet during Pregnancy on Children's Health: A Systematic Review. *Nutrients* **2019**, *11*, 997. [CrossRef]
28. Jin, Q.; Black, A.; Kales, S.N.; Vattem, D.; Ruiz-Canela, M.; Sotos-Prieto, M. Metabolomics and Microbiomes as Potential Tools to Evaluate the Effects of the Mediterranean Diet. *Nutrients* **2019**, *11*, 207. [CrossRef]

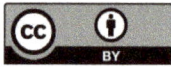

© 2019 by the author. Licensee MDPI, Basel, Switzerland. This article is an open access article distributed under the terms and conditions of the Creative Commons Attribution (CC BY) license (http://creativecommons.org/licenses/by/4.0/).

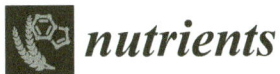

Opinion

A Mediterranean Diet Model in Australia: Strategies for Translating the Traditional Mediterranean Diet into a Multicultural Setting

Elena S. George [1,2,*], Teagan Kucianski [1], Hannah L. Mayr [1], George Moschonis [1], Audrey C. Tierney [1,3] and Catherine Itsiopoulos [1]

1. Department of Rehabilitation, Nutrition and Sport, La Trobe University, Health Sciences 3, Kingsbury Drive, Bundoora, VIC 3086, Australia; T.Kucianski@latrobe.edu.au (T.K.); H.Mayr@latrobe.edu.au (H.L.M.); G.Moschonis@latrobe.edu.au (G.M.); A.Tierney@latrobe.edu.au (A.C.T.); C.Itsiopoulos@latrobe.edu.au (C.I.)
2. School of Exercise and Nutrition Sciences, Deakin University, Building J, 221 Burwood Hwy, Burwood, VIC 3125, Australia
3. School of Allied Health, University of Limerick, Castletroy, Limerick V94 T9PX, Ireland
* Correspondence: Elena.George@deakin.edu.au; Tel.: +61-3-924-68622

Received: 2 March 2018; Accepted: 8 April 2018; Published: 9 April 2018

Abstract: Substantial evidence supports the effect of the Mediterranean Diet (MD) for managing chronic diseases, although trials have been primarily conducted in Mediterranean populations. The efficacy and feasibility of the Mediterranean dietary pattern for the management of chronic diseases has not been extensively evaluated in non-Mediterranean settings. This paper aims to describe the development of a MD model that complies with principles of the traditional MD applied in a multiethnic context. Optimal macronutrient and food-based composition was defined, and a two-week menu was devised incorporating traditional ingredients with evidence based on improvements in chronic disease management. Strategies were developed for the implementation of the diet model in a multiethnic population. Consistent with the principles of a traditional MD, the MD model was plant-based and high in dietary fat, predominantly monounsaturated fatty acids from extra virgin olive oil. Fruits, vegetables and wholegrains were a mainstay, and moderate amounts of nuts and seeds, fish, dairy and red wine were recommended. The diet encompassed key features of the MD including cuisine, biodiversity and sustainability. The MD model preserved traditional dietary components likely to elicit health benefits for individuals with chronic diseases, even with the adaptation to an Australian multiethnic population.

Keywords: Mediterranean diet; dietary intervention; diet; nutrition; translation; non-alcoholic fatty liver disease; cardiovascular disease

1. Introduction

There is a substantial body of evidence to support the efficacy of the Mediterranean Diet (MD) in chronic disease prevention and management [1]. In this regard, results from several intervention studies support the efficacy of a MD for individuals with cardiovascular disease (CVD) as well as a broad range of associated disease states, including metabolic syndrome, type 2 diabetes mellitus (T2DM), cognitive function decline, depression and anxiety, autoimmune diseases, cancer and non-alcoholic fatty liver disease (NAFLD) [2–4]. As inflammation drives insulin resistance and oxidative stress [5,6], the anti-inflammatory and antioxidant properties of the MD pattern are proposed to slow the progression of some of the oxidative damage associated with the aforementioned clinical conditions [7,8].

Some of the proposed benefits of the MD pertain to the dietary pattern as a whole. This encompasses overall macro and micronutrient composition, the variety of foods included as well as the combination, preparation and consumption of these foods which contribute to the synergistic effect of the food matrix [9]. The combination of foods and how these are traditionally prepared is often referred to as cuisine, and this is a key element of the MD that is likely to contribute to added health benefits [10].

The majority of clinical trials which have assessed the efficacy of the MD have been conducted in Mediterranean populations, where this dietary pattern and these types of foods are familiar [1]. Embedding the principles of a MD in non-Mediterranean populations worldwide with different habitual food cultures remains a great challenge. Australia is a culturally diverse nation, with almost half the population (49%) having either been born overseas or with at least one parent born overseas [11]. Given the high prevalence of chronic disease in Australia, and the scientific evidence base of the MD, assessing the efficacy of the diet for the prevention and management of these diseases in this population group is warranted. However, given the heterogeneity around the definitions and interpretations of what constitutes a MD intervention, researchers need to be transparent about the exact methods and dietary prescriptions used to ensure reproducibility and translation of favourable effects for other research studies and to drive practice change [12].

The current paper provides the rationale and process undertaken for the development of a MD model intervention in two clinical trials, currently underway. Protocols for each study are presented elsewhere Papamiltiadous et al. [13] and Itsiopoulos et al. [14]. In this context, the specific aims of the present study were (1) to identify the nutrient composition profiles of previous MD interventions delivered to Mediterranean and Australian populations; (2) to identify the key dietary and food-based components within the MD (with evidence-based health benefits) and to use these to develop key food intake recommendations; (3) to develop a two-week meal plan based on the nutrient composition profile and the key food intake recommendations identified in the previous steps; and (4) to assess the barriers to translatability of this dietary pattern to multiethnic Australian populations with chronic disease and to develop strategies to overcome these.

2. Methodological Steps to Address Each Specific Aim

A MD intervention for provision in an Australian, multiethnic population with diagnosed NAFLD and CVD, undergoing clinical trial conditions, was developed using the below steps which are summarized in Figure 1.

2.1. Step One: Identification of the Nutrient Composition Profile of Previous MD Interventions Delivered to Mediterranean and Australian Populations

In determining the key nutrients required to achieve a MD, it was important to establish a clear definition of a 'MD pattern' using a strong evidence base. This included using MD interventions that have successfully translated this dietary pattern and achieved health benefits. There have been a number of trials published, which refer to and apply a MD intervention; however, the nutrient composition across the literature remains inconsistent [12]. Therefore, the authors used the Cretan MD as the definition for this MD model, which was determined using published data from trials based on the archetypal traditional Cretan (Greek) MD [15]. These dietary practices have been the most pivotal in demonstrating prevention and management of chronic disease [16–18].

A comprehensive assessment of MD studies, including seminal MD trials in Mediterranean regions and smaller clinical trials implemented in the Australian context, was conducted. Nutrient composition data is depicted in Table 1. From this assessment the nutrient compositions for this intervention were derived and are discussed below.

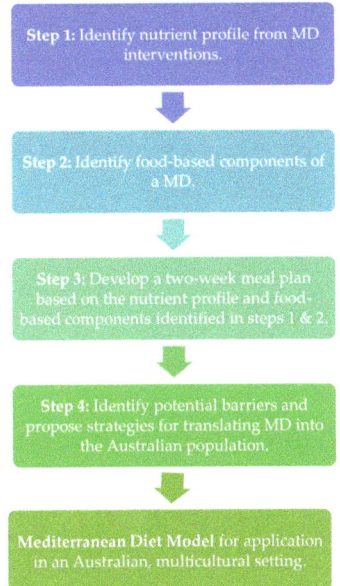

Figure 1. A schematic summarising the key methodological steps taken to develop a Mediterranean Diet model for an Australian multicultural setting. MD: Mediterranean Diet.

Table 1. Nutrient data from the seminal Keys study and subsequent clinical trials within Mediterranean regions and clinical trials using a Mediterranean diet in Australian populations.

Trials	7 Countries Study	Diabetes Cross Over	PREDIMED	The Medi-RIVAGE	NAFLD Cross Over
	Keys et al. [15] (Cohort)	Itsiopoulos et al. [19] (Intervention)	Estruch et al. [20] (Intervention)	Vincent et al. [21] (Intervention)	Ryan et al. [4] (Intervention)
Dietary data	Prospective cohort	Feeding trial, full provision of diet. Data is recommended diet ^	Data is from diet consumed *	Data is from recommended diet ^	Feeding trial, full provision of diet. Data is the recommended diet ^
Population	Mediterranean	Non-Mediterranean (Australia)	Mediterranean (Spain)	Mediterranean (Spain)	Non-Mediterranean (Australia)
Nutrients					
Energy (MJ)	-	11.9	9.2	-	11.3
Protein (%E)	10.5	12.0	16.3	12–15	15.8
CHO (%E)	-	44.3	40.1	50	33.6
Total Fat (%E)	36.1	40.2	41.3	35–38	44.3
SFA (%E)	7.7	7.5	9.3	8–10	13.6
MUFA (%E)	25.8	22.9	21.5	18–20	22.8
PUFA (%E)	2.5	5.6	6.9	8–10	7.9
Alcohol (%E)	4	4	-	≤5%	1.5
Fibre (g/d)	-	46.7	-	>25 g	36.4
Linoleic acid n-6 (g)	-	15.6	14.1	-	15.1
α-linolenic acid n-3 (g)	-	1.5	1.6	-	1.6
EPA (g)	-	0.44	-	-	-
DHA (g)	-	0.48	-	-	-
Total LCN3s (mg)	-	-	-	-	200.3
Key outcome	All-cause mortality CHD	HbA1c	↓CVD complications	↓CVD risk	liver fat insulin resistance

Abbreviations: PREDIMED: Prevención con Dieta Mediterráne, Medi-RIVAGE: Mediterranean Diet, Cardiovascular Risks and Gene Polymorphisms, CHO: carbohydrates; SFA: saturated fatty acids; MUFA: monounsaturated fatty acids; PUFA: polyunsaturated fatty acids; EPA: eicosapentaenoic acid; DHA: docosahexaenoic acid; LCN3s: long chain omega 3 fatty acids; CHD: coronary heart disease; CVD: cardiovascular disease; NAFLD: non-alcoholic fatty liver disease. -: indicates that values were not published and/or measured; * The PREDIMED trial included two Mediterranean Diet (MD) arms; one with the provision of extra virgin olive oil (EVOO) and the other with nuts. Results presented are a mean of the consumption data presented from the two groups; ^ Recommended diet refers to the diet prescribed; therefore, a participant would receive the described macro- and micronutrient composition if they were 100% adherent.

Table 1 captures the nutrient composition from trials where substantial benefits were demonstrated with the prescription of the MD. Benefits were defined as improvements in outcome measures in a range of chronic diseases or where feasibility in an Australian population was shown.

Of note, the landmark LYON diet heart study was clearly the most impressive secondary prevention trial using a Mediterranean style diet to prevent secondary myocardial infarcts; however, the dietary intervention model of this trial was not used to inform our intervention model due to major differences in fat type. The LYON heart study had a heavy reliance on high alpha-linolenic acid (ALA) canola oil and margarine which are not documented traditional fats used in the MD [22]. Clinical trials encompassing traditional MD principles that have been carried out in non-Mediterranean regions, namely Australia, were feeding trials that provided all meals to participants for the study duration [4,19]. These trials demonstrated 'proof of concept' that positive health outcomes can be achieved for chronic disease states in Australian populations with consumption of a MD. Ongoing provision of complete meals is not achievable and is cost prohibitive in clinical trials and does not adequately represent the feasibility of implementing this dietary pattern in a free living population. Therefore, the Australian dietary intervention developed and described herein encompasses the traditional MD patterns for application in free living participants [13].

2.2. Step Two: Identification of the Key Food-Based Components of a MD with Strong Published Evidence of Health Benefits

Using the nutrient profile derived in step one, food components with health promoting effects were used to formulate a meal plan. When translating optimal levels of essential nutrients into food-based recommendations, references in Table 1 were used as a guide, as were the Hellenic dietary guidelines [23]. It is worth noting that since the development of this MD model intervention model, the Hellenic dietary guidelines have been updated. Cross referencing with published MD food group recommendations, labelled 'commandments', was also carried out [24]. Determination of key food-based recommendations and a review of the evidence-based mechanisms surrounding these dietary components were conducted; these are summarised in Table 2.

Table 2. Nutrient composition of the Australian Mediterranean Diet *.

Nutrients	Australian Mediterranean Diet Composition
Energy (MJ)	9.4
Protein (%E)	15.8
CHO (%E)	33.8
Added sugar (%E)	5.2
Total fat (%E)	41.8
SFA (%E)	8.9
MUFA (%E)	22.3
PUFA (%E)	10.6
Alcohol (%E)	2.4
Fibre (g/d)	41.1
Linoleic acid n-6 (g)	18.7
α linolenic acid n-3 (g)	4.9
Total LCN3s (mg)	932

* This nutrient profile was calculated by entering two-week food diaries into the software program Foodworks 7™ (Xyris software Australia Pty Ltd.). Abbreviations: CHO: carbohydrates; SFA: saturated fatty acids; MUFA: monounsaturated fatty acids; PUFA: polyunsaturated fatty acids, LCN3s: long chain omega 3 fatty acids.

For both steps one and two, there was also consideration of other evidence-based, disease specific dietary recommendations. For example, for CVD patients, the National Heart Foundation guidelines were incorporated, and for NAFLD patients, alcohol recommendations were kept to the lower end of the suggested range. This was important to ensure that the MD model dietary model did not was consistent with established clinical guidelines for these medical conditions.

2.3. Step Three: Development of a Two-Week Meal Plan Based on the Nutrient Composition Profile and the Key Food Intake Recommendations Identified in the Previous Steps

Based on steps one and two, a two-week meal plan, suitable for an Australian multiethnic population was developed (Figure S1). The meal plan was based on the macro and micronutrients and food-based components consistent with a traditional MD. These meal plans were analyzed using a standard food analysis program, Foodworks 7™, to ensure nutrient composition was consistent with the desired profile as identified in step one. The two-week meal plan also incorporated other key elements of the MD highlighted in step two, including combinations and preparation of foods described as part of the MD cuisine.

2.4. Step Four: Identification of Potential Barriers and Proposal of Strategies for Translating MD into the Australian Population

The studies presented are summarized in Tables 1 and 2 and were used to determine the perceived feasibility of the intervention through highlighting potential barriers for the translation of a MD into the Australian population. To overcome these barriers, a theoretical framework encompassing a SWOT (strengths, weaknesses, opportunities, threats) analysis was conducted. This was carried out to identify barriers that were likely to occur and embed strategies within the MD model to overcome these. This SWOT analysis was conducted alongside the experience and expertise of practising dietitians and researchers to ensure appropriate strategies were embedded into the intervention with the aim of addressing the perceived barriers identified.

3. Practical Strategies Related to Each Specific Aim

3.1. Nutrient Composition Profiles of Other MD Interventions Delivered to Mediterranean and Australian Populations

The rationale for the MD intervention model, including the composition, specific ingredients and cooking methods, is discussed throughout this section. As described in step one of the previous section, a prospective cohort trial as well as four other clinical trials [4,19–21] were used to document the ideal nutrient components of the MD, and their reported nutrient data is summarised in Table 1. The single observational study and the four clinical trials identified in step one were used to derive desirable macro and micronutrient ranges to inform the dietary prescription of the MD model.

The application of this Mediterranean diet model will determine whether this diet can be translated to the Australian, multiethnic population and whether a MD pattern is sustainable in the long term. Furthermore, the MD model intervention is being tested within two clinical trials that are currently underway [13] to determine the efficacy, feasibility and sustainability of delivering this intervention in Australian cohorts with chronic diseases, such as Coronary Heart Disease (CHD) and NAFLD.

3.2. Macronutrient Profile of the MD Model

As well as the nutrient compositions described in Table 1, this section provides an overview of the macronutrient composition and corresponding foods for the MD model intervention. The MD model intervention is a 'high fat' diet, with fat comprising, at the macronutrient level, between 35% and 45% of energy intake. At least 50% of the energy from fat is from monounsaturated fatty acids (MUFAs) and the remaining energy contribution comes from polyunsaturated fatty acids (PUFAs) and saturated fatty acids (SFAs). Protein contributes 15–20% of total energy, and carbohydrates contribute 35–40%. This MD intervention also includes moderate amounts of alcohol which may contribute up to 5% of total energy, which is within the recommendations set by the Australian National Health and Medical Research Council (NHMRC) [25]. The importance of the specific nutrient profiles within the MD model and how they impact on chronic disease risk factors are described below.

3.2.1. Fats

Monounsaturated Fatty Acids

This MD model intervention emulates the traditional MD in that it is high in MUFAs, mainly due to the daily consumption of Extra Virgin Olive Oil (EVOO), the predominant culinary fat used in the diet. While there are other oils that are classed as high MUFA, they do not contain the same level of MUFA as EVOO. Importantly, EVOO contains an abundance of polyphenols which are thought to drive the anti-inflammatory and antioxidant benefits attributed to the MD diet [26,27].

Polyunsaturated Fatty Acids

PUFAs are also a key nutrient encompassed in the MD intervention. These are sourced from a variety of foods, including nuts, seeds, olive oil and fish. Long chain omega-3 fatty acids, namely eicosapentaenoic acid (EPA) and docosahexaenoic acid (DHA), are particularly abundant in marine dietary sources. The plant-derived essential PUFA, alpha linoleic acid, is derived from staple dietary components, such as wild edible greens and nuts and seeds. These omega-3 rich PUFAs are critical for achieving a more favourable omega-6 (n-6) to omega-3 (n-3) ratio within the diet. A traditional Cretan (Greek) MD is characterised by a 2:1 ratio, while Western diets are closer to 20:1 [28]. An elevated n-6:n-3 ratio mediates detrimental vascular changes and limits anti-inflammatory processes, which likely exacerbates oxidative stress, increasing the risk and severity of chronic diseases [29]. The MD model diet developed for our dietary interventions and presented in this manuscript achieved a favourable n-6:n-3 ratio close to 3:1, reflected in Table 2.

Saturated Fatty Acids

SFAs constitute a small proportion of the overall MD model intervention—less than a 10% contribution to total energy consumption. The small SFA component of the diet is derived from staple MD components, such as EVOO, nuts and seeds and animal-based products, such as yogurt and small amounts of meat. SFA-rich products such as processed foods and large amounts, or frequent consumption of, animal products are not a feature of the traditional MD, nor were these foods incorporated into our MD model [30].

3.2.2. Carbohydrates

Carbohydrates contribute between 35–40% of energy in the MD model intervention. The focus is on whole grains which are processed minimally and never refined. Traditionally, these included sourdough bread, potatoes, rice and pasta. The accessibility of 'true' sourdough bread is not readily available in Australian supermarkets. Thus, soy and linseed bread was recommended as an alternative which also served to increase dietary alpha-linoleic acid. The traditional MD was consumed *ad libitum*; therefore, portions are not a key feature of the MD model intervention. However, given the quantities of carbohydrate consumed in Australian populations [31], to achieve the desired macronutrient contribution, examples of appropriate portions for carbohydrate-based foods were provided within the principles of the MD intervention to moderate intake.

3.2.3. Protein

The MD model is a predominantly plant-based diet, and animal proteins are consumed in small amounts [28]. Thus, a lot of dietary protein is sourced from a variety of plant-based protein sources, including legumes, lentils, nuts and seeds. The MD also includes moderate consumption of fish and animal protein, including dairy, eggs and white meat, and red meat is recommended for less frequent consumption. The traditional MD included infrequent and small portions of white meat and even less red meat. However, to ensure acceptability, the MD model intervention allows a maximum quantity of 450 g/week (white and red meat varieties). In the MD model intervention, recommended dairy sources are predominantly fermented, including yogurt and white cheese, especially feta (Table 2). Of note, low fat/skim or light dairy alternatives were not traditionally part of a MD; however, modern dairy production does not follow traditional methods, whereby some full fat options contain additional fat as cream to enhance 'creaminess'. Therefore, low fat options were used in the MD intervention (analysis described in Table 3) to achieve the desired SFA composition as per Table 1 and to ensure that the Australian National Heart Foundation (NHF) Guidelines were maintained, as appropriate. This was especially important given that participant cohorts targeted for the application of the MD model intervention were at risk of, or had CVD [32].

3.2.4. Alcohol

Alcohol, traditionally from red wine, is included and recommended to be consumed with meals in the MD model. However, individuals not previously consuming alcohol were not encouraged to commence drinking. The quantity recommended is one to two standard glasses of red wine per day, which is within the Australian NHMRC alcohol recommendations of <20 g ethanol per day [25]. The maximum contribution of energy from alcohol included in the composition is approximately 5% of total energy. In some instances, alcohol was not recommended. For example, patients who had progressed NAFLD were advised to avoid alcohol due to the increased risk of hepatocellular carcinoma [33].

Table 3. The 12 components of a Mediterranean diet and the proposed mechanisms of effect.

Recommendation	Practical Dietary Applications	Key Components	Evidence Based Benefits
Use extra virgin olive oil (EVOO) as the main added fat.	Minimum 3–4 tablespoons (60–80 mL) per day	The highest proportions of MUFAs and polyphenols squalene and α-tocopherol are available in extra virgin olive oil.	Prevention of CHD, cancers and modification to immune and inflammatory responses have been attributed to EVOO. The high antioxidant content of EVOOs contributes to health of the vascular system through improved endothelial function [34] and has been shown to inhibit LDL oxidation [35]. EVOO consumption has also been proposed to improve bone mineralisation [36].
Eat vegetables with every meal.	Include 100 g leafy greens, and 200 g all other vegetables daily (cauliflower, zucchini, eggplant, capsicum etc.). use onion and garlic daily; include 100 g tomatoes daily; fresh or sofrito (tomato-based sauce).	Vegetables are the most significant source of phenolic compounds. They contain carotenoids, folic acid, fibre and phytosterols. Garlic, onion, herbs and spices also have key benefits. See Section 3.3.2 for importance of combining and/or cooking ingredients.	Flavonoids, are essential bioactive compounds that provide health benefits due to their antioxidant effects and have been associated with improvements in cognitive function and mood [37]. Traditional diets which are predominantly plant-based are associated with lower rates of chronic diseases and increased longevity [38]. Carotenoids, folic acid and fibre play important roles in CHD prevention [38]. Phytosterols contribute to reduced serum cholesterol and CVD risk [39]. Garlic, onions, herbs and spices contain large amounts of flavonoids or allicin which have cardiovascular benefits and also improve cognitive function [40]. Vegetables which are high in potassium, magnesium and calcium tend to reduce arterial blood pressure [34,36].
Include at least two legume meals per week.	Canned or dry legumes are acceptable; this may include tofu (1 serve = 250 g). This should replace meat on days when meat is not consumed.	Legumes are high in fibre, protein, B vitamins, iron, zinc, calcium, magnesium, selenium, phosphorus, copper and potassium [41]. They provide a nutritious, nourishing meat alternative.	Legumes are linked to longevity, and are a strong predictor of survival [42]. Vegetables have been shown to reduce serum homocysteine concentrations and thus coronary events, especially in high risk individuals [43]. An inverse association between the risk of T2DM and CHD and legume intake has been reported [44,45].

Table 3. Cont.

Recommendation	Practical Dietary Applications	Key Components	Evidence Based Benefits
Eat at least three servings of fish or shellfish per week.	Fish (1 serve = 100–150 g); shellfish (1 serve = 200 g). Include oily fish at least 1–2 times per week.	Marine long chain omega-3 polyunsaturated fatty acids provide eicosapentaenoic acid (EPA) and docosahexaenoic acid (DHA).	EPA and DHA effectively regulate haemostatic factors and protect against cardiac arrhythmias, cancer and hypertension and help to maintain neural functions [34,40]. A high intake of fish and seafood has also been shown to reduce systolic blood pressure [34,36]. Immunomodulatory effects may improve inflammatory conditions [46].
Eat red meat less often and choose smaller portions. Choose white meat.	150–200 g weekly of beef, lamb and, pork. 200–250 g per week of poultry. Choose lean varieties, wild, free range and grass fed varieties are encouraged.	Meat is a bioavailable source of vitamin B12, and iron, selenium, and zinc and are a good source of protein. Excessive amounts of red meat have been linked to adverse health outcomes and excess saturated fatty acids—unfavourable fat ratios and displacement of more nutritious alternatives. Wild, free range and grass fed varieties are preferred due to the improved n-6:n-3 ratio [29].	Red meat is a good source of protein which assists with satiety [47]. Red and processed meats, especially when consumed in excess, are associated with total CVD and cancer mortality [48]. Excessive SFA intake from meat is also linked to adverse health outcomes [1].
Eat fresh fruit every day.	300g or 2 serves.	Fruit provides fibre, potassium, vitamins A and C, B vitamins, folate, flavonoids and terpenes providing protection against oxidative processes.	Consumption of fruit has been shown to reduce the risk of CVD and cancers [49]. Fibre, vitamins, minerals, flavonoids and terpenes may provide protection against oxidative processes which drive the onset and exacerbate chronic diseases [40]. Flavonoids have also been associated with improvements in cognitive function and mood [37].
Eat a serve of nuts every day and dried fruit as a snack or dessert.	Nuts-1 serve = ~30 g or 1/4 cup or a small handful daily. Dried fruit—2 tablespoons or 30 g.	Nuts are a good source of monounsaturated fats, fibre, vitamin C and E, selenium, magnesium, providing an abundance of antioxidants including flavonoids, resveratrol, polyphenols and tocopherols [50].	Monounsaturated fats, phenols, phytosterols, phytic acid and fibre are abundant in nuts and are associated with a reduction in plasma lipids and reduced incidence of CVD [40]. Nut consumption has been associated with the prevention and reversal of oxidative stress [50,51].
Eat dairy every day.	2 serves per day including milk-1 serve = 250 mL or 1 cup. Yoghurt preferably Greek style yoghurt 1 serve = 150 g or $\frac{3}{4}$ cup.	Dairy is a good source of calcium, vitamin D, phosphorus, magnesium, zinc, potassium, vitamins A and B12, and lactic acid bacteria confer probiotic effects [52]. Choose mostly fermented dairy which are higher in potent beneficial bioactive compounds from milk such as lactic acid bacteria [53].	Bioactive milk components have been shown to be protective in several diseases, including hypertension, coronary vascular diseases, obesity, osteoporosis and cancer [53]. Lactic acid bacteria confer probiotic effects, including improvements in gastrointestinal health and immune response. Yogurt, specifically, may induce desirable changes in faecal bacterial flora, potentially reducing the risk of colon cancer. Yoghurt is also likely to regulate mouth-to-caecum transit time [54].
Eat cheese in moderation, about 3 times per week and preferably feta.	1 serve = 30 g or the size of a matchbox.		
Include wholegrain breads and cereals with meals, such as wholegrain bread, rice, pasta and potato.	1 serve = 1 slice of bread or; $\frac{1}{2}$ cup or; 50–60 g cooked pasta/rice or; 1 small 100 g potato.	Wholegrains are a good source of fermentable carbohydrates including fibre, resistant starch, and oligosaccharides. They contain phytochemicals, antioxidants including trace minerals, phenolic compounds, lignans and B group vitamins including folate, vitamin E, minerals iron, magnesium, copper and selenium [55].	Components such as fibre, antioxidants and vitamins and minerals promote health and may be protective against cancer, CVD, T2DM and obesity [56,57]. Production of short chain fatty acids through indigestible carbohydrates promote reduced serum cholesterol levels and decrease cancer risk [58].

Table 3. Cont.

Recommendation	Practical Dietary Applications	Key Components	Evidence Based Benefits
Have sweets or sweet drinks in moderate amounts and on special occasions only.	Preferably home made.	Homemade varieties have key ingredients that are encouraged in the MD, such as nuts, EVOO and milk and are less refined and lower in SFA.	Liver fat accumulation may be attributed, at least in part, to excess dietary sugar consumption, especially from fructose, which increases the levels of enzymes involved in hepatic de-novo lipogenesis [59,60].
Consume up to 3 eggs per week.	Free range or omega-3 varieties.	Eggs are a good source of protein, choline, selenium, vitamin B12, riboflavin, phosphorus and fat soluble vitamins A, D and E. They are a bioavailable source of carotenoids; lutein and zeaxanthin, [61]. Free range and omega-3 enriched varieties have higher amounts of omega-3 fatty acids [62].	The benefits of eggs, including the provision of protein and micronutrients including vitamins, minerals and carotenoids may prevent age related macular degeneration and some cancers [61]. A limit to egg consumption is set to achieve the desired fat ratios in line with other MD guidelines [23].
OPTIONAL Consume wine in moderation.	Choose red wine. Have 0–2 glasses per day, (100 mL per glass) and always with meals. Do not get drunk.	Red wine contains phenolic compounds with high antioxidant properties. For example, red wine has higher amounts of the stilbene polyphenol, resveratrol, compared with white wine [63].	Red wine provides polyphenols whose antioxidant activity may contribute to the cytoprotective effects. Resveratrol has been found to protect the heart and kidneys from ischaemia-reperfusion injury and has a likely positive effect on endothelial function (vasodilation) with prolonged moderate consumption [64,65].

3.3. Identification of the Key Food-Based Components of a MD with Strong Published Evidence of Health Benefits

The food-based recommendations developed in step two are presented in Table 2. Scientific literature was used to support the development of these recommendations, and identification of components which include key mechanisms that drive optimal health outcomes for the management of chronic diseases are also highlighted in Table 2.

3.3.1. Food Groups

The food group recommendations in Table 2 are based upon documented MD 'commandments' [24]. Table 2 highlights these adapted food-based recommendations which were designed to be easy for participants to understand and interpret. Education material outlining these dietary recommendations and how they could be applied has been designed to be provided to participants in the initial dietary consultation, with accompanying pictures to aid translatability (Figures S2 and S3). Table 2 also highlights the proposed mechanisms and evidence-based benefits of each recommendation—these were not included in patient resources.

3.3.2. Cuisine

The term cuisine refers to the method of cooking which is often characteristic to a country or region [10]. Cooking includes the fusion of different ingredients, which has been shown to have additional nutritional benefits compared with its isolated and/or uncooked counterparts. Specifically, the addition of olive oil to tomatoes during cooking considerably increases the absorption of lycopene (a carotenoid linked to reduced rates of certain cancers and heart disease) [10]. Furthermore, the antioxidant capacity of salads has been assessed with and without the addition of aromatic herbs. Lemon balm and marjoram (1.5% (w/w)) increased antioxidant capacity by 150% and 200%, respectively [66]. In terms of salad dressings, the combination of EVOO and wine or apple vinegar gave the greatest increase in antioxidant capacity [66].

Given the benefits of cuisine in the MD pattern, it was important that cooking and preparation methods were captured in this MD model diet intervention. When providing dietary recommendations concerning cuisine for participants in this intervention there were two key areas embedded into the dietary intervention design, and these were emphasised during consultations: (1) herbs and spices and (2) cooking. These are elaborated upon below.

3.3.3. Herbs and Spices

Culinary herbs and spices are a part of the traditional MD, where they are used to flavour most dishes, and many are thought to have medicinal properties based on their ability to heal [28]. It is thought that the enhancement and depth of flavour resulting from the addition of herbs and spices contributes, at least in part, to the enjoyment and palatability of MD meals and may therefore encourage sustainability. The evidence in modern science for the benefits of the phytonutrients found in culinary herbs and spices continues to grow. Polyphenols have been associated with improved health outcomes due to the antioxidant capacity of these phytonutrients and thus, an increased quantity and improved bioavailability of polyphenols through dietary cuisine is desirable [27]. It is well established that herbs and spices are a concentrated source of polyphenols; for example, the polyphenol contents in 100 g of both oregano and carrot are 935 vs. 58 mg gallic acid equivalents (GAE), respectively [67,68]. It is also well accepted through other dietary guidelines, such as those endorsed by the Australian NHF, that flavour enhancement using herbs and spices can reduce the addition of excessive salt (sodium) to meals, which is associated with hypertension [32]. The element of cuisine was a key consideration within the development of the MD intervention to ensure replication of these health benefits. To encourage the addition of herbs and spices in meal preparation, recipes and meal plans were provided to illustrate how to cook with these ingredients.

3.3.4. Cooking

In order to achieve the benefits of combining ingredients and replicating the benefits of a 'cuisine' from the MD dietary pattern, traditional cooking practices are encouraged. In addition, cooking skills and cooking itself are linked to improved health outcomes [69,70]. Encouraging participants to cook facilitates dietary changes becoming part of lifestyle and behaviour, assisting in sustaining the changes, and thus achieving benefits.

Of note, many participants who are involved in clinical trials are either not willing to, or unable to prepare foods and cook meals for a range of reasons. The need for fast and convenient foods is well recognised in today's busy lifestyles. To accommodate for such lifestyles, resources were provided to assist participants to 'assemble' meals with choices that required minimal preparation. These convenient options enabled nutritious choices, while retaining key elements of the MD model without the need for expansive cooking skills or equipment. These quick and easy meal options were designed within a resource that could be provided to all participants but was emphasised to those who had limited cooking skills or for meals such as lunch at work where there was limited time and/or access to cooking equipment. Figure 2 highlights how these types of nutritious, MD-inspired cook-free meals were modelled in the resource developed for provision to participants (Figure S4)). This resource was supplied to participants as part of a toolkit to enable them to implement the principles of this diet within their own diet and lifestyle.

3.3.5. Eating Together

A key aspect of the traditional MD pattern is the emphasis of eating together. Food pyramids which depict MD often include a component showing people sharing meals [30]. This element is featured because it is the essence of the MD culture. It is thought that the table acts as a unifier and gives a sense of community [30,71,72]. This ideology was captured within our dietary intervention by recommending social interaction such as family meals or eating with others.

3.3.6. Being Mindful

A key part of the traditional MD is the notion of eating to appetite. Thus, to assist in facilitating the inclusion of this *ad libitum* approach, elements of mindfulness are included as a part of the

MD intervention delivery. As well as eating with others, participants are encouraged to practice mindfulness between and during meals, avoid electronic devices and screen time during meals, and be more aware of what they are eating through slower eating, chewing thoroughly and understanding their hunger and fullness cues [73].

Vegetables	Carbohydrate	Protein	Condiments
Green salad mix	Whole grain crackers	Canned lentils or legumes	EVOO*
Frozen vegetables	Microwavable rice	Canned chicken	Salt (minimal) +/- pepper
Cucumber, tomato and carrot	Wholegrain bread	Canned fish (e.g. tuna, sardines, salmon, mackerel, herring)	Lemon juice
Cabbage and carrot shredded	Potato (all varieties) – small for microwaving	Boiled egg (s)	Vinegar
Rocket and/or spinach leaves	Cous-cous (add boiling water, cover for 3 min)	Nuts or nut butter	Herbs +/- spices

*EVOO should be added to all meals

Figure 2. A summary of the MD inspired 'Cook free' meals based on the resource provided to study participants. EVOO: extra virgin olive oil.

3.3.7. Biodiversity and Seasonality, Local and Eco Friendly

Including a predominantly plant-based varied diet is a key component of the MD pattern. In addition, the MD traditionally focused on local, accessible and seasonal produce. This is important, as accessible produce is (1) environmentally and eco-friendly due to reduced emissions in production, storage and transportation; (2) often provides a more nutrient-dense food source; and (3) is usually more abundant and therefore affordable [30,74]. With regard to the practical application of this aspect of the dietary intervention, food variety and choices are adapted for the Australian context. The example provided in Figure 2 extrapolates the key points addressed during a dietary consultation to achieve practical application of biodiversity and seasonality in the Australian context.

The example shown in Figure 3 for traditional MD and modifications for the Australian context is by no means exhaustive. It simply showcases one example of flexible implementation of the dietary intervention. This flexibility allows for seasonal and accessible produce in the Australian context and accommodates different cultural preferences including what is familiar and acceptable to individuals. This substitution example is important to ensure that the diet model is feasible and translatable into multiethnic populations.

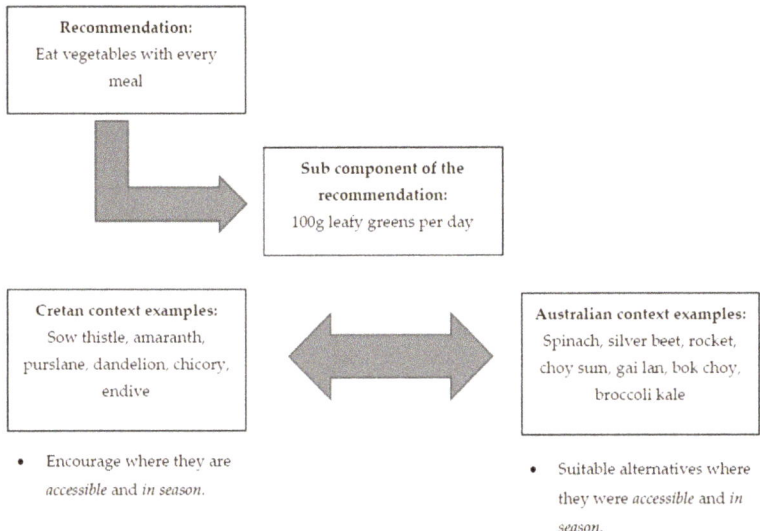

Figure 3. An example which models the practical dietary application of a recommendation from the traditional Cretan MD in an Australian context. Biodiversity and seasonality are considered.

3.4. A Two-Week Meal Plan Based on the Nutrient Composition Profile and the Key Food Intake Recommendations Identified in the Previous Steps

The nutrient ranges described in Table 1 in conjunction with the key principles of a MD described in Table 2 guided the development of the MD model intervention and the two week meal plans discussed in this section. The two-week meal plan was analysed in Foodworks™ version 7 and the macro- and micronutrients that were derived from these menus are reported in Table 3. These meal plans are available in Figure S1. There were three main meals and three snacks provided per day. A recipe book [24] detailing the preparation of all the meals and a shopping list (Figure S5) accompanied the meal plans. So, while the meal plan was designed to model optimal consumption of MD, composition was assumed to deviate from this based on individuals' preferences, satiety, cooking skills, culture, etc. The recommended meal pattern is an important component of the dietary model and is described here explicitly to clarify the purpose of each recommendation.

3.4.1. Breakfast

For the first meal of the day, the diet plan aimed to incorporate wholegrains and high contents of MUFAs and antioxidants while considering what was easily accessible. The options ranged from porridge with fruit as well as including more traditional components, such as honey and cinnamon. Soy and linseed bread with either chopped tomatoes, onion, herbs, EVOO and lemon juice or eggs with stewed tomatoes or avocado were also included. Greek style yogurt with fruit, honey, cinnamon and nuts were also incorporated into the meal plan. Herbal tea or coffee were included daily. Less traditional components, such as using low fat dairy, soy and linseed bread, were substituted to ensure an optimal fat ratio for the meal plan was reached.

3.4.2. Lunch/Dinner

Lunch meals were intended to be high in vegetables, wholegrains and MUFAs. Options ranged from soy and linseed bread, fish and salad or roast vegetables and feta cheese with EVOO, lentil/legume-based soups, or leftover dinner meals. Smaller meals were also accompanied by a piece of fruit. Canned fish, for example, is a less traditional component of the meals which was included to meet desirable fatty acid profiles while maintaining the convenience often desired in Western societies.

Dinner meals were also high in vegetables, wholegrains and MUFAs. Most of the meals at dinner required some cooking, but, as previously mentioned, convenient meal resources could be used in place of this. Furthermore there were tips on how main meals could be altered or made more convenient. The main meals at dinner included fish, small portions of white meat twice per week, and red meat, which was limited to once per week. There were at least two vegetarian days per week and at least two lentil dishes per week. Meal plans were designed so that meals could be moved around between meal times, days and weeks to suit individual preferences and time commitments.

3.4.3. Snacks

Snacks primarily composed of Greek yogurt, fresh or dried fruit and/or raw unsalted nuts providing a source of antioxidants as well as wholegrains, MUFAs and/or protein. There was an allowance for a small, homemade sweets after dinner twice per week. Snacks provided an opportunity to include important elements of the MD, such as fermented dairy and healthy fats from nuts, and were not just 'fillers'.

3.5. Potential Barriers and Proposed Strategies for Translating MD into the Australian Population

When designing the MD intervention for Australians, a key consideration was whether the diet would be feasible in a non-Mediterranean population. It is generally easy to replicate desirable macronutrient contributions such as those described for the MD as macronutrients are broad and non-specific. However, the task becomes more multifaceted when foods and their combination through cuisine is considered, to replicate the synergistic effects of the food matrix. When drawing on more customary recipes from various cuisines, each meal has its own unique flavour profile based on the region from which it originates. It is therefore important to model how the key elements of cuisine within the MD could be replicated across a variety of culturally-specific dishes. Table 4 provides an example of a traditional Cretan (Greek) Mediterranean dish called Fasolatha, and models popular multicultural alternatives which include similar key ingredients and combinations in cooking. This example demonstrates that macronutrients and foods, even when combined as part of cuisine from the MD, can be captured and translated across other traditional recipes. This demonstrates that the MD principles shown to improve health, can be replicated for a multicultural setting, which is both important and relevant due to the multiethnic landscape of Australia. This also ensures flexibility can be achieved through individualised dietary advice that can accommodate individual eating preferences. This substitution therefore enables the MD to be translatable across multiple ethnic groups.

Table 4. Replicating the cuisine in a traditional Cretan Mediterranean dish across different cultures and cuisines.

Cuisine	Greek (Cretan)	Middle Eastern	Indian	Chinese	Western
Meal	Fasolatha	Mujadara	Dhal	Mapo Tofu	Homemade Baked beans
Key ingredients	Legumes, onions, garlic, tomato, herbs, EVOO	Lentils, rice, onions, spices, EVOO	Lentils onion, garlic, tomatoes, ghee	Tofu, garlic scallions, peppers, ginger, soy sauce +/− pork, peanut +/− sesame oils	Legumes, onion, garlic, tomato, vegetable oil
Fat Modifications	-	-	Replace *part or all* added fat with EVOO		

Abbreviations: EVOO: extra virgin olive oil, -: indicates no change was made or required.

4. General Overview and Future Implications

This paper described the nutrient and food-based components of a traditional Mediterranean diet using data from seminal trials and a cohort trial including dietary intakes of people from Crete in the

1950s, considered the archetypal traditional Mediterranean diet. This information was used to model the development of a MD model for specific use in two multiethnic cohorts with chronic diseases: CVD [14] and NAFLD [13].

The MD model intervention includes specific dietary prescription, including a breakdown of macro and micronutrients and food components. This allows for transparency when reviewing literature and thus optimal analysis of dietary adherence and translation into other research trials and clinical practice. This belief around ensuring transparency was inherent in the modelling of this paper through the development and design of the MD model intervention and showed that the components of the Mediterranean cuisine [20,30] could be maintained across a number of different cultural cuisines. There is a strong rationale for assessing the efficacy of the MD in a Western, multicultural population where there is a need to identify a superior dietary pattern that can prevent and manage the growing epidemic of chronic diseases. This dietary pattern should also be assessed for its ability to be achieved and sustained by individuals. Furthermore, the MD model described herein has been developed for application within free living populations. This is an important strength of this dietary intervention model because theoretically, if adopted by individuals, it is more likely to be sustained. Sustainability is an outcome that is critical for the management of chronic diseases.

Having comprehensively reviewed the key nutrients, foods and mechanisms which facilitate health benefits, the development of this MD model intervention is anticipated to be comparable to interventions delivered in the Mediterranean basin. The MD model intervention is consistent with the traditional MD, being a predominantly plant-based diet high in dietary fat, predominantly from MUFA from EVOO consumption. The MD model intervention reported in this paper also features moderate amounts of fermented dairy, fish and white meat with minimal amounts of red meat. White and red meat portions are higher than those consumed as part of a traditional MD, where an allowance of 450 g/week was developed in accordance with successful clinical trials described in Tables 1 and 2. This resulted in a slightly higher total protein recommendation in the MD model (Table 3) compared with percentages reported in the traditional MD counterpart. Furthermore, there is an increased amount of prescribed α-linoleic acid and total long chain n-3s included within the MD model intervention model in an effort to improve the n6:n3 ratio consumed, which is indicated in clinical practice guidelines for CVD.

This intervention is in line with the whole diet approach for MD, which has been shown to be more healthful compared to isolated nutrients [9]. As well as a whole of diet approach, the inclusion of cuisine means that the MD model intervention incorporates a combination of foods and optimises health outcomes based on the enhanced benefits of the food matrix and the preparation of these combinations.

Incorporating elements of cuisine such as combining EVOO with herbs and tomatoes resulted in the improved bioavailability of antioxidants and micronutrients; however, preparation may be considered challenging or not suitable for individuals who seek or require convenient options. To overcome this potential barrier the MD model intervention includes a range of non-cooking meal options for participants to ensure convenience, optimise consistency amongst dietary adherence and to enable sustainability. To date we are not aware of any direct comparison surrounding the effects of cuisine in cooked and raw meals. It is also likely that given the complexity around food and its constituents, results would be variable across specific foods and antioxidants.

One of the other key predicted barriers with application of a MD in non-Mediterranean countries, such as Australia, is the adaptability to other cultural preferences. This has been highlighted as a perceived barrier in other countries who have considered the application of a MD for the prevention and management of chronic diseases [75]. This paper showcased some practical solutions surrounding how to apply MD principles within other cultural dishes. In particular, the demonstration of the commonalities between ingredients and combinations from traditional dishes from range of countries was presented and how the composition and cuisine could be optimised with only minor recipe changes.

5. Conclusions

The MD model intervention maintained traditional dietary components to ensure that reported health benefits could be preserved while the context was adapted and evolved to suit an Australian multiethnic population. There were multiple factors that were considered, and thus, steps were developed to include strong evidence base and strategies surrounding potential barriers were applied to achieve this. Firstly, an optimal evidence-based dietary prescription which encompassed nutrition composition, ingredients and food combinations which were likely to elicit health benefits was adopted. Next, the dietary prescriptions were designed in a way that could be implemented across multiple cultures. This MD model is currently being assessed for acceptability and feasibility for participants with chronic diseases in two clinical trials. This MD model intervention demonstrates that it is possible to translate the key elements of the traditional MD to populations outside the Mediterranean region to increase the likelihood of acceptability and sustainability. Furthermore, this paper indicates the need for a consistent definition to describe the MD to ensure the key elements are captured and translated so that the translated MD model retains authenticity. The MD model and accompanying resources described herein can be used by nutrition researchers for future clinical trials adopting a MD. In addition, they may be used by health practitioners in the care of their patients with chronic diseases and by policy makers to provide evidence-based food guidelines for the prevention and management of many chronic diseases.

Supplementary Materials: The following are available online at http://www.mdpi.com/2072-6643/10/4/465/s1, Figure S1: Mediterranean Diet: two week cycle menu, Figure S2: Mediterranean Dietary Guidelines- Summary, Figure S3: Mediterranean Diet Pyramid, Figure S4: "No Cooking" Meal Options, Figure S5: Shopping List.

Acknowledgments: This work was supported by an Australian Government Research Training Program Scholarship (ESG).

Author Contributions: E.S.G. and T.K. designed the dietary intervention and resources with the support of A.C.T. and C.I., E.S.G. and H.L.M. delivered the dietary intervention and application of the intervention design. E.S.G. drafted the manuscript. All authors contributed to the critical review and approval of the final manuscript.

Conflicts of Interest: The authors declare no conflict of interest.

References

1. Sofi, F.; Macchi, C.; Abbate, R.; Gensini, G.F.; Casini, A. Mediterranean diet and health status: An updated meta-analysis and a proposal for a literature-based adherence score. *Public Health Nutr.* **2014**, *17*, 2769–2782. [CrossRef] [PubMed]
2. Sofi, F.; Abbate, R.; Gensini, G.F.; Casini, A. Accruing evidence on benefits of adherence to the mediterranean diet on health: An updated systematic review and meta-analysis. *Am. J. Clin. Nutr.* **2010**, *92*, 1189–1196. [CrossRef] [PubMed]
3. Itsiopoulos, C.; Hodge, A.; Kaimakamis, M. Can the mediterranean diet prevent prostate cancer? *Mol. Nutr. Food Res.* **2009**, *53*, 227–239. [CrossRef] [PubMed]
4. Ryan, M.C.; Itsiopoulos, C.; Thodis, T.; Ward, G.; Trost, N.; Hofferberth, S.; O'Dea, K.; Desmond, P.V.; Johnson, N.A.; Wilson, A.M. The Mediterranean diet improves hepatic steatosis and insulin sensitivity in individuals with non-alcoholic fatty liver disease. *J. Hepatol.* **2013**, *59*, 138–143. [CrossRef] [PubMed]
5. Dhalla, N.S.; Temsah, R.M.; Netticadan, T. Role of oxidative stress in cardiovascular diseases. *J. Hypertens.* **2000**, *18*, 655–673. [CrossRef] [PubMed]
6. Khansari, N.; Shakiba, Y.; Mahmoudi, M. Chronic inflammation and oxidative stress as a major cause of age-related diseases and cancer. *Recent Pat. Inflamm. Allergy Drug Discov.* **2009**, *3*, 73–80. [CrossRef] [PubMed]
7. Esposito, K.; Marfella, R.; Ciotola, M.; Di Palo, C.; Giugliano, F.; Giugliano, G.; D'Armiento, M.; D'Andrea, F.; Giugliano, D. Effect of a Mediterranean-style diet on endothelial dysfunction and markers of vascular inflammation in the metabolic syndrome: A randomized trial. *JAMA* **2004**, *292*, 1440–1446. [CrossRef] [PubMed]

8. Estruch, R. Anti-inflammatory effects of the Mediterranean diet: The experience of the PREDIMED study. *Proc. Nutr. Soc.* **2010**, *69*, 333–340. [CrossRef] [PubMed]
9. Widmer, R.J.; Flammer, A.J.; Lerman, L.O.; Lerman, A. The mediterranean diet, its components, and cardiovascular disease. *Am. J. Med.* **2015**, *128*, 229–238. [CrossRef] [PubMed]
10. Fielding, J.M.; Rowley, K.G.; Cooper, P.; O'Dea, K. Increases in plasma lycopene concentration after consumption of tomatoes cooked with olive oil. *Asia Pac. J. Clin. Nutr.* **2005**, *14*, 131–136. [PubMed]
11. Australian Bureau of Statistics. *Census Reveals a Fast Changing, Culturally Diverse Nation*; Australian Government: Canberra, Australia, 2017.
12. Dinu, M.; Pagliai, G.; Casini, A.; Sofi, F. Mediterranean diet and multiple health outcomes: An umbrella review of meta-analyses of observational studies and randomised trials. *Eur. J. Clin. Nutr.* **2018**, *72*, 30–43. [CrossRef] [PubMed]
13. Papamiltiadous, E.S.; Roberts, S.K.; Nicoll, A.J.; Ryan, M.C.; Itsiopoulos, C.; Salim, A.; Tierney, A.C. A randomised controlled trial of a Mediterranean dietary intervention for adults with non alcoholic fatty liver disease (MEDINA): Study protocol. *BMC Gastroenterol.* **2016**, *16*, 14. [CrossRef] [PubMed]
14. Itsiopoulos, C.; Kucianski, T.; Mayr, H.L.; van Gaal, W.J.; Martinez-Gonzalez, M.; Vally, H. The AUStralian MEDiterranean Diet Heart Trial (AUSMED Heart Trial): A randomised clinical trial in secondary prevention of coronary heart disease in a multi-ethnic Australian population: Study Protocol. *Am. Heart J.* **2018**. under review.
15. Keys, A.; Mienotti, A.; Karvonen, M.J.; Aravanis, C.; Blackburn, H.; Buzina, R.; Djordjevic, B.; Dontas, A.; Fidanza, F.; Keys, M.H.; et al. The diet and 15-year death rate in the seven countries study. *Am. J. Epidemiol.* **1986**, *124*, 903–915. [CrossRef] [PubMed]
16. Keys, A.; Menotti, A.; Aravanis, C.; Blackburn, H.; Djordevič, B.S.; Buzina, R.; Dontas, A.S.; Fidanza, F.; Karvonen, M.J.; Kimura, N.; et al. The seven countries study: 2,289 deaths in 15 years. *Prev. Med.* **1984**, *13*, 141–154. [CrossRef]
17. Trichopoulou, A.; Vasilopoulou, E.; Lagiou, A. Mediterranean diet and coronary heart disease: Are antioxidants critical? *Nutr. Rev.* **1999**, *57*, 253–255. [PubMed]
18. Trichopoulou, A.; Lagiou, P. Healthy traditional mediterranean diet: An expression of culture, history, and lifestyle. *Nutr. Rev.* **1997**, *55*, 383–389. [CrossRef] [PubMed]
19. Itsiopoulos, C.; Brazionis, L.; Kaimakamis, M.; Cameron, M.; Best, J.D.; O'Dea, K.; Rowley, K. Can the mediterranean diet lower HbA1c in type 2 diabetes? Results from a randomized cross-over study. *Nutr. Metab. Cardiovasc. Dis.* **2011**, *21*, 740–747. [CrossRef] [PubMed]
20. Estruch, R.; Ros, E.; Salas-Salvadó, J.; Covas, M.-I.; Corella, D.; Arós, F.; Gómez-Gracia, E.; Ruiz-Gutiérrez, V.; Fiol, M.; Lapetra, J.; et al. Primary prevention of cardiovascular disease with a Mediterranean diet. *N. Engl. J. Med.* **2013**, *368*, 1279–1290. [CrossRef] [PubMed]
21. Vincent-Baudry, S.; Defoort, C.; Gerber, M.; Bernard, M.C.; Verger, P.; Helal, O.; Portugal, H.; Planells, R.; Grolier, P.; Amiot-Carlin, M.J.; et al. The MEDI-RIVAGE study: Reduction of cardiovascular disease risk factors after a 3-mo intervention with a Mediterranean-type diet or a low-fat diet. *Am. J. Clin. Nutr.* **2005**, *82*, 964–971. [CrossRef] [PubMed]
22. Leaf, A. Dietary prevention of coronary heart disease: The lyon diet heart study. *Circulation* **1999**, *99*, 733–735. [CrossRef] [PubMed]
23. Ministry of Health and Welfare. Dietary Guidelines for Adults in Greece. *Arch. Hell. Med.* **1999**, *16*, 516–524.
24. Itsiopoulos, C. *The Mediterranean Diet*; Macmillan Publishers: Melbourne, Australia, 2013.
25. National Health and Medical Research Council. Australian Guidelines to Reduce Health Risks from Drinking Alcohol. Available online: https://www.nhmrc.gov.au/health-topics/alcohol-guidelines (accessed on 25 May 2016).
26. Meschino, J.P. How components of the Mediterranean diet reduce heart disease and stroke risk. *Dyn. Chiropr.* **2013**, *31*, 8.
27. Ross, S.M. Effects of extra virgin olive oil phenolic compounds and the Mediterranean diet on cardiovascular health. *Holist. Nurs. Pract.* **2013**, *27*, 303–307. [CrossRef] [PubMed]
28. Simopoulos, A.P.; Sidossis, L. What is so special about the traditional diet of Greece. *World Rev. Nutr. Diet.* **2000**, *87*, 24–42. [PubMed]
29. Simopoulos, A.P. The importance of the ratio of omega-6/omega-3 essential fatty acids. *Biomed. Pharmacother.* **2002**, *56*, 365–379. [CrossRef]

30. Bach-Faig, A.; Berry, E.M.; Lairon, D.; Reguant, J.; Trichopoulou, A.; Dernini, S.; Medina, F.X.; Battino, M.; Belahsen, R.; Miranda, G.; et al. Mediterranean diet pyramid today. Science and cultural updates. *Public Health Nutr.* **2011**, *14*, 2274–2284. [CrossRef] [PubMed]
31. McNaughton, S.A.; Ball, K.; Crawford, D.; Mishra, G.D. An index of diet and eating patterns is a valid measure of diet quality in an Australian population. *J. Nutr.* **2008**, *138*, 86–93. [CrossRef] [PubMed]
32. Aroney, C.; Aylward, P.; Kelly, A.; Chew, D.; Clune, E. National Heart Foundation of Australia Cardiac Society of Australia and New Zealand guidelines for the management of acute coronary syndromes 2006. *Med. J. Aust.* **2006**, *184*, S1–S32.
33. Wang, C.H.; Wey, K.C.; Mo, L.R.; Chang, K.K.; Lin, R.C.; Kuo, J.J. Current trends and recent advances in diagnosis, therapy, and prevention of hepatocellular carcinoma. *Asian Pac. J Cancer Prev.* **2015**, *16*, 3595–3604. [CrossRef] [PubMed]
34. Psaltopoulou, T.; Naska, A.; Orfanos, P.; Trichopoulos, D.; Mountokalakis, T.; Trichopoulou, A. Olive oil, the Mediterranean diet, and arterial blood pressure: The Greek European prospective investigation into cancer and nutrition (EPIC) study. *Am. J. Clin. Nutr.* **2004**, *80*, 1012–1018. [CrossRef] [PubMed]
35. Lamuela-Raventós, R.M.; Gimeno, E.; Fito, M.; Castellote, A.-I.; Covas, M.; de la torre-boronat, M.C.; López-Sabater, M.C. Interaction of olive oil phenol antioxidant components with low-density lipoprotein. *Biol. Res.* **2004**, *37*, 247–252. [CrossRef] [PubMed]
36. Stark, A.H.; Madar, Z. Olive oil as a functional food: Epidemiology and nutritional approaches. *Nutr. Rev.* **2002**, *60*, 170–176. [CrossRef] [PubMed]
37. Kinoshita, T.; Lepp, Z.; Chuman, H. Approach to novel functional foods for stress control 1. Toward structure-activity relationship and data mining of food compounds by chemoinformatics. *J. Med. Investig.* **2005**, *52*, 240–241. [CrossRef]
38. Kushi, L.H.; Lenart, E.B.; Willett, W.C. Health implications of mediterranean diets in light of contemporary knowledge. 1. Plant foods and dairy products. *Am. J. Clin. Nutr.* **1995**, *61*, 1407S–1415S. [CrossRef] [PubMed]
39. Ortega, R.M.; Palencia, A.; López-Sobaler, A.M. Improvement of cholesterol levels and reduction of cardiovascular risk via the consumption of phytosterols. *Br. J. Nutr.* **2006**, *96*, S89–S93. [CrossRef] [PubMed]
40. Serra Majem, L.; García Alvarez, A.; Ngo de la Cruz, J. Dieta Mediterránea: Características y beneficios para la salud. *Arch. Latinoam. Nutr.* **2004**, *54*, 44–51. [PubMed]
41. Kouris-Blazos, A.; Belski, R. Health benefits of legumes and pulses with a focus on Australian sweet lupins. *Asia Pac. J. Clin. Nutr.* **2016**, *25*, 1–17. [PubMed]
42. Darmadi-Blackberry, I.; Wahlqvist, M.L.; Kouris-Blazos, A.; Steen, B.; Lukito, W.; Horie, Y.; Horie, K. Legumes: The most important dietary predictor of survival in older people of different ethnicities. *Asia Pac. J. Clin. Nutr.* **2004**, *13*, 217–220. [PubMed]
43. Samman, S.; Sivarajah, G.; Man, J.C.; Ahmad, Z.I.; Petocz, P.; Caterson, I.D. A mixed fruit and vegetable concentrate increases plasma antioxidant vitamins and folate and lowers plasma homocysteine in men. *J. Nutr.* **2003**, *133*, 2188–2193. [CrossRef] [PubMed]
44. Bazzano, L.A.; He, J.; Ogden, L.G.; Loria, C.; Vupputuri, S.; Myers, L.; Whelton, P.K. Legume consumption and risk of coronary heart disease in US men and women: NHANES I epidemiologic follow-up study. *Arch. Intern. Med.* **2001**, *161*, 2573–2578. [CrossRef] [PubMed]
45. Becerra-Tomás, N.; Díaz-López, A.; Rosique-Esteban, N.; Ros, E.; Buil-Cosiales, P.; Corella, D.; Estruch, R.; Fitó, M.; Serra-Majem, L.; Arós, F.; et al. Legume consumption is inversely associated with type 2 diabetes incidence in adults: A prospective assessment from the PREDIMED study. *Clin. Nutr.* **2017**. [CrossRef]
46. Ruxton, C.; Reed, S.C.; Simpson, M.; Millington, K. The health benefits of omega-3 polyunsaturated fatty acids: A review of the evidence. *J. Hum. Nutr. Diet.* **2004**, *17*, 449–459. [CrossRef] [PubMed]
47. Biesalski, H.-K. Meat as a component of a healthy diet—Are there any risks or benefits if meat is avoided in the diet? *Meat Sci.* **2005**, *70*, 509–524. [CrossRef] [PubMed]
48. Sinha, R.; Cross, A.J.; Graubard, B.I.; Leitzmann, M.F.; Schatzkin, A. Meat intake and mortality: A prospective study of over half a million people. *Arch. Intern. Med.* **2009**, *169*, 562–571. [CrossRef] [PubMed]
49. John, J.; Ziebland, S.; Yudkin, P.; Roe, L.; Neil, H. Effects of fruit and vegetable consumption on plasma antioxidant concentrations and blood pressure: A randomised controlled trial. *Lancet* **2002**, *359*, 1969–1974. [CrossRef]
50. Blomhoff, R.; Carlsen, M.H.; Andersen, L.F.; Jacobs, D.R. Health benefits of nuts: Potential role of antioxidants. *Br. J. Nutr.* **2006**, *96*, S52–S60. [CrossRef] [PubMed]

51. Sabaté, J.; Ang, Y. Nuts and health outcomes: New epidemiologic evidence. *Am. J. Clin. Nutr.* **2009**, *89*, 1643S–1648S. [CrossRef] [PubMed]
52. Panesar, P.S. Fermented dairy products: Starter cultures and potential nutritional benefits. *Food Nutr. Sci.* **2011**, *2*, 47–51. [CrossRef]
53. Ebringer, L.; Ferenčík, M.; Krajčovič, J. Beneficial health effects of milk and fermented dairy products—Review. *Folia Microbiol.* **2008**, *53*, 378–394. [CrossRef] [PubMed]
54. Bartram, H.-P.; Scheppach, W.; Gerlach, S.; Ruckdeschel, G.; Kelber, E.; Kasper, H. Does yogurt enriched with bifidobacterium longum affect colonic microbiology and fecal metabolites in health subjects? *Am. J. Clin. Nutr.* **1994**, *59*, 428–432. [CrossRef] [PubMed]
55. Slavin, J.L.; Jacobs, D.; Marquart, L.; Wiemer, K. The role of whole grains in disease prevention. *J. Am. Diet. Assoc.* **2001**, *101*, 780–785. [CrossRef]
56. Slavin, J. Whole grains and human health. *Nutr. Res. Rev.* **2004**, *17*, 99–110. [CrossRef] [PubMed]
57. Slavin, J.L.; Martini, M.C.; Jacobs, D.R.; Marquart, L. Plausible mechanisms for the protectiveness of whole grains. *Am. J. Clin. Nutr.* **1999**, *70*, 459s–463s. [CrossRef] [PubMed]
58. Cook, S.I.; Sellin, J.H. Review article: Short chain fatty acids in health and disease. *Aliment. Pharmacol. Ther.* **1998**, *12*, 499–507. [CrossRef] [PubMed]
59. Goran, M.I.; Walker, R.; Allayee, H. Genetic-related and carbohydrate-related factors affecting liver fat accumulation. *Curr. Opin. Clin. Nutr. Metab. Care* **2012**, *15*, 392–396. [CrossRef] [PubMed]
60. Jin, R.; Welsh, J.A.; Le, N.-A.; Holzberg, J.; Sharma, P.; Martin, D.R.; Vos, M.B. Dietary fructose reduction improves markers of cardiovascular disease risk in Hispanic-American adolescents with NAFLD. *Nutrients* **2014**, *6*, 3187–3201. [CrossRef] [PubMed]
61. Handelman, G.J.; Nightingale, Z.D.; Lichtenstein, A.H.; Schaefer, E.J.; Blumberg, J.B. Lutein and zeaxanthin concentrations in plasma after dietary supplementation with egg yolk. *Am. J. Clin. Nutr.* **1999**, *70*, 247–251. [CrossRef] [PubMed]
62. Anderson, K.E. Comparison of fatty acid, cholesterol, and vitamin a and e composition in eggs from hens housed in conventional cage and range production facilities. *Poult. Sci.* **2011**, *90*, 1600–1608. [CrossRef] [PubMed]
63. Wallerath, T.; Deckert, G.; Ternes, T.; Anderson, H.; Li, H.; Witte, K.; Förstermann, U. Resveratrol, a 'polyphenolic phytoalexin present in red wine, enhances expression and activity of endothelial nitric oxide synthase. *Circulation* **2002**, *106*, 1652–1658. [CrossRef] [PubMed]
64. Echeverry, C.; Blasina, F.; Arredondo, F.; Ferreira, M.; Abin-Carriquiry, J.A.; Vasquez, L.; Aspillaga, A.A.; Diez, M.S.; Leighton, F.; Dajas, F. Cytoprotection by neutral fraction of tannat red wine against oxidative stress-induced cell death. *J. Agric. Food chem.* **2004**, *52*, 7395–7399. [CrossRef] [PubMed]
65. Ortega, R. Importance of functional foods in the mediterranean diet. *Public Health Nutr.* **2006**, *9*, 1136–1140. [CrossRef] [PubMed]
66. Ninfali, P.; Mea, G.; Giorgini, S.; Rocchi, M.; Bacchiocca, M. Antioxidant capacity of vegetables, spices and dressings relevant to nutrition. *Br. J. Nutr.* **2005**, *93*, 257–266. [CrossRef] [PubMed]
67. Bower, A.; Marquez, S.; de Mejia, E.G. The health benefits of selected culinary herbs and spices found in the traditional Mediterranean diet. *Crit. Rev. Food Sci. Nutr.* **2016**, *56*, 2728–2746. [CrossRef] [PubMed]
68. Stahl, W. Carrots, tomatoes and cocoa: Research on dietary antioxidants in dusseldorf. *Arch. Biochem. Biophys.* **2016**, *595*, 125–131. [CrossRef] [PubMed]
69. Wolfson, J.A.; Bleich, S.N. Is cooking at home associated with better diet quality or weight-loss intention? *Public Health Nutr.* **2015**, *18*, 1397–1406. [CrossRef] [PubMed]
70. Garcia, A.L.; Reardon, R.; McDonald, M.; Vargas-Garcia, E.J. Community interventions to improve cooking skills and their effects on confidence and eating behaviour. *Curr. Nutr. Rep.* **2016**, *5*, 315–322. [CrossRef] [PubMed]
71. Hoffman, R.; Gerber, M. Evaluating and adapting the mediterranean diet for non-mediterranean populations: A critical appraisal. *Nutr. Rev.* **2013**, *71*, 573–584. [CrossRef] [PubMed]
72. Radd-Vagenas, S.; Kouris-Blazos, A.; Singh, M.F.; Flood, V.M. Evolution of mediterranean diets and cuisine: Concepts and definitions. *Asia Pac. J. Clin. Nutr.* **2013**, 1–32. [CrossRef]
73. Jordan, C.H.; Wang, W.; Donatoni, L.; Meier, B.P. Mindful eating: Trait and state mindfulness predict healthier eating behavior. *Pers. Indiv. Differ.* **2014**, *68*, 107–111. [CrossRef]

74. Burlingame, B.; Dernini, S. Sustainable diets: The mediterranean diet as an example. *Public Health Nutr.* **2011**, *14*, 2285–2287. [CrossRef] [PubMed]
75. Moore, S.; McEvoy, C.; Prior, L.; Lawton, J.; Patterson, C.; Kee, F.; Cupples, M.; Young, I.; Appleton, K.; McKinley, M.; et al. Barriers to adopting a mediterranean diet in northern European adults at high risk of developing cardiovascular disease. *J. Hum. Nutr. Diet.* **2017**. [CrossRef] [PubMed]

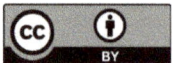

© 2018 by the authors. Licensee MDPI, Basel, Switzerland. This article is an open access article distributed under the terms and conditions of the Creative Commons Attribution (CC BY) license (http://creativecommons.org/licenses/by/4.0/).

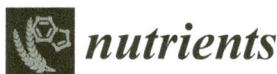

Article

Adherence to the Mediterranean Diet Is Associated with Physical Activity, Self-Concept and Sociodemographic Factors in University Student

Félix Zurita-Ortega [1], Silvia San Román-Mata [2], Ramón Chacón-Cuberos [3], Manuel Castro-Sánchez [4,*] and José Joaquín Muros [1]

1. Department of Didactics of Musical, Plastic and Corporal Expression, University of Granada, 18071 Granada, Spain; felixzo@ugr.es (F.Z.-O.); jjmuros@ugr.es (J.J.M.)
2. Department of Nursing, University of Granada, 18071 Granada, Spain; silviasanroman@ugr.es
3. Department of Integrated Didactics, University of Huelva, 21007 Huelva, Spain; ramon.chacon@ddi.uhu.es
4. Department of Education, University of Almería, 04120 Almería, Spain
* Correspondence: mcastros@ual.es; Tel.: +34-958-248-949

Received: 21 June 2018; Accepted: 23 July 2018; Published: 26 July 2018

Abstract: (1) Background: The aim of this study was to assess adherence to the Mediterranean diet (MD) and to examine the relationship between MD adherence, physical activity, self-concept, and other sociodemographic factors; (2) Methods: A cross-sectional study ($N = 597$; 18.99 ± 0.64 years) was conducted in a sample of university students from Ceuta, Melilla, and Granada (Spain). Religious beliefs and place of residence were directly reported, while physical activity and adherence to the MD were self-reported using the Physical Activity Questionnaire for Adolescents (PAQ-A) and the Mediterranean Diet Quality Index (KIDMED) respectively. Self-concept was evaluated using the Five-Factor Self-Concept Scale; (3) Results: Of those students reporting high levels of habitual physical activity, 82.3% also reported high adherence to the MD, with 17.7% reporting a medium adherence. Of students reporting no physical activity, 25.7% also reported medium adherence to the MD. No significant associations were found between the MD and religious beliefs. It was observed that the university campus was associated with the level of adherence to the MD ($p = 0.030$), with adherence being lowest in Ceuta and Melilla. Finally, the MD was associated with academic ($p = 0.001$) and physical self-concept ($p = 0.005$); 4) Conclusions: The MD should be promoted to university students, particularly those studying at Ceuta and Melilla, given the present findings of lower MD adherence. In addition, as higher MD adherence was also highlighted with more positive self-concept, its promotion would be beneficial in wider educational contexts.

Keywords: Mediterranean diet; physical activity; self-concept; socioeconomic factors

1. Introduction

Considerable research has addressed the beneficial effects of the Mediterranean diet (MD) on life expectancy and quality of life [1], since it has a positive effect on public health, and reduces the risk of suffering cardiovascular diseases, Alzheimer's, depression, diabetes, and cancer, as well as many others [2–7]. In addition, the MD is associated with better cognitive and emotional functioning [6,7]. In addition, higher socioeconomic status and living in the family home is associated with a better quality of diet [8–10].

The composition of the MD is based on the consumption of food cultivated around the Mediterranean Sea, which contain a high amount of natural antioxidants. It is characterized by a high intake of olive oil, cereals, fruits, vegetables, and legumes, with also a moderate consumption of fish, eggs, and dairy products. Red and processed meats, saturated fats, and alcoholic drinks are consumed in low amounts [3,11,12]. Following a balanced diet, the MD has been shown to provide essential macronutrients and demonstrates important health benefits, such as improved body composition and the prevention of cardiovascular diseases [4–6,10].

The benefits of adhering to a MD have been studied for young people living in Mediterranean areas are shown in countries, such as Italy [13,14], Turkey [15,16], Cyprus and Greece [17,18], Spain [19,20], Lebanon [11], and Croatia [21]. Additionally, studies have been conducted in countries with cultural and linguistic influence, such as Chile [4,10], Brazil [22], or the south of the United States [23].

Arnet describes university students as being in an "emerging adulthood stage [24] during which they possess the biological maturation of an adult, but have not yet achieved comparable psychosocial development [19]. These young adults, often during the first years of study, live outside of the family home, often with negative implications for the quality of their diet [24,25]. Unhealthy habits appearing during this life stage often persist into adulthood, for example, previous research has linked poor nutrition with the use of harmful substances and negative repercussions later in life [25,26].

Diet is one of the cornerstones of a healthy lifestyle, and it is sometimes characterised in university students by a lack of meals and essential foods, and by the intake of large amounts of sugar, alcohol, and saturated fats [27]. These facets may be influenced by the place in which the student lives (e.g., shared flat, halls of residence), with moving away from home to live in the city of the university being a potentially important factor [11,25,28,29]. Further, university students often show reduced levels of physical activity and greater engagement in sedentary behaviour [24]. It should be noted that this is not the case for all students, with one study of students enrolled in nursing and teaching courses showing a higher adherence to the MD [30,31]. Studying subjects related to nutrition may, therefore, be a protective factor for some of the previously identified negative habits.

Self-concept is defined as the collection of beliefs about oneself and is also associated with health behaviours [32]. For instance, diets with an excess of fat and sugar can lead to increased overweight indices and a negative belief about oneself [33,34]. Moreover, several studies have shown that a worse adherence to the MD is associated with academic performance and subsequent negative academic self-concept [35], and negative emotions, such as higher levels of stress and anxiety, and a subsequent negative emotional self-concept [36].

Students' religious beliefs might also have an influence, since the Mediterranean Sea is surrounded by countries that are traditionally Catholic and Islamic [37]. The Islamic religion associated with Arabian culture does not allow the consumption of some food, such as pork or alcohol. It could be thought that Spain, since it is so near to Africa, could have similar food and cooking traditions. However, the norms associated with both regions are very different. The cities of Ceuta and Melilla, for example, are Spanish, but are in Africa, thus, being highly influenced by Arabian culture [38].

Although the MD has been studied in relation to physical activity and healthy lifestyles, research in relation to self-concept, place of residence [24,39], and cultural-religion [38] is scarce. Thus, the present study will present novel data on the MD and its association with sociodemographic, physical, and emotional factors within a sample of university students enrolled in social and health science courses based at three campuses of the University of Granada (Ceuta, Melilla, and Granada).

The present study will address the following research question and associated hypotheses: Is adherence to the MD related to religion, place of residence, physical activity, and self-concept of university students from different parts of Spain?

Hypothesis 1 (H1). *The university students from Ceuta and Melilla will present a lower adherence to the MD. In addition, those who do not live in a shared flat and report Christian beliefs will follow a better-quality diet.*

Hypothesis 2 (H2). *University students reporting higher levels of physical activity will also report greater adherence to the MD.*

Hypothesis 3 (H3). *Higher adherence to the MD will be associated with more positive self-concept both overall and for all its associated dimensions.*

The main aims of the present study are: (a) To assess adherence to the MD within a population of students from Ceuta, Melilla, and Granada (Spain); and (b) to examine the relationship between adherence to the MD, physical activity, self-concept, religion, and place of residence.

2. Materials and Methods

2.1. Subjects

The present research reports a cross-sectional study with a sample of 636 university students aged between 18 and 20 (18.99 ± 0.64 years) enrolled in education or health-related degree programmes in Granada, Ceuta, and Melilla (Spain). Of these, 39 participants did not meet the inclusion criteria (i.e., incomplete questionnaires, failure to complete informed consent forms) and so could not be included. The final sampled, therefore, consisted of 597 participants (156 males and 441 females): Granada ($n = 103$); Ceuta ($n = 138$); and Melilla ($n = 356$).

2.2. Instruments

The Mediterranean Diet Quality Index (KIDMED) [40] was used to determine the level of adherence to the MD. This questionnaire consists of sixteen items that relate to Mediterranean dietary patterns. Four items denote negative connotations with respect to the MD (e.g., do you eat sweets daily?) and are scored as a −1, while twelve items relate to positive connotations (e.g., do you use olive oil for cooking at home?) and are scored as a +1. All items are then summed to produce a total score, which ranges from −4 to 12. Adherence to the MD can then be classified as high (≥8), medium (2–7), or low (≤1). The KIDMED demonstrates reliable psychometric properties using Cronbach's alpha ($\alpha = 0.836$).

To estimate physical activity levels, the Physical Activity Questionnaire for Adolescents (PAQ-A) was used, which has been previously validated by Kowalski et al. [41] and adapted to Spanish by Martínez-Gómez et al. [42]. The instrument asks participants to retrospectively report the frequency and type of physical activity engaged in on each of the seven days preceding administration. The questionnaire comprises ten items (e.g., last weekend, how many times did you do sports, dance, or play games in which you were very active?), rated using a five-point Likert scale. Individual items are then summed to create a variable, which describes overall physical activity levels. The PAQ-A demonstrates reliable psychometric properties using Cronbach's alpha ($\alpha = 0.874$).

Self-concept was assessed using the Five-Factor Self-Concept Questionnaire (AF-5) [43]. The AF-5 is formed according to the dimensions of academic self-concept (A-SC), social self-concept (S-SC), emotional self-concept (E-SC), family self-concept (F-SC), and physical self-concept (P-SC). The test includes thirty items (e.g., I am a friendly person), which are rated on a five-point Likert scale ranging from never (1) to always (5). Each dimension is described by six items (A-SC: Items 1, 6, 11, 16, 21, 26; S-SC: Items 2, 7, 12, 17, 22, 27; E-SC: Items 3, 8, 13, 18, 23, 28; F-SC: Items 4, 9, 14, 19, 24, 29; P-SC: Items 5, 10, 15, 20, 25, 30). The AF-5 demonstrates reliable psychometric properties using Cronbach's alpha ($\alpha = 0.800$). This replicates earlier reports by García and Musitu [43] ($\alpha = 0.810$).

Socioeconomic factors were directly reported by participants using a self-registration sheet. Participants reported their gender, age, religious belief (Catholic, Muslim, Atheist-Agnostic, and other), and place of residence (family home, shared flat, or university residence).

2.3. Procedure

Eligible participants were provided a detailed explanation of the aims and implications of the research. Those who decided to participate then provided written informed consent. Participants were instructed on how to fill out the questionnaires. All tests were conducted during a non-teaching lesson at the student's university. No incentives were provided for participation. A research assistant attended all data collection sessions to provide guidance on the completion of questionnaires. Ethical principles of the Declaration of Helsinki were adhered to and ethical approval was granted by the Ethics Committee of the University of Granada.

2.4. Statistical Analysis

Data were analysed using SPSS® version 24.0 (IBM Corp, Armonk, NY, USA) for Windows. Means for all quantitative variables (self-concept) are reported alongside the standard deviation. Averages and percentages are presented for all qualitative variables (MD, physical activity, gender, religious belief, university campus, and place of residence). Normality of the data was tested using the Kolmogorov-Smirnov test with Lilliefors correction, and homoscedasticity was assessed using the Levene test. The association between variables was determined using chi-square analysis and ANOVA. The level of significance was set at 0.05.

3. Results

Table 1 shows the proportion of the sample attending the university campuses of Granada, Ceuta, and Melilla. A total of 636 university students were invited to participate in the study. Of these, 39 students were excluded for not meeting inclusion criteria, leaving a final sample of 597 participants. Of the final sample, 17.3% (n = 103) were attending the university campus in Granada, 23.1% (n = 138) were attending in Ceuta, and 59.6% (n = 356) were attending in Melilla.

Table 1. Proportion of the sample (eligible sample, excluded participants, and final sample) attending the university campuses of Granada, Ceuta, and Melilla.

University Campus	Eligible Sample % (n)	Excluded Participants % (n)	Final Sample % (n)
Granada	17.6% (n = 112)	23.1% (n = 9)	17.3% (n = 103)
Ceuta	23.4% (n = 149)	28.2% (n = 11)	23.1% (n = 138)
Melilla	59.0% (n = 375)	48.7% (n = 19)	59.6% (n = 356)
Total	100.0% (n = 636)	100.0% (n = 39)	100.0% (n = 597)

As shown in Table 2, adherence to the MD was high, medium, and low for 77.6%, 21.9%, and 0.5% of the sample, respectively. The percentage of participants who reported engaging in physical activity was similar to those reporting not engaging in physical activity (52.8% vs. 47.2%). A total of 54.9% of participants reported being of Catholic faith, 27.5% were atheist or agnostic, and 16.3% identified themselves as Muslim. A total of 63.8% of the participants reported residing with their family, while only 6.7% reported residing in student housing. Self-concept was reported most positively for the dimension relating to family (Mean (M) = 4.36) followed by the social dimension. Academic, emotional, and physical self-concept were rated less positively, with average scores being lower than 3.65 for these dimensions.

As shown in Table 3, there were significant associations between MD adherence and physical activity (p = 0.014). Students who reported practicing physical activity were more likely to report a high adherence to the MD (82.3% of the active participants), while only 73.3% of participants who reported not engaging in physical activity reported a high adherence to the MD.

As shown in Table 4, the MD was associated with academic self-concept (p = 0.001), which was more positive in students with high MD adherence (M = 3.67) relative to those reporting only a medium adherence (M = 3.45). The same tendency was observed with regards to physical self-concept (p = 0.005), with higher scores reported by students with high MD adherence (M = 3.39) compared with those who had a medium adherence (M = 3.16). No differences were found with regards to social, emotional, and family self-concept ($p \geq 0.050$).

Finally, no significant differences ($p \geq 0.050$) were found in the associations between MD, religious belief, and place of residence (Table 5). It was observed that the university campus was associated with adherence to the MD (p = 0.030). The percentage of students who had a high adherence was 90.2% in Granada, 74.7% in Ceuta, and 72.5% in Melilla. Medium adherence was reported by 10.7% in Granada, 23.9% in Ceuta, and 26.7% in Melilla.

Table 2. Characteristics of study sample according to sex.

Variables		All (n = 597)	Sex Male (n = 156)	Female (n = 441)
MD	High	77.6% (n = 463)	33.3% (n = 118)	66.7% (n = 345)
	Medium	21.9% (n = 131)	28.2% (n = 37)	71.8% (n = 94)
	Low	0.5% (n = 3)	0.6% (n = 1)	0.5% (n = 2)
Campus	Granada	17.3% (n = 103)	18.4% (n = 19)	81.6% (n = 84)
	Ceuta	23.1% (n = 138)	26.8% (n = 37)	73.2% (n = 101)
	Melilla	59.6% (n = 356)	28.1% (n = 100)	71.9% (n = 256)
Physical Activity	Yes	47.2% (n = 282)	39.4% (n = 111)	60.6% (n = 171)
	No	52.8% (n = 315)	14.3% (n = 45)	85.7% (n = 270)
Religious Belief	Catholic	54.9% (n = 328)	25.3% (n = 83)	74.7% (n = 245)
	Muslim	16.3% (n = 97)	13.4% (n = 13)	86.6% (n = 84)
	Atheist-Agnostic	27.5% (n = 164)	34.1% (n = 56)	65.9% (n = 108)
	Other	1.3% (n = 8)	50.0% (n = 4)	50.0% (n = 4)
Place of Residence	Family Home	63.8% (n = 381)	24.9% (n = 95)	75.1% (n = 286)
	Shared Flat	29.5% (n = 176)	26.7% (n = 47)	73.3% (n = 129)
	University Residence	6.7% (n = 40)	35.0% (n = 14)	65.0% (n = 26)
Self-Concept	A-SC	M = 3.62 SD = 0.601	M = 3.48 SD = 0.600	M = 3.67 SD = 0.595
	S-SC	M = 3.91 SD = 0.660	M = 3.94 SD = 0.661	M = 3.90 SD = 0.659
	E-SC	M = 3.31 SD = 0.440	M = 3.43 SD = 0.407	M = 3.27 SD = 0.444
	F-SC	M = 4.36 SD = 0.626	M = 4.23 SD = 0.664	M = 4.41 SD = 0.605
	P-SC	M = 3.34 SD = 0.741	M = 3.64 SD = 0.681	M = 3.23 SD = 0.733

MD, Mediterranean diet; A-SC, academic self-concept; S-SC, social self-concept; E-SC, emotional self-concept; F-SC, family self-concept; P-SC, physical self-concept.

Table 3. Adherence to the MD according to self-reported physical activity level ($p = 0.014$).

MD	Physical Activity [% (n)] Yes	No	Total [% (n)]
Low adherence	0.0% (n = 0)	1.0% (n = 3)	0.5% (n = 3)
Medium adherence	17.7% (n = 50)	25.7% (n = 81)	21.9% (n = 131)
High adherence	82.3% (n = 232)	73.3% (n = 231)	77.6% (n = 463)
Total	100.0% (n = 232)	100.0% (n = 315)	100.0% (n = 567)

Table 4. Dimensions of self-concept according to adherence to the MD.

Self-Concept	MD	M	SD	F	P
A-SC	Low	3.50	1.25	6.744	0.001
	Medium	3.45	0.62		
	High	3.67	0.58		
S-SC	Low	3.83	1.15	2.181	0.114
	Medium	3.80	0.62		
	High	3.94	0.66		
E-SC	Low	3.13	0.64	0.420	0.657
	Medium	3.29	0.40		
	High	3.31	0.45		
F-SC	Low	4.67	0.44	1.926	0.147
	Medium	4.28	0.69		
	High	4.39	0.60		
P-SC	Low	3.11	0.94	5.296	0.005
	Medium	3.16	0.73		
	High	3.39	0.73		

Table 5. Adherence to the MD according to religious belief, campus, and place of residence.

Variables		MD Adherence			P
		Low	Medium	High	
Religious belief	Catholic	0.6% (n = 2)	23.5% (n = 77)	75.9% (n = 249)	0.762
	Muslim	0.0% (n = 0)	22.7% (n = 22)	77.3% (n = 75)	
	Atheist-Agnostic	1.2% (n = 2)	20.1% (n = 33)	78.7% (n = 129)	
	Other	0.0% (n = 0)	25.0% (n = 2)	75.0% (n = 6)	
Place Residence	Family Home	0.8% (n = 3)	20.7% (n = 79)	78.5% (n = 299)	0.881
	Shared Flat	1.2% (n = 2)	25.5% (n = 45)	73.3% (n = 129)	
	University Residence	0.0% (n = 0)	20.0% (n = 8)	80.0% (n = 32)	
Campus	Granada	0.0% (n = 0)	9.8% (n = 10)	90.2% (n = 93)	0.030
	Ceuta	1.4% (n = 2)	23.9% (n = 33)	74.7% (n = 103)	
	Melilla	0.8% (n = 3)	26.7% (n = 95)	72.5% (n = 258)	

4. Discussion

The main objective of the present study was to identify the relationships between adherence to the MD, physical activity, self-concept, and selected sociodemographic factors. High adherence to a MD was reported by almost 80% of the included participants. One factor that could contribute to this high level of adherence is the relatively young age of the participants (none of whom were older than 20 years of age), making it likely these participants were still highly influenced by their family with regards to their eating behavior, a suggestion supported by previous research conducted by San Mauro et al. [44]. On the other hand, previous research conducted with samples of older university students has failed to support these suggestions [26,29,45].

More participants in the present study were attending the campus in Melilla than Ceuta or Granada. At this particular campus, all of the degrees pertained to the fields of social sciences or health. While the campus of Granada is the biggest of the three, it also has the greatest variety of available courses. The present study chose to focus on students studying courses previously identified by Rodrigo et al. [31] as being disciplines with likely associations with adherence and understanding of the MD. Further, it is also important to highlight the greater participation of women in the present study, which is because these areas of study are more popular amongst women than men [29].

Findings relating to the practice of physical activity are similar to those obtained in other studies, which have shown physical activity engagement to decrease upon reaching adulthood and starting university. This may at least be partly caused by the change in social tendencies and the development of habits leading to weight gain, stress, and anxiety [46–48]. This life period is, therefore, critical and the promotion of healthy habits in relation to nutrition and physical activity is necessary [49].

Associations were established between adherence to the MD and the practice of physical activity, with the conclusion that those who exercise regularly have better nutritional levels. Students with low adherence to the MD tended also to not engage in physical activity, whilst those typically adhering to a MD diet also show higher levels of physical activity [50–52]. One potential explanation for this is that young people who practice physical activity tend to consume a nutritious diet to obtain greater results in terms of performance, body image, or wellbeing [53,54].

In the present study, academic self-concept was higher in students who reported high adherence to the MD than in those who reported low adherence. This suggests that diet influences academic achievement, as has been suggested by Unal et al. [55] who discuss the importance of breakfast and the MD as a contributor to academic success. Since a better academic performance is related to a more positive perception of the individual in the university environment, their academic self-concept could improve [55,56]. In this sense, these results are similar to those reported in other teenage populations [56] and corroborate previous research conducted by Inauen et al. [57], which discussed the benefits of exercise on nutritional behavior.

Contrary to research suggesting an increase in the amount of people who do not practise any religion in Spain [37], Catholicism is still followed in southern areas. However, in the areas of Ceuta and Melilla, the Islamic faith is widely practiced. In recent years, the number of degrees studied at the three university campuses has increased, leading to more students studying locally and living in their family home. Resultantly, the family dimension of self-concept becomes highly valued and has a clear effect on improving nutritional consumption.

In the present study, religious and cultural tendencies were not associated with diet, which is contrary to previous findings reported by Navarro-Prado et al. [38] suggesting that Muslims had a lower quality diet than Christians due to their regular omission of breakfast and dinner. The present study suggests that culinary cultures in the south of Spain and the north of Africa influence one another, thus, masking differences. Age is likely a stronger influence on eating behaviours than place of residence as almost 70% of the participants still lived at home, reducing the variability of this variable. Furthermore, several studies, such as those developed by Donnelly et al. [58] and Bernardo et al. [59], demonstrate that the cost of healthy food inhibits the ability of university students to adhere to a MD.

Higher MD adherence was reported by participants studying at the campus in Granada than the other two included campuses. As this city is inside the Peninsula, it has an enhanced supply of good quality food in comparison to those cities outside of the Peninsula. This, alongside the previously mentioned culture of Arabian food in Ceuta and Melilla, [38], can help to explain the lower adherence to the MD in these regions.

The present study also has a number of limitations. The cross-sectional design prevents any conclusions pertaining to causality from being made. This type of study provides preliminary evidence, which should now be followed by longitudinal research. Other limitations relate to the scales used. For instance, errors caused by poor comprehension of the KIDMED test and the self-report questionnaire were identified, though evidence suggests that such errors should not impede their application [8,60]. Finally, while the PAQ-A demonstrates good internal consistency within samples of university students and Arnet [24] has highlighted similarities during emerging adulthood and this period of adolescence, it should be noted that this instrument has only been validated within samples of adolescents and older adolescents, and so could present adjustment errors within this sample.

In consideration of the limitations and findings of the present study, the following suggestions are made for future research. Future studies should seek to apply the present self-report instruments to more areas of knowledge and within samples of adults. Moreover, the PREDIMED and GPAQ questionnaires may be more appropriately used to measure adherence to the MD and physical activity behaviour in future research as they have been validated amongst young adults. Finally, an intervention using nutritional talks and practical activity should be developed to improve the level of adherence to the MD of university students, particularly in the cities of Ceuta and Melilla. This should also include periodic measurement of psychosocial factors and health indices to ascertain relationships with adherence to the MD.

5. Conclusions

Adherence to the MD was related to certain socioeconomic factors, such as the university campus attended, the practice of physical activity, and some dimensions of self-concept. The following conclusions can, therefore, be made regarding the study hypotheses:

- Hypothesis 1 (H1) was partially supported as university students from Ceuta and Melilla reported a lower adherence to the MD. However, statistically significant differences were not found according to the place of residence and religious belief;
- Hypothesis 2 (H2) was completely supported. The results showed the practice of physical activity to be associated with a higher adherence to the MD; and
- Hypothesis 3 (H3) was partially supported, since adherence to the MD was only associated with the physical and academic dimensions of self-concept.

The main conclusions established from the present study were that participating students at the three included campuses typically reported moderate levels of MD adherence, with adherence being higher amongst students at the Granada campus. No relationships were identified between MD and the place of residence or religious belief, while physical activity was positively associated with MD adherence. Finally, adherence to the MD was positively associated with the physical and academic self-concept. Given the relationships observed, the MD should be promoted in university students, with a view to improving psychosocial factors. The lower quality of diet prevalent at the campuses of Ceuta and Melilla highlights these areas as important contexts for intervention. A main strength of the present analysis of the MD in a population with particular social and cultural characteristics is the highlighting of relevant social factors, such as religion, and psychological factors of well-being, such as self-concept. Future research should now build on this to replicate the present study within other populations of relevance, such as children or adolescents, and to include other key factors for health, such as overweight or substance consumption.

Author Contributions: F.Z.-O., R.C.-C., M.C.-S. and J.J.M. conceived the hypothesis of this study. F.Z.-O., S.S.R.-M., R.C.-C., M.C.-S. and J.J.M. participated in data collection. R.C.-C., M.C.-S. and S.S.R.-M. analysed the data. All authors contributed to data interpretation of statistical analysis. F.Z.-O., S.S.R.-M., R.C.-C., M.C.-S. and J.J.M. wrote the paper. All authors read and approved the final manuscript.

Funding: This research received no external funding.

Conflicts of Interest: The authors declare no conflict of interest.

References

1. García, S.; Herrera, N.; Rodríguez, C.; Nissensohn, M.; Román, B.; Serra-Majem, L. KIDMED test; prevalence of low adherence to the Mediterranean diet in children and young; a systematic review. *Nutr. Hosp.* **2015**, *32*, 2390–2399. [CrossRef]
2. De la Montaña, J.; Castro, L.; Cobas, N.; Rodríguez, M.; Miguez, M. Adherence to the Mediterranean diet and its relation to the body mass index in university students of Galicia. *Nutr. Clín. Diet. Hosp.* **2012**, *32*, 72–80.
3. Baldini, M.; Pasqui, F.; Bordoni, A.; Maranesi, M. Is the Mediterranean lifestyle still a reality? Evaluation of food consumption and energy expenditure in Italian and Spanish university students. *Public Health Nutr.* **2008**, *12*, 148–155. [CrossRef] [PubMed]
4. Rodríguez, F.J.; Espinoza, L.R.; Gálvez, J.; Macmillan, N.G.; Solis, P. Nutritional status and lifestyles in university students of the Pontificia Universidad Católica de Valparaiso. *Rev. Univ. Salud* **2013**, *15*, 123–135.
5. Grao-Cruces, A.; Nuviala, A.; Fernández-Martínez, A.; Porcel-Gálvez, A.M.; Moral-García, J.E.; Martínez-López, E.J. Adherence to the Mediterranean diet in rural and urban in the south of Spain, satisfaction with life, anthropometry and physical and sedentary activities. *Nutr. Hosp.* **2013**, *28*, 1129–1135. [CrossRef] [PubMed]
6. Sánchez-Villegas, A.; Ruiz-Canela, M.; Gea, A.; Lahortiga, F.; Martínez-González, M.A. The association between the Mediterranean lifestyle and depression. *Clin. Psychol. Sci.* **2016**, *4*, 1085–1093. [CrossRef]
7. Mosconi, L.; Walters, M.; Sterling, J.; Quinn, C.; McHugh, P.; Andrews, R.E.; Matthews, D.C.; Ganzer, C.; Osorio, R.S. Lifestyle and vascular risk effects on MRI-based biomarkers of Alzheimer´s disease: A cross-sectional study of middle-aged adults from the broader New York City area. *BMJ Open* **2018**, *8*, e019362. [CrossRef] [PubMed]
8. Muros, J.J.; Cofre-Bolados, C.; Arriscado, D.; Zurita-Ortega, F.; Knox, E. Mediterranean diet adherence is associated with lifestyle, physical fitness, and mental wellness among 10-y-olds in Chile. *Nutrition* **2017**, *35*, 87–92. [CrossRef] [PubMed]
9. Papadaki, S.; Mavrikaki, E. Greek adolescents and the Mediterranean diet: Factors affecting quality and adherence. *Nutrition* **2015**, *31*, 345–349. [CrossRef] [PubMed]
10. Darmon, N.; Drewnowski, A. Contribution of food prices and diet cost to socioeconomic disparities in diet quality and health: A systematic review and analysis. *Nutr. Rev.* **2015**, *73*, 643–660. [CrossRef] [PubMed]
11. Yahia, N.; Achkar, A.; Abdallah, A.; Rizk, S. Eating habits and obesity among Lebanese university students. *Nutr. J.* **2008**, *7*, 1–6. [CrossRef] [PubMed]
12. Ortiz-Moncada, R.; Norte, A.I.; Zaragoza, A.; Fernández, J.; Davo, M.C. Mediterranean diet patterns follow Spanish university students. *Nutr. Hosp.* **2012**, *27*, 1952–1959. [CrossRef] [PubMed]

13. Roccaldo, R.; Censi, L.; D'Addezio, L.; Toti, E.; Martone, D.; D'Addesa, D.; Cernigliaro, A.; ZOOM8 Study Group; Censi, L.; D'Addesa, D.; et al. Adherence to the Mediterranean diet in Italian school children (the ZOOM8 study). *Int. J. Food Sci. Nutr.* **2014**, *65*, 621–628. [CrossRef] [PubMed]
14. Forleo, M.B.; Tamburro, M.; Mastronard, L.; Giaccio, V.; Ripabelli, G. Food consumption and eating habits: A segmentation of university students from Central-South Italy. *New Medit.* **2017**, *16*, 56–65.
15. Santomauro, F.; Lorini, C.; Tanini, T.; Indiani, L.; Lastrucci, V.; Comodo, N.; Bonaccorsi, G. Adherence to Mediterranean diet in a simple of Tuscan adolescents. *Nutrition* **2014**, *30*, 1379–1383. [CrossRef] [PubMed]
16. Baydemir, C.; Ozgur, E.G.; Balci, S. Evaluation of adherence to Mediterranean diet in medical students at Kocaeli University, Turkey. *J. Int. Med. Res.* **2018**, *46*, 1585–1594. [CrossRef] [PubMed]
17. Kyriacou, A.; Evans, J.M.; Economides, N.; Kyriacou, A. Adherence to the Mediterranean diet by the Greek and Cypriot population: A systematic review. *Eur. J. Public Health* **2015**, *25*, 1012–1018. [CrossRef] [PubMed]
18. Hadjimbei, E.; Botsaris, G.; Gekas, V.; Panayiotou, A.G. Adherence to the Mediterranean diet and lifestyle characteristics of university students in Cyprus: A cross-sectional survey. *Clin. Nutr. ESPEN* **2018**, *2016*, 2742841. [CrossRef] [PubMed]
19. Chacón-Cuberos, R.; Castro-Sánchez, M.; Muros-Molina, J.J.; Espejo-Garcés, T.; Zurita-Ortega, F.; Linares-Manrique, M. Adherence to Mediterranean diet in university students and its relationship with digital leisure habits. *Nutr. Hosp.* **2016**, *33*, 405–410. [CrossRef]
20. Padial-Ruz, R.; Viciana-Garófano, V.; Palomares. Adherence to the Mediterranean diet, physical activity and its relationship with the BMI, in university students of the grade of Primary, mention in Physical Education of Granada. *ESHPA* **2018**, *2*, 30–49.
21. Stefan, L.; Cule, M.; Milinovic, I.; Juranko, D.; Sporis, G. The relationship between lifestyle factors and body composition young adults. *Int. J. Environ. Res. Public Health* **2017**, *14*, 893. [CrossRef] [PubMed]
22. Dare, C.; Viebig, R.F.; Batista, N.S. Body composition and components of Mediterranean diet in Brazilian and European University Students. *Rev. Bras. Obes. Nutr. Emag.* **2017**, *11*, 557–566.
23. Bottcher, M.R.; Marincic, P.Z.; Nahay, K.L.; Baerlocher, B.E.; Willis, A.W.; Park, J. Nutrition knowledge and Mediterranean diet adherence in the southeast United States: Validation of a field-based survey instrument. *Appetite* **2017**, *111*, 166–176. [CrossRef] [PubMed]
24. Chacón-Cuberos, R.; Zurita-Ortega, F.; Castro-Sánchez, M.; Espejo-Garcés, T.; Martínez-Martínez, A.; Lucena-Zurita, M. Descriptive analysis of the consumption of harmful substances, adherence to the Mediterranean diet and type of residence in university students of Granada. *Rev. Commun. Educ.* **2017**, *28*, 823–837. [CrossRef]
25. Arnett, J.J. *Adolescence and Emerging Adulthood*; Pearson: Boston, MA, USA, 2014; pp. 102–111.
26. Cervera, F.; Serrano, R.; Vico, C.; Milla, M.; García, M.J. Food habits and nutritional assessment in a university population. *Nutr. Hosp.* **2013**, *28*, 438–446. [CrossRef]
27. Papadaki, A.; Hondros, G.; Scott, J.A.; Kapsokefalou, M. Eating habits of University students living at, or away from home in Greece. *Appetite* **2007**, *49*, 169–176. [CrossRef] [PubMed]
28. Harford, T.; Wechsler, H.; Muthen, B. The impact of current residence and high school drinking on alcohol problems among college students. *J. Stud. Alcohol.* **2002**, *63*, 271–279. [CrossRef] [PubMed]
29. Martínez-González, L.; Fernández Villa, T.; Molina de la Torre, A.J.; Ayán Pérez, C.; Bueno Cavanillas, A.; Capelo Álvarez, R.; Mateos Campos, R.; Martín Sánchez, V. Prevalence of eating behavior disorders in Spanish University Students and associated factors: Project uniHcos. *Nutr. Hosp.* **2014**, *30*, 927–934. [CrossRef] [PubMed]
30. Torres-Luque, G.; Molero, D.; Lara, A.; Latorre-Román, P.; Cachón-Zagalaz, J.; Zagalaz-Sánchez, M.L. Influence of the environment where people live (rural vs. urban) on the physical condition of students of Primary Education. *Apunts. Med. Sport* **2014**, *49*, 105–111. [CrossRef]
31. Rodrigo, M.; Ejeda, J.M.; González, M.P.; Mijancos, M.T. Changes in adherence to the Mediterranean diet in students of the Nursing and Teaching degrees after taking a nutrition course. *Nutr. Hosp.* **2014**, *30*, 1173–1180. [CrossRef]
32. Babic, M.J.; Morgan, P.J.; Plotnikoff, R.C.; Lonsdale, C.; White, R.L.; Lubans, D.R. Physical activity and physical self-concept in youth: Systematic review and meta-analysis. *Sport Med.* **2014**, *44*, 1589–1601. [CrossRef] [PubMed]
33. López, G.F.; Ahmed, D.; Díaz, A. Level of habitual physical activity among 13-year-old adolescents from Spain and India. A cross-cultural study. *SPORT-TK* **2017**, *6*, 67–74.

34. Martín, D.; González, C.; Zagalaz, M.L.; Chinchilla, J.J. Extracurricular physical activities: Motivational climate, sportspersonship, disposition and context. A study with primary 6th grade students. *J. Hum. Sport Exerc.* **2018**, *13*, 466–486.
35. Esteban-Cornejo, I.; Izquierdo-Gomez, R.; Gómez-Martínez, S.; Padilla-Moledo, C.; Castro-Piñero, J.; Marcos, A.; Veiga, O.L. Adherence to the Mediterranean diet and academic performance in youth: The UP&DOWN study. *Eur. J. Nutr.* **2016**, *55*, 1133–1140. [CrossRef] [PubMed]
36. Mamplekou, E.; Bountziouka, V.; Psaltopoulou, T.; Zeimbekis, A.; Tsakoundakis, N.; Papaerakleous, N.; Lionis, C. Urban environment, physical inactivity and unhealthy dietary habits correlate to depression among elderly living in eastern Mediterranean islands: The MEDIS study. *J. Nutr. Health Aging* **2010**, *14*, 449–455. [CrossRef] [PubMed]
37. García-Alandete, J.; Pérez-Delgado, E. Religious attitudes and values in a group of Young Spanish university students. *Ann. Psychol.* **2005**, *21*, 149–169.
38. Navarro-Prado, S.; González-Jiménez, E.; Perona, J.; Montero-Alonso, M.A.; López-Bueno, M.; Schmidt-Rio, J. Need of improvement of diet and life habits among university student regardless of religion professed. *Appetite* **2017**, *114*, 6–14. [CrossRef] [PubMed]
39. Zurita-Ortega, F.; Castro-Sánchez, M.; Álvaro-Rodríguez, J.I.; Rodríguez-Fernandez, S.; Pérez-Cortés, A. Self-concept, physical activity and family: Analysis of a structural equation model. *Int. J. Sport Psychol.* **2016**, *25*, 97–101.
40. Serra-Majem, L.; Ribas, L.; Ngo, J.; Ortega, R.M.; Garcia, A.; Pérez-Rodrigo, C.; Aranceta, J. Food, youth and the Mediterranean diet in Spain. Development of KIDMED, Mediterranean diet quality index in children and adolescents. *Public Health Nutr.* **2004**, *7*, 931–935. [CrossRef] [PubMed]
41. Kowalski, K.C.; Crocker, P.R.; Donen, R.M. *The Physical Activity Questionnaire for Older Children (PAQ-C) and Adolescents (PAQ-A) Manual*; College of Knesiology University of Saskatchewan: Saskatchewan, SK, Canada, 2004; pp. 1–38.
42. Martínez-Gómez, D.; Martínez-de-Haro, V.; Pozo, T.; Welk, G.J.; Villagra, A.; Calle, M.E. Fiabilidad y validez del cuestionario de actividad física PAQ-A en adolescentes españoles. *Span. J. Public Health* **2009**, *83*, 427–439. [CrossRef]
43. García, F.; Musitu, G. *AF5: Autoconcepto Forma 5*; TEA Ediciones: Madrid, Spain, 1999.
44. San Mauro, I.; Megias, A.; García, B.; Bodega, P.; Rodríguez, P.; Grande, G. Influence of healthy habits in the weight status of children and adolescents of school age. *Nutr. Hosp.* **2015**, *31*, 1996–2005. [CrossRef] [PubMed]
45. Deliens, T.; Clarys, P.; Bourdeaudhuij, I.; Deforche, B. Determinants of eating behavior in university students: A qualitative study using focus group discussions. *BMC Public Health* **2014**, *14*, 1–12. [CrossRef] [PubMed]
46. Hootman, K.C.; Guertin, K.A.; Cassano, P.A. Stress and psychological constructs related to eating behavior are associated with anthropometry and body composition in young adults. *Appetite* **2018**, *125*, 287–294. [CrossRef] [PubMed]
47. Lee, E.; Kim, Y. Effect of university student´s sedentary behavior on stress, anxiety and depression. *Perspect. Psychiatr. Care* **2018**, 1–6. [CrossRef] [PubMed]
48. Walsh, A.; Taylor, C.; Brennick, D. Factors that influence campus dwelling University Student´s facility to practice healthy living guidelines. *Can. J. Nurs. Res.* **2018**, *50*, 57–63. [CrossRef] [PubMed]
49. Plotnikoff, R.C.; Costigan, S.A.; Williams, R.L.; Hutchesson, M.J.; Kennedy, S.G.; Robards, S.L.; Germov, J. Effectiveness of interventions targeting physical activity, nutrition and healthy weight for university and college students: A systematic review and meta-analysis. *Int. J. Behav. Nutr. Phys.* **2015**, *12*, 45. [CrossRef] [PubMed]
50. Redondo, M.P.; De Mateo, B.; Enciso, L.; Marugan, J.M.; Fernández, M.; Camina, M.A. Dietary intake and adherence to the Mediterranean diet in a group of university students depending on the sports practice. *Nutr. Hosp.* **2016**, *33*, 1172–1178. [CrossRef]
51. Cuervo, C.; Cachón, J.; González, C.; Zagalaz, M.L. Eating habits and sport practice in a simple of teenagers of a city on the north of Spain. *J. Sport Health Res.* **2017**, *9*, 75–84.
52. López, G.F.; González, S.; Díaz, A. Level of habitual physical activity in children and adolescents from the Region of Murcia (Spain). *SpringerPlus* **2016**, *5*, 386. [CrossRef] [PubMed]
53. Smith, L.; López, G.F.; Díaz, A.; Stubbs, B.; Dowling, M.; Scruton, A. Barriers and Facilitators of Physical Activity in Children of a South Asian Ethnicity. *Sustainability* **2018**, *10*, 761. [CrossRef]

54. Pinel, C.; Chacón, R.; Castro, M.; Espejo, T.; Zurita, F.; Cortés, A. Differences between gender in relation with Body Mass Index, diet quality and sedentary activies on children from 10 to 12 year. *Retos* **2017**, *31*, 176–180.
55. Unal, G.; Uzdil, Z.; Kokdener, M.; Ozenoglu, A. Breakfast habits and diet quality among university students and its effect on anthropometric measurements and academic success. *Prog. Nutr.* **2017**, *19*, 154–162. [CrossRef]
56. Zurita-Ortega, F.; Álvaro-González, J.I.; Castro-Sánchez, M.; Knox, E.; Muros, J.J.; Viciana-Garófano, V. The influence of exercise on adolescents' self-concept. *Int. J. Sport Psychol.* **2015**, *46*, 67–80.
57. Inauen, J.; Radtke, T.; Rennie, L.; Scholz, U.; Orbell, S. Transfer or compensation? An experiment testing the effects of actual and imagined exercise on eating behavior. *Swiss J. Psychol.* **2018**, *77*, 59–67. [CrossRef]
58. Donnelly, T.T.; Fung, T.S.; Al Thani, A.B. Fostering active living and healthy eating through understanding physical activity and dietary behaviors of Arabic-speaking adults: A cross-sectional study from the Middle East. *BMJ Open* **2018**, *8*, e019980. [CrossRef] [PubMed]
59. Bernardo, G.L.; Jomori, M.M.; Fernandes, A.C.; Proenca, R.P. Food intake of university students. *Rev. Nutr.* **2017**, *30*, 847–865. [CrossRef]
60. Mariscal-Arcas, M.; Rivas, A.; Velasco, J.; Ortega, M.; Caballero, A.M.; Olea, F. Evaluation of the Mediterranean diet quality index (KIDMED) in children and adolescents in Southern Spain. *Public Health Nutr.* **2009**, *14*, 1408–1412. [CrossRef] [PubMed]

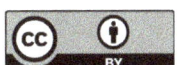

© 2018 by the authors. Licensee MDPI, Basel, Switzerland. This article is an open access article distributed under the terms and conditions of the Creative Commons Attribution (CC BY) license (http://creativecommons.org/licenses/by/4.0/).

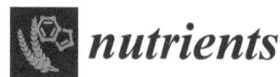

Article

Impact of a Mediterranean Dietary Pattern and Its Components on Cardiovascular Risk Factors, Glucose Control, and Body Weight in People with Type 2 Diabetes: A Real-Life Study

Marilena Vitale [1], Maria Masulli [1], Ilaria Calabrese [1], Angela Albarosa Rivellese [1], Enzo Bonora [2], Stefano Signorini [3], Gabriele Perriello [4], Sebastiano Squatrito [5], Raffaella Buzzetti [6], Giovanni Sartore [7], Anna Carla Babini [8], Giovanna Gregori [9], Carla Giordano [10], Gennaro Clemente [11], Sara Grioni [12], Pasquale Dolce [13], Gabriele Riccardi [1], Olga Vaccaro [1,*] and on behalf of the TOSCA.IT Study Group [†]

[1] Department of Clinical Medicine and Surgery, Federico II University of Naples, 80131 Naples, Italy; marilena.vitale@unina.it (M.V.); maria.masulli@unina.it (M.M.); ilariacalabrese@live.it (I.C.); rivelles@unina.it (A.A.R.); riccardi@unina.it (G.R.)
[2] Division of Endocrinology, Diabetes and Metabolism, University and Hospital Trust of Verona, 37134 Verona, Italy; enzo.bonora@univr.it
[3] University Department Laboratory Medicine, Hospital of Desio, 20832 Monza, Italy; s.signorini@asst-monza.it
[4] Endocrinology and Metabolism, University of Perugia, 06126, Perugia, Italy; gabriele.perriello@gmail.com
[5] Diabetes Unit, University Hospital Garibaldi-Nesima of Catania, 95122 Catania, Italy; squatrit@unict.it
[6] Department of Experimental Medicine, Sapienza University, 04100 Rome, Italy; raffaella.buzzetti@uniroma1.it
[7] Department of Medicine, University of Padua, 35100 Padova, Italy; g.sartore@unipd.it
[8] Medical Division, Rimini Hospital, 47900 Rimini, Italy; acbabini@auslrn.net
[9] Diabetes Unit, Azienda Sanitaria Toscana Nord-Ovest, Massa Carrara, 54100 Massa Carrara, Italy; g.gregori@usl1.toscana.it
[10] Section of Endocrinology, Diabetology and Metabolic Diseases, University of Palermo, 90127 Palermo, Italy; carlagiordano53@gmail.com
[11] Institute for Research on Population and Social Policies—National Research Council, 84084 Fisciano, Italy; gennaro.clemente@cnr.it
[12] Unità di Epidemiologia e Prevenzione, Fondazione IRCCS, Istituto Nazionale Tumori, 20133 Milano, Italy; sara.grioni@istitutotumori.mi.it
[13] Department of Public Health, Federico II University of Naples, 80131 Naples, Italy; pasquale.dolce@unina.it
* Correspondence: ovaccaro@unina.it; Tel.: +39-081-746-3665
[†] The complete list of Investigators and participating centers is available in the online Supplementary Materials.

Received: 24 July 2018; Accepted: 7 August 2018; Published: 10 August 2018

Abstract: This study evaluates the relation of a Mediterranean dietary pattern and its individual components with the cardiovascular risk factors profile, plasma glucose and body mass index (BMI) in people with type 2 diabetes. We studied 2568 participants at 57 diabetes clinics. Diet was assessed with the EPIC (European Prospective Investigation into Cancer and Nutrition) questionnaire, adherence to the Mediterranean diet was evaluated with the relative Mediterranean diet score (rMED). A high compared to a low score was associated with a better quality of diet and a greater adherence to the nutritional recommendations for diabetes. However, even in the group achieving a high score, only a small proportion of participants met the recommendations for fiber and saturated fat (respectively 17% and 30%). Nonetheless, a high score was associated with lower values of plasma lipids, blood pressure, glycated hemoglobin, and BMI. The relationship of the single food items components of the rMED score with the achievement of treatment targets for plasma lipids, blood pressure, glucose, and BMI were also explored. The study findings support the Mediterranean dietary model as a suitable model for type 2 diabetes and the concept that the beneficial health effects of the Mediterranean diet lie primarily in its synergy among various nutrients and foods rather than on any individual component.

Keywords: Mediterranean diet; diabetes; cardiovascular risk; glucose control; plasma lipids; relative Mediterranean diet score

1. Introduction

Diet remains the cornerstone of effective type 2 diabetes management; the aim of promoting nutritional changes in people with diabetes is to optimize metabolic control and overall health. Nutritional recommendations have been issued by several scientific societies to support clinicians in the choice of the most suitable dietary intervention(s) in people with diabetes [1]. However, adherence to these recommendations in real life clinical practice is generally poor [2–4] and partly reflects the wider problem of the overabundance of saturated fat and refined cereals in the western diet [5]. Furthermore, nutritional recommendations are based on nutrients, which might hamper patients' understanding and compliance. Last but not least, nutritional recommendations have been criticized as being scarcely based on evidence, and there is debate in the literature regarding the optimal dietary macronutrient composition of the diet in people with type 2 diabetes under energy balanced conditions [1,6,7].

In the last decades, human nutrition science has shifted from a reductionist approach focused on specific nutrients to a broader view emphasizing the concepts of overall dietary quality and patterns that promote metabolic health [8]. This paradigm change is supported by convincing evidence that food exposure is complex and its impact on health is influenced not only by single nutrients, but also by their interplay and by the interactions of the bioactive non-nutrients present in food (i.e., fiber, antioxidants, minerals, etc.). Therefore, the relationship between nutrition and health may not be fully appreciated unless evaluated within the context of the whole diet.

The Mediterranean diet is among the most widely studied dietary patterns. The traditional Mediterranean diet is characterized by the consumption of whole grains, legumes, fruits, vegetables, nuts, fish and olive oil, wine in moderation, and a moderate intake of meat, dairy products, processed foods and sweets. The Mediterranean dietary pattern is also an important source of vitamins, minerals, antioxidants, mono- and poly-unsaturated fatty acids, and fiber—all of which provide a wide range of health benefits. There is abundant evidence of its health benefits [9–12]; in addition, this type of diet has also a great potential for long-term adherence and sustainability [13]. However, data in populations with diabetes are scant; available information is mostly restricted to the experimental setting of controlled trials whereas little is known on the impact of a Mediterranean like dietary pattern on metabolic outcomes in real life clinical practice [14,15]. Furthermore, Mediterranean diet is a broad term used to describe the traditional food choices of people living around the Mediterranean basin, but there is remarkably little information on the protective/detrimental health impact of specific food groups. In particular, it is unclear whether the beneficial health effects of the Mediterranean diet are due to the diet as a whole or are driven by key food/food components that could also be provided as supplements.

Against this background, the aims of the study were to analyze the food and nutrient intake of a large cohort of people with type 2 diabetes in real-life clinical practice, to explore the impact of a Mediterranean-like dietary pattern on major cardiovascular risk factors, glucose control and body weight, and identify whether and to what extent the beneficial effect of the Mediterranean diet are driven by some food items/components which may be particularly beneficial for people with type 2 diabetes.

2. Materials and Methods

2.1. Study Population

To explore the study questions, we used data collected within the framework of the TOSCA.IT study—a randomized controlled trial (NCT00700856) designed to compare the effects of a sulfonylurea or pioglitazone, in add-on to metformin, on cardiovascular events in people with type 2 diabetes inadequately controlled with metformin monotherapy. Details on inclusion and exclusion criteria are reported elsewhere [16,17]. Briefly men and women with type 2 diabetes, aged 50–75 years, with glycated hemoglobin 7.0–9.0%, were recruited in 57 centers distributed throughout Italy. People with impaired renal function (serum creatinine $\geq$ 1.5 mg/dL), a cardiovascular event in the previous six months, and conditions other than diabetes requiring special dietary treatment were excluded from the study. The study protocol was approved by the Ethics Review Board of the Coordinating Center and of each participating center, and written informed consent was obtained from all participants before entering the study. For the purposes of this study, only baseline data, collected prior to the randomization to the study treatments, were used. The present analyses include 2568 men and women with a complete data set.

2.2. Measurements

Body weight, height, waist and hip circumference were measured with standard procedures, body mass index (BMI) was calculated as weight (kg)/height (m^2). Sitting blood pressure was measured according to a standard protocol. Blood samples were obtained in the morning after an overnight fast, all biochemical analyses were performed in a central laboratory. Total and HDL cholesterol, triglycerides and high sensitivity C-reactive protein (CRP) were measured by standard methods. LDL cholesterol was calculated according to the Friedewald equation only for triglyceride values <400 mg/dL. Glycated hemoglobin (HbA1c) was measured with high liquid performance chromatography standardized according to IFCC.

2.3. Evaluation of Eating Habits

Eating habits were assessed with the European Prospective Investigation into Cancer and Nutrition (EPIC) questionnaire, a validated method frequently used in large epidemiological studies [18,19]; details have been given elsewhere [3,6]. Briefly, the questionnaire contained 248 items on 188 different foods including the type of fat used as condiment or added after cooking. People were asked to indicate the absolute frequency of consumption of each item (per day, week, month or year), and the quantity of the food consumed by selection of pictures showing a small, medium and large portion size, with additional quantifiers (e.g., "smaller than the small portion" or "between the small and medium portion", etc.). Incomplete questionnaires and questionnaires with implausible data (i.e., energy intake less than 800 or greater than 5000 kcal/day) were excluded from the analyses. A specific software (Nutrition Analysis of food frequency questionnaire—FFQ), developed by the Epidemiology and Prevention Unit, Fondazione IRCCS, Istituto Nazionale dei Tumori, Milan, was used to convert dietary data from the questionnaire into average daily amounts of foods (g/day) [18,19]. Nutrition analysis of FFQ was linked to the Italian Food Composition Tables (FCTs) for nutrients and energy assessment [20,21]. The intake of polyphenols was evaluated using the USDA database [22] in combination with the Phenol-Explorer®database [23] to enable the examination of the polyphenol content of as many foods as possible. Details have been given elsewhere [24,25].

2.4. Adherence to the Mediterranean Diet

The adherence to the Mediterranean dietary model was evaluated with the rMED score (relative Mediterranean diet score), a variation of the original Mediterranean diet score, proposed by Buckland [26] and based on the intake of 9 key food groups: fruits, vegetables, legumes, cereals, fish, olive oil, meat and meat products, dairy products, and alcohol. The consumption of each food group (except alcohol) was measured as grams per 1000 kcal/day to adjust for energy density and divided into tertiles. A score of 0, 1, or 2 was assigned to the first, second, or third tertile of intake, assigning a positive score for high intakes for the 6 food groups fitting the Mediterranean model: fruit (including nuts and seeds but excluding fruit juices), vegetables (excluding potatoes), legumes, cereals (including whole-grain and refined flour, pasta, rice, other grains, and bread), fish and seafood, olive oil. The scoring was reversed for meat (including fresh and processed meat) and dairy products (including high- and low-fat milk, cheese, cream desserts, and dairy and nondairy creams), assigning a positive score for lower intakes. Alcohol was scored as a dichotomous variable as in prior studies: two points were assigned for moderate consumption—defined as 5–25 g/day for women and 10–50 g/day for men—and 0 points were assigned for a consumption above or below the sex-specific range. For each participant a total score was calculated by summing the scores obtained for each of the 9 food groups. Values for the rMED score ranged from 0 to 18; based on this score, three groups with low (score 0–6), intermediate (score 7–10) or high (score 11–18) were created [26]. The rMED score was selected among others for this study as it excludes sweetened beverages and potatoes which are foods restricted in people with diabetes.

2.5. Statistical Analysis

Data are shown as mean and standard deviation (M ± SD) or number and proportions, as appropriate. The analysis of variance (ANOVA) with linear term and the *post-hoc* test adjusted for multiple comparisons (Bonferroni test) were used to test for the differences in the composition of the habitual diet, blood pressure and metabolic parameters across categories of adherence to the Mediterranean Diet and between the highest vs. lowest rMED score, respectively. The χ^2 test was used to compare proportions. A binary logistic regression analysis was performed to evaluate the association of total rMED score and single food groups components of the rMED score with the achievement of treatment targets for the major cardiovascular risk factors (i.e., LDL cholesterol, triglycerides, HDL cholesterol, blood pressure), measures of glucose control—glycated hemoglobin—and BMI. A *p*-value < 0.05 (two-tailed) was considered statistically significant. All analyses were conducted with the SPSS Statistics software for Windows (version 20.0; SPSS Inc., Chicago, IL, USA).

3. Results

The study population consists of 1534 males and 1034 females with mean age 62.1 ± 6.5 years and BMI 30.3 ± 4.4 kg/m^2. Table 1 shows the general features of the study participants according to the rMED score groups. A high adherence score was significantly more frequent among females (*p* = 0.002), older people (*p* = 0.027) and residents of the southern regions (*p* < 0.0001). No relation was found with education, smoking, or marital status.

Tables 2 and 3 report the average food consumption and nutrient composition of the diet in the three rMED score groups. By definition, people with a high adherence score consumed substantially more fruit, vegetables, legumes, cereals, fish, olive oil, and alcohol, and substantially less meat, and dairy products (Table 2).

Eating a high rMED diet was characterized by a lower energy content, a lower intake of proteins from animal food sources, saturated fat and cholesterol, added sugars, a higher intake of fiber and a lower glycemic index and glycemic load (Table 3). As for micronutrients, a high rMED score was associated with a significantly lower intake of calcium and sodium and a significantly higher intake of total polyphenols (Table 3); no significant difference was detected for potassium intake.

We also evaluated the adherence to the current nutritional recommendation for people with diabetes in the participants with low, intermediate or high rMED score (Figure 1). Increasing rMED score values were associated with higher adherence to the nutritional recommendations. Interestingly, whereas the adherence to the nutritional recommendations for added sugar and carbohydrates was good in all three groups, the adherence to the recommendations for fiber and saturated fat remained low even in the high rMED score group. In this group, the proportion of adherence was respectively

31% for saturated fat and 17% for fiber, which is significantly higher than in the low rMED score group, although still far from optimal.

With regard to the cardiovascular risk factors profile, a high versus low rMED score was associated with a more favorable plasma lipid profile—i.e., lower LDL cholesterol (101.5 ± 31.2 vs. 105.1 ± 31.9 mg/dL, $p = 0.035$) and triglycerides (146.7 ± 71.0 vs. 156.2 ± 78.6 mg/dL, $p = 0.040$), and higher HDL cholesterol (46.8 ± 12.4 vs. 45.3 ± 11.6 mg/dL, $p = 0.032$), significantly lower blood pressure—systolic (133.3 ± 23.7 vs. 135.3 ± 14.9 mmHg, $p = 0.045$) and diastolic (78.6 ± 8.5 vs. 80.7 ± 8.7 mmHg, $p < 0.0001$)—lower HbA1c (7.63 ± 0.48 vs. 7.69 ± 0.52%, $p = 0.038$), lower BMI (30.0 ± 4.2 vs. 30.6 ± 4.5 kg/m^2, $p = 0.020$), and lower C-reactive protein (3.12 ± 4.8 vs. 3.79 ± 6.7 mg/L, $p = 0.029$) (Table 4). Of note, the proportion of people on lipid- or blood pressure-lowering drugs was not significantly different across the three groups (Table 4), thus suggesting a significant effect of diet beyond the effect of drugs.

Finally, we explored the association of the rMED score globally and for the single food groups with the achievement of treatment targets for plasma lipids, blood pressure, HbA1c, and BMI (Table 5). The odds of reaching the treatment target for LDL cholesterol increased by 13% per unit increase in the rMED score for fruit and nuts (OR 1.134; CI 1.006–1.277); for triglycerides, there was a significant association with fish consumption (OR 1.128; CI 1.003–1.269), and for HDL cholesterol a significant association was found for fruit and nuts (OR 1.142; CI 1.016–1.283) and alcohol (moderate consumption) (OR 1.206; CI 1.090–1.335). As for systolic blood pressure, the score for fruit and nuts (OR 1.174; CI 1.034–1.333), legumes (OR 1.259; CI 1.106–1.433), cereals (OR 1.133; CI 1.001–1.284), fish (OR 1.146; CI 1.013–1.297) and meat (inverse) (OR 1.170; CI 1.035–1.323) were all significantly associated with achievement of treatment targets; data for diastolic blood pressure were similar (not shown). The score for meat (low consumption) (OR 1.141; CI 1.035–1.258), fish (OR 1.109; CI 1.004–1.225), and alcohol (moderate consumption) (OR 1.183; CI 1.090–1.284) were also significantly associated with likelihood of a BMI below 30 kg/m^2. For HbA1c, a significant association was found for fish (inverse) (OR 0.888; CI 0.803–0.981) and dairy products (low consumption) (OR 1.154; CI 1.045–1.273).

Table 1. Characteristics of the study participants by rMED score groups.

	rMED Score Groups			p-Value
	Low (Score 0–6) (n = 834)	Intermediate (Score 7–10) (n = 1029)	High (Score 11–18) (n = 705)	
Age (years)				
<60 years (%)	316 (37.9)	355 (34.5)	221 (31.3)	0.027
≥60 years (%)	518 (62.1)	674 (65.5)	484 (68.7)	
Sex				
Men (%)	537 (64.4)	601 (58.4)	396 (56.2)	0.002
Women (%)	297 (35.6)	428 (41.6)	309 (43.8)	
Geographical Area				
North (%)	369 (44.2)	349 (33.9)	175 (24.8)	
Centre (%)	219 (26.3)	287 (27.9)	171 (24.3)	<0.0001
South (%)	246 (29.5)	393 (38.2)	359 (50.9)	
Education				
Secondary/University (%)	261 (31.3)	326 (31.7)	232 (33.0)	0.607
None/Primary (%)	573 (68.7)	703 (68.3)	472 (67.0)	
Smoking status [1]				
Never smoker (%)	388 (46.5)	510 (49.6)	341 (48.4)	
Current Smoker (%)	152 (18.2)	182 (17.7)	110 (15.6)	0.376
Former Smoker (%)	294 (35.3)	337 (32.8)	254 (36.0)	
Marital status				
Married (%)	697 (83.6)	868 (84.3)	615 (87.2)	0.112
Single or widowed (%)	137 (16.4)	161 (15.6)	90 (12.8)	

Data are expressed as number and percentage. Subjects are classified as "current smokers" if they smoke ≥5 cigarettes/day, and "former smokers" if they had smoked in the past and had stopped smoking for at least 1 year.

Table 2. Consumption of food groups (expressed as g/1000 kcal/day) by rMED score groups.

Food Item	rMED Score Groups			p-Value for Trend
	Low (Score 0–6) (n = 834)	Intermediate (Score 7–10) (n = 1029)	High (Score 11–18) (n = 705)	
Fruit & Nuts	125.8 ± 79.6	161.2 ± 93.2	200.7 ± 84 *	<0.0001
Vegetables	66.7 ± 36.1	96.9 ± 46.2	124 ± 44.6 *	<0.0001
Legumes	8.2 ± 7.2	13.5 ± 10.5	19.3 ± 12.1 *	<0.0001
Cereals	90.3 ± 35.5	95.8 ± 36.7	95.6 ± 32.6 *	0.033
Fish	16.9 ± 13.1	22.8 ± 16.4	28.9 ± 18.1 *	<0.0001
Olive oil	9.4 ± 4.7	13 ± 5.6	16.4 ± 5.6 *	<0.0001
Meat	76.4 ± 28.2	68 ± 27.8	58.7 ± 24.5 *	<0.0001
Dairy products	24.8 ± 14.5	20.3 ± 12.2	14.8 ± 10.2 *	<0.0001
Alcohol	0.27 ± 0.44	0.41 ± 0.50	0.50 ± 0.50 *	<0.0001

Data are expressed as mean ± standard deviation; * $p < 0.001$ vs. low score, *post-hoc* test adjusted for multiple comparisons (Bonferroni Test).

Table 3. Energy and nutrient composition of the diet by rMED score groups.

	rMED Score Groups			p-Value for Trend
	Low (Score 0–6) (n = 834)	Intermediate (Score 7–10) (n = 1029)	High (Score 11–18) (n = 705)	
Total Energy (kcal/day)	2093 ± 773	1890 ± 638	1718 ± 561 *	<0.0001
Proteins (% TE)	18.6 ± 2.5	18.3 ± 2.6	17.7 ± 2.3 *	<0.0001
Animal sources (% TE)	13.4 ± 3	12.55 ± 3.2	11.6 ± 2.8 *	<0.0001
Vegetable sources (% TE)	5.2 ± 1.1	5.7 ± 1.1	6.1 ± 1 *	<0.0001
Lipids (% TE)	37.0 ± 5.8	36.5 ± 6.3	36.5 ± 5.6	0.166
SFA (% TE)	13.4 ± 2.5	12.1 ± 2.3	10.9 ± 2 *	<0.0001
MUFA (% TE)	16.9 ± 3.3	17.9 ± 3.9	19.0 ± 3.7 *	<0.0001
PUFA (% TE)	4.3 ± 1.1	4.4 ± 1.2	4.5 ± 1.0 *	0.034
Cholesterol (mg/die)	379 ± 162	325 ± 133	272 ± 111 *	<0.0001
Carbohydrates (% TE)	44.3 ± 7.2	45.1 ± 7.6	45.8 ± 6.5 *	<0.0001
Added sugars (% TE)	3.0 ± 3.7	2.2 ± 3.0	2.0 ± 2.7 *	<0.0001
Fiber (g/1000 kcal/day)	8.8 ± 2.0	10.8 ± 2.3	12.8 ± 2.4 *	<0.0001
Glycaemic Index	52.7 ± 3.7	51.8 ± 3.5	51.3 ± 3.2*	<0.0001
Glycaemic load	143.4 ± 68.2	113.8 ± 46.8	98.9 ± 37.5 *	<0.0001
Alcohol (g/die)	12.9 ± 20.5	10.2 ± 13.5	10.4 ± 12.2 *	<0.0001
Calcium (mg)	1007 ± 476	880 ± 370	759 ± 333 *	<.0001
Sodium (mg)	2453 ± 1132	2077 ± 938	1758 ± 752 *	<0.0001
Potassium (mg)	3045 ± 1087	3045 ± 946	3072 ± 984	0.832
Total Polyphenols (mg)	653 ± 317	674 ± 289	733 ± 280 *	<0.0001

Data are expressed as mean ± standard deviation; * $p < 0.001$ vs. low score, *Post-hoc* test adjusted for multiple comparisons (Bonferroni Test). TE: Total Energy; SFA: Saturated fatty acids; MUFA: Monounsaturated fatty acids; PUFA: Polyunsaturated fatty acids.

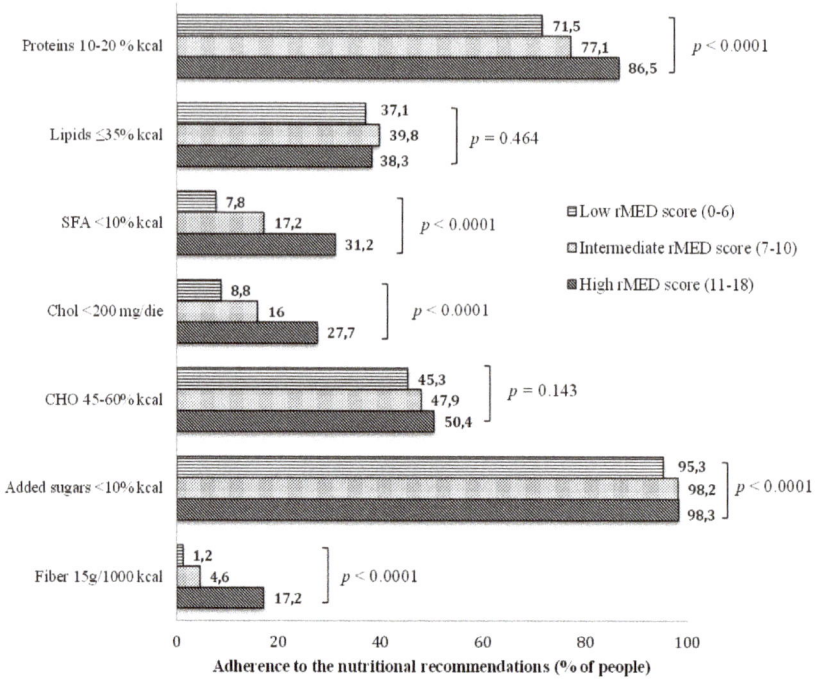

Figure 1. Adherence to the nutritional recommendations for people with diabetes (DNSG [27] and SID [28]) by rMED score. DNSG: Diabetes and Nutrition Study Group; SID: Italian Diabetes Society; SFA: Saturated Fatty Acids; Chol: Cholesterol; CHO: Carbohydrates.

Table 4. Cardiovascular risk factors profile by rMED score groups.

	rMED Score Groups			*p*-Value for Trend
	Low (Score 0–6) (n = 834)	Intermediate (Score 7–10) (n = 1029)	High (Score 11–18) (n = 705)	
BMI (kg/m^2)	30.6 ± 4.5	30.1 ± 4.4	30.0 ± 4.2 *	0.020
HbA1c (%)	7.69 ± 0.52	7.67 ± 0.49	7.63 ± 0.48 *	0.038
LDL cholesterol (mg/dL)	105.1 ± 31.9	101.8 ± 30.8	101.5 ± 31.2 *	0.035
HDL cholesterol (mg/dL)	45.3 ± 11.6	45.8 ± 11.4	46.8 ± 12.4 *	0.032
Triglycerides (mg/dL)	156.2 ± 78.6	150.2 ± 73.9	146.7 ± 71.0 *	0.040
Systolic blood pressure (mmHg)	135.3 ± 14.9	133.5 ± 14.4	133.3 ± 23.7 *	0.045
Diastolic blood pressure (mmHg)	80.7 ± 8.7	79.3 ± 8.4	78.6 ± 8.5 *	<0.0001
C-reactive protein [1] (mg/L)	3.79 ± 6.7	3.23 ± 4.7	3.12 ± 4.8 *	0.029
People on blood pressure lowering drugs (%)	73.7	71.9	68.4	0.063
People on lipid lowering drugs (%)	65.1	66.6	67.0	0.702

M ± SD or %. * $p < 0.05$ vs. low score. *Post-hoc* test adjusted for multiple comparisons (Bonferroni Test). [1] Excluding subjects with C-reactive protein value >100 mg/L.

Table 5. Odds ratio (95% CI) for the achievement of treatment target for LDL cholesterol, triglycerides, HDL-cholesterol, systolic blood pressure, BMI, and HbA1c associated to one-point increase of the total rMED score and of the score for each food item component of the score.

	Odd Ratio (95% CI)					
	LDL-Chol <100 mg/dL	Triglycerides <150 mg/dL	HDL-Chol >40 M or 50 F mg/dL	Systolic BP <130 mmHg	HbA1c <7.5%	BMI <30 kg/m²
Total rMED Score	1.119 (1.002–1.250) *	1.128 (1.036–1.228) *	1.150 (1.006–1.315) *	1.305 (1.100–1.548) *	1.087 (1.001–1.180) *	1.097 (1.005–1.197) *
Mediterranean food item						
Fruits and Nuts	1.134 (1.006–1.277) *	1.024 (0.908–1.155)	1.142 (1.016–1.283) *	1.174 (1.034–1.333) *	1.041 (0.941–1.152)	0.997 (0.902–1.102)
Vegetables	0.979 (0.848–1.132)	1.017 (0.879–1.177)	0.948 (0.821–1.094)	1.074 (0.921–1.252)	1.056 (0.928–1.202)	0.901 (0.793–1.024)
Legumes	1.015 (0.898–1.146)	1.004 (0.888–1.136)	1.013 (0.897–1.144)	1.259 (1.106–1.433) *	1.057 (0.954–1.171)	0.981 (0.874–1.010)
Cereals	0.953 (0.848–1.070)	1.009 (0.897–1.135)	0.917 (0.816–1.030)	1.133 (1.001–1.284) *	0.924 (0.834–1.024)	1.049 (0.947–1.161)
Meat and meat products (low intake)	1.051 (0.936–1.180)	1.003 (0.892–1.127)	1.020 (0.909–1.145)	1.170 (1.035–1.323) *	1.082 (0.981–1.194)	1.141 (1.035–1.258) *
Fish	1.073 (0.955–1.205)	1.128 (1.003–1.269) *	0.978 (0.871–1.098)	1.146 (1.013–1.297) *	0.888 (0.803–0.981) *	1.109 (1.004–1.225) *
Dairy products (low intake)	1.036 (0.922–1.165)	0.958 (0.851–1.078)	1.006 (0.895–1.131)	1.044 (0.922–1.182)	1.154 (1.045–1.273) *	1.005 (0.911–1.108)
Olive oil	0.928 (0.806–1.068)	1.053 (0.914–1.214)	0.975 (0.847–1.122)	0.982 (0.845–1.140)	0.974 (0.858–1.107)	1.066 (0.939–1.210)
Moderate alcohol consumption	1.052 (0.951–1.165)	1.075 (0.970–1.191)	1.206 (1.090–1.335) *	1.061 (0.952–1.182)	1.019 (0.939–1.106)	1.183 (1.090–1.284) *

* $p < 0.05$.

4. Discussion

Several scores have been developed to evaluate the degree of adherence to the Mediterranean Diet, but none has been validated so far for the use in people with diabetes, for whom nutritional therapy and, hence, food choice restrictions and limited consumption of selected food is recommended. The reason we selected the rMED score for this study [26] is because it excludes sweetened beverages and potatoes which are foods restricted in people with diabetes.

Although not specifically validated for people with diabetes, the rMED score efficiently identified three groups with substantially different eating habits. The study results show that in real-life clinical practice, the dietary habits of people with type 2 diabetes vary significantly with gender, age, and area of residence. In particular, females, older people, and residents of the southern regions tend to adhere more to a Mediterranean eating pattern.

The habitual diet of people with a high rMED score, as compared to that of people with a low score, was characterized by a lower energy intake, a lower intake of saturated fat and cholesterol, a higher intake of fish, vegetable proteins and fiber; glycemic index and glycemic load were also significantly lower, as was the intake of sodium and calcium, whereas the intake total polyphenols was significantly higher. On the overall, this group had a significantly less atherogenic and less proinflammatory diet. Nevertheless, even in the group with the highest score, the intake of fiber and saturated fat remained respectively lower and higher than recommended by the European and Italian nutritional guidelines for people with diabetes [27,28].

A low consumption of fiber and a relatively high intake of saturated fat have been reported by other studies in type 1 and type 2 diabetes [2–4] and most likely reflect the wider problem of a progressive shifting towards more western dietary models in all cultures, including countries with strong Mediterranean roots like Italy [29,30]. This notwithstanding, a high rMED score is associated with a more favorable cardiovascular risk factors profile, lower BMI, lower HbA1c, and lower subclinical inflammation. The magnitude of the differences between the high and low rMED score group may seem trivial, but if translated at the population level, may considerably impact on the absolute cardiovascular risk of the study population. Based on prior observational and intervention studies exploring the impact of the modification of major cardiovascular risk factors on the absolute cardiovascular risk [31–35], it can be estimated that combining the differences between the high and low rMED score groups in LDL cholesterol, triglycerides, HDL cholesterol, blood pressure, and HbA1c could result in a 21% reduction of the estimated absolute cardiovascular risk. Thus, emphasizing that the individual effects of the Mediterranean diet are small but taken as a whole the effects are large.

To our knowledge, this is one of the very few studies exploring the impact of a Mediterranean-like dietary pattern on glucose control and major cardiovascular risk factors in people with type 2 diabetes in real-life conditions. Most prior evidence on the beneficial effects of a Mediterranean diet model in people with diabetes comes from intervention trials, often of short duration, some of which have used food supplements [14,15,36]. The results of this study are in line with observational studies conducted in people without diabetes, and with a recent observational study conducted in a community-based sample of people with type 2 diabetes showing a significant reduction of all cause and cardiovascular deaths in patients who adhered most to the Mediterranean diet [37]. However, the lack of data on intermediate outcomes in this study does not allow comparisons with our findings. In addition, there is no standard definition for the Mediterranean diet, and adherence scores are based on population specific cut-off values for food consumption; this makes them poorly reproducible when utilized in different population groups, and further limits comparison between different studies.

We also explored the relation between scores of each individual food group component of the Mediterranean diet and the achievement of treatment targets for individual risk factors. Based on these analyses, a differential effect of single food groups was observed with regard to different risk factors (i.e., increasing the scores for fruit and vegetables significantly improved the probability of reaching the treatment target for LDL cholesterol; increasing the consumption of fish significantly improve the likelihood of reaching the target for triglycerides; the scores for legumes and vegetables were the main drivers for the achievement of treatment targets for blood pressure, etc.). All together, these data point to the conclusion that the beneficial health effects of the Mediterranean diet are largely due to the overall diet rather than being driven by single components, as different food items target different risk factors.

The major study strengths rely on the large sample size, the selection of a study population representative of real-life clinical practice, the standardized collection of nutritional and clinical data and the centralized biochemical measurements. Among the study limitations, we acknowledge the cross-sectional design and the use of intermediate endpoints. In addition, the dietary data were collected only once and could be prone to recall bias and seasonal variation, which might, however, bias the findings towards null, thus leading to the underestimation of the effect size. Finally, the extensive use of hypolipidemic and antihypertensive drugs could have partly offset the quantitative effect of nutritional factors. In this regard, the appreciation of the impact of dietary adherence in the face of pharmacological treatment was even more relevant.

5. Conclusions

In conclusion, a dietary pattern mimicking the Mediterranean model in people with type 2 diabetes is associated with more favorable cardiovascular risk factors profile, better glucose control and lower BMI and it is therefore a valid and sustainable nutritional strategy for people with diabetes in real-life clinical practice. However, a high rMED score in this population does not guarantee an ideal adherence to the nutritional recommendations for the management of diabetes, in fact, the intake of saturated fat and fiber in the highest rMED score group remain respectively higher and lower than recommended. These findings together with available evidence from other observational and intervention studies emphasize the need to reinforce the importance of higher fiber, low glycemic index foods such as legumes, fruit and vegetables, wholegrain cereals, and the substitution of monounsaturated for saturated fat sources, in energy balanced conditions, in people with diabetes.

Large-scale primary prevention trials focused on dietary patterns and cardiovascular disease risk in people with diabetes are unlikely to be undertaken; hence, observational findings such as these represent an important basis for dietary recommendations, government programs, and negotiations with industry to help people make healthy food choices.

Supplementary Materials: The following are available online at http://www.mdpi.com/2072-6643/10/8/1067/s1, complete list of collaborators, members of the TOSCA.IT Study Group (surname is reported in bold).

Author Contributions: O.V., G.R., A.A.R., M.M., E.B., and S.S. designed the study; G.P., S.S., R.B., G.S., A.C.B., G.G., C.G., and G.C. conducted the research; S.G. and S.S. provided essential materials; M.V., P.D. and I.C. analyzed data and performed statistical analysis; M.V. and O.V. drafted the paper; M.V. and O.V. had primary responsibility for final content. All authors read and approved the final manuscript.

Funding: The study is supported by the Italian Medicines Agency (AIFA) within the Independent Drug Research Program—contract N. FARM6T9CET—and by Diabete Ricerca, the nonprofit Research Foundation of the Italian Diabetes Society. The funding agency played no role in the study design; in the collection, analysis, and interpretation of data; in the writing of the manuscript; or in the decision to submit the manuscript for publication.

Acknowledgments: The participation of the patients in the study is gratefully acknowledged. We thank all the investigators and the dietitians in the TOSCA.IT centers for their excellent cooperation. We are also indebted to the administrative personnel of the Italian Diabetes Society (SID) for their support.

Conflicts of Interest: The authors declare no conflicts of interest.

References

1. Ajala, O.; English, P.; Pinkney, J. Systematic review and meta-analysis of different dietary approaches to the management of type 2 diabetes. *Am. J. Clin. Nutr.* **2013**, *97*, 505–516. [CrossRef] [PubMed]
2. Rivellese, A.A.; Boemi, M.; Cavalot, F.; Costagliola, L.; De Feo, P.; Miccoli, R.; Patti, L.; Trovati, M.; Vaccaro, O.; Zavaroni, I.; et al. Dietary habits in type ii diabetes mellitus: How is adherence to dietary recommendations? *Eur. J. Clin. Nutr.* **2008**, *62*, 660–664. [CrossRef] [PubMed]

3. Vitale, M.; Masulli, M.; Cocozza, S.; Anichini, R.; Babini, A.C.; Boemi, M.; Bonora, E.; Buzzetti, R.; Carpinteri, R.; Caselli, C.; et al. Sex differences in food choices, adherence to dietary recommendations and plasma lipid profile in type 2 diabetes—The TOSCA.IT study. *Nutr. Metab. Cardiovasc. Dis.* **2016**, *26*, 879–885. [CrossRef] [PubMed]
4. Toeller, M.; Klischan, A.; Heitkamp, G.; Schumacher, W.; Milne, R.; Buyken, A.; Karamanos, B.; Gries, F.A. Nutritional intake of 2868 iddm patients from 30 centres in europe. Eurodiab iddm complications study group. *Diabetologia* **1996**, *39*, 929–939. [CrossRef] [PubMed]
5. Breen, C.; Ryan, M.; McNulty, B.; Gibney, M.J.; Canavan, R.; O'Shea, D. High saturated-fat and low-fibre intake: A comparative analysis of nutrient intake in individuals with and without type 2 diabetes. *Nutr. Diabetes* **2014**, *4*, e104. [CrossRef] [PubMed]
6. Vitale, M.; Masulli, M.; Rivellese, A.A.; Babini, A.C.; Boemi, M.; Bonora, E.; Buzzetti, R.; Ciano, O.; Cignarelli, M.; Cigolini, M.; et al. Influence of dietary fat and carbohydrates proportions on plasma lipids, glucose control and low-grade inflammation in patients with type 2 diabetes—The TOSCA.IT study. *Eur. J. Nutr.* **2016**, *55*, 1645–1651. [CrossRef] [PubMed]
7. Franz, M.J. Diabetes nutrition therapy: Effectiveness, macronutrients, eating patterns and weight management. *Am. J. Med. Sci.* **2016**, *351*, 374–379. [CrossRef] [PubMed]
8. Fardet, A.; Rock, E. From a reductionist to a holistic approach in preventive nutrition to define new and more ethical paradigms. *Healthcare (Basel)* **2015**, *3*, 1054–1063. [CrossRef] [PubMed]
9. Trichopoulou, A.; Costacou, T.; Bamia, C.; Trichopoulos, D. Adherence to a mediterranean diet and survival in a Greek population. *N. Engl. J. Med.* **2003**, *348*, 2599–2608. [CrossRef] [PubMed]
10. Sofi, F.; Abbate, R.; Gensini, G.F.; Casini, A. Accruing evidence on benefits of adherence to the mediterranean diet on health: An updated systematic review and meta-analysis. *Am. J. Clin. Nutr.* **2010**, *92*, 1189–1196. [CrossRef] [PubMed]
11. Martinez-Gonzalez, M.A.; Bes-Rastrollo, M. Dietary patterns, mediterranean diet, and cardiovascular disease. *Curr. Opin. Lipidol.* **2014**, *25*, 20–26. [CrossRef] [PubMed]
12. Martinez-Lacoba, R.; Pardo-Garcia, I.; Amo-Saus, E.; Escribano-Sotos, F. Mediterranean diet and health outcomes: A systematic meta-review. *Eur. J. Public Health* **2018**. [CrossRef] [PubMed]
13. Dernini, S.; Berry, E.M.; Serra-Majem, L.; La Vecchia, C.; Capone, R.; Medina, F.X.; Aranceta-Bartrina, J.; Belahsen, R.; Burlingame, B.; Calabrese, G.; et al. Med diet 4.0: The mediterranean diet with four sustainable benefits. *Public Health Nutr.* **2017**, *20*, 1322–1330. [CrossRef] [PubMed]
14. Schwingshackl, L.; Chaimani, A.; Hoffmann, G.; Schwedhelm, C.; Boeing, H. A network meta-analysis on the comparative efficacy of different dietary approaches on glycaemic control in patients with type 2 diabetes mellitus. *Eur. J. Epidemiol.* **2018**, *33*, 157–170. [CrossRef] [PubMed]
15. Sleiman, D.; Al-Badri, M.R.; Azar, S.T. Effect of mediterranean diet in diabetes control and cardiovascular risk modification: A systematic review. *Front. Public Health* **2015**, *3*, 69. [CrossRef] [PubMed]
16. Vaccaro, O.; Masulli, M.; Bonora, E.; Del Prato, S.; Giorda, C.B.; Maggioni, A.P.; Mocarelli, P.; Nicolucci, A.; Rivellese, A.A.; Squatrito, S.; et al. Addition of either pioglitazone or a sulfonylurea in type 2 diabetic patients inadequately controlled with metformin alone: Impact on cardiovascular events. A randomized controlled trial. *Nutr. Metab. Cardiovasc. Dis.* **2012**, *22*, 997–1006. [CrossRef] [PubMed]
17. Vaccaro, O.; Masulli, M.; Nicolucci, A.; Bonora, E.; Del Prato, S.; Maggioni, A.P.; Rivellese, A.A.; Squatrito, S.; Giorda, C.B.; Sesti, G.; et al. Effects on the incidence of cardiovascular events of the addition of pioglitazone versus sulfonylureas in patients with type 2 diabetes inadequately controlled with metformin (TOSCA.IT): A randomised, multicentre trial. *Lancet Diabetes Endocrinol.* **2017**, *5*, 887–897. [CrossRef]
18. Pala, V.; Sieri, S.; Palli, D.; Salvini, S.; Berrino, F.; Bellegotti, M.; Frasca, G.; Tumino, R.; Sacerdote, C.; Fiorini, L.; et al. Diet in the Italian epic cohorts: Presentation of data and methodological issues. *Tumori J.* **2003**, *89*, 594–607. [CrossRef]
19. Pisani, P.; Faggiano, F.; Krogh, V.; Palli, D.; Vineis, P.; Berrino, F. Relative validity and reproducibility of a food frequency dietary questionnaire for use in the Italian epic centres. *Int. J. Epidemiol.* **1997**, *26*, S152–S160. [CrossRef] [PubMed]
20. Salvini, S.; Parpinel, M.; Gnagnarella, P.; Maisonneuve, P.; Turrini, A. Banca Dati Di Composizione Degli Alimenti per Studi Epidemiologici in Italia. Available online: http://agris.fao.org/agris-search/search.do?recordID=XF2015019268 (accessed on 24 July 2018).

21. Carnovale, E.; Marletta, L. Tabella di Composizione Degli Alimenti. Available online: http://nut.entecra.it/646/tabelle_di_composizione_degli_alimenti.html (accessed on 24 July 2018).
22. USDA Special Interest Databases on Flavonoids. Available online: http://www.ars.usda.gov/nutrientdata/flav (accessed on 24 July 2018).
23. Phenol-Explorer: Database on Polyphenol Content in Foods. Available online: http://phenolexplorer.eu/ (accessed on 24 July 2018).
24. Vitale, M.; Vaccaro, O.; Masulli, M.; Bonora, E.; Del Prato, S.; Giorda, C.B.; Nicolucci, A.; Squatrito, S.; Auciello, S.; Babini, A.C.; et al. Polyphenol intake and cardiovascular risk factors in a population with type 2 diabetes: The TOSCA.IT study. *Clin. Nutr.* **2017**, *36*, 1686–1692. [CrossRef] [PubMed]
25. Vitale, M.; Masulli, M.; Rivellese, A.A.; Bonora, E.; Cappellini, F.; Nicolucci, A.; Squatrito, S.; Antenucci, D.; Barrea, A.; Bianchi, C.; et al. Dietary intake and major food sources of polyphenols in people with type 2 diabetes: The TOSCA.IT study. *Eur. J. Nutr.* **2018**, *57*, 679–688. [CrossRef] [PubMed]
26. Buckland, G.; González, C.A.; Agudo, A.; Vilardell, M.; Berenguer, A.; Amiano, P.; Ardanaz, E.; Arriola, L.; Barricarte, A.; Basterretxea, M.; et al. Adherence to the mediterranean diet and risk of coronary heart disease in the spanish epic cohort study. *Am. J. Epidemiol.* **2009**, *170*, 1518–1529. [CrossRef] [PubMed]
27. Mann, J.I.; De Leeuw, I.; Hermansen, K.; Karamanos, B.; Karlström, B.; Katsilambros, N.; Riccardi, G.; Rivellese, A.A.; Rizkalla, S.; Slama, G.; et al. Evidence-based nutritional approaches to the treatment and prevention of diabetes mellitus. *Nutr. Metab. Cardiovasc. Dis.* **2004**, *14*, 373–394. [CrossRef]
28. SID, AMD—Standard Italiani per la Cura del Diabete Mellito. Available online: http://aemmedi.it/wp-content/uploads/2009/06/AMD-Standard-unico1.pdf (accessed on 24 July 2018).
29. Vitale, M.; Racca, E.; Izzo, A.; Giacco, A.; Parente, E.; Riccardi, G.; Giacco, R. Adherence to the traditional mediterranean diet in a population of south of italy: Factors involved and proposal of an educational field-based survey tool. *Int. J. Food Sci. Nutr.* **2018**, 1–7. [CrossRef] [PubMed]
30. Benhammou, S.; Heras-González, L.; Ibáñez-Peinado, D.; Barceló, C.; Hamdan, M.; Rivas, A.; Mariscal-Arcas, M.; Olea-Serrano, F.; Monteagudo, C. Comparison of mediterranean diet compliance between european and non-european populations in the mediterranean basin. *Appetite* **2016**, *107*, 521–526. [CrossRef] [PubMed]
31. Turnbull, F.; Neal, B.; Ninomiya, T.; Algert, C.; Arima, H.; Barzi, F.; Bulpitt, C.; Chalmers, J.; Fagard, R.; Gleason, A.; et al. Effects of different regimens to lower blood pressure on major cardiovascular events in older and younger adults: Meta-analysis of randomised trials. *BMJ* **2008**, *336*, 1121–1123. [PubMed]
32. Genser, B.; März, W. Low density lipoprotein cholesterol, statins and cardiovascular events: A meta-analysis. *Clin. Res. Cardiol.* **2006**, *95*, 393–404. [CrossRef] [PubMed]
33. National Cholesterol Education Program (NCEP) Expert Panel on Detection, Evaluation, and Treatment of High Blood Cholesterol in Adults (Adult Treatment Panel III). Third report of the national cholesterol education program (ncep) expert panel on detection, evaluation, and treatment of high blood cholesterol in adults (adult treatment panel iii) final report. *Circulation* **2002**, *106*, 3143–3421.
34. Miller, M.; Stone, N.J.; Ballantyne, C.; Bittner, V.; Criqui, M.H.; Ginsberg, H.N.; Goldberg, A.C.; Howard, W.J.; Jacobson, M.S.; Kris-Etherton, P.M.; et al. Triglycerides and cardiovascular disease: A scientific statement from the american heart association. *Circulation* **2011**, *123*, 2292–2333. [CrossRef] [PubMed]
35. Eeg-Olofsson, K.; Cederholm, J.; Nilsson, P.M.; Zethelius, B.; Svensson, A.M.; Gudbjörnsdóttir, S.; Eliasson, B. New aspects of hba1c as a risk factor for cardiovascular diseases in type 2 diabetes: An observational study from the swedish national diabetes register (ndr). *J. Intern. Med.* **2010**, *268*, 471–482. [CrossRef] [PubMed]
36. Estruch, R.; Ros, E.; Salas-Salvadó, J.; Covas, M.I.; Corella, D.; Arós, F.; Gómez-Gracia, E.; Ruiz-Gutiérrez, V.; Fiol, M.; Lapetra, J.; et al. Primary prevention of cardiovascular disease with a mediterranean diet supplemented with extra-virgin olive oil or nuts. *N. Engl. J. Med.* **2018**, *378*, e34. [CrossRef] [PubMed]
37. Bonaccio, M.; Di Castelnuovo, A.; Costanzo, S.; Persichillo, M.; De Curtis, A.; Donati, M.B.; de Gaetano, G.; Iacoviello, L.; Investigators, M.-S.S. Adherence to the traditional mediterranean diet and mortality in subjects with diabetes. Prospective results from the moli-sani study. *Eur. J. Prev. Cardiol.* **2016**, *23*, 400–407. [CrossRef] [PubMed]

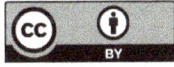

© 2018 by the authors. Licensee MDPI, Basel, Switzerland. This article is an open access article distributed under the terms and conditions of the Creative Commons Attribution (CC BY) license (http://creativecommons.org/licenses/by/4.0/).

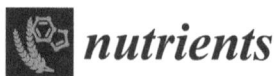

Article

Adherence to the Mediterranean Diet among School Children and Adolescents Living in Northern Italy and Unhealthy Food Behaviors Associated to Overweight

Francesca Archero [1], Roberta Ricotti [1], Arianna Solito [1], Deborah Carrera [2], Federica Civello [1], Rosina Di Bella [1], Simonetta Bellone [1,3] and Flavia Prodam [1,3,4,]*

1. SCDU of Pediatrics, Department of Health Sciences, University of Piemonte Orientale, 28100 Novara, Italy; francesca.archero@gmail.com (F.A.); robertaricotti@gmail.com (R.R.); arianna.solito@hotmail.it (A.S.); federicacivello@hotmail.it (F.C.); rosina.dibella@med.uniupo.it (R.D.B.); simonetta.bellone@med.uniupo.it (S.B.)
2. SCDO of Clinical Nutrition and Dietetics, Maggiore della Carità Hospital, 28100 Novara, Italy; carrera.deborah@gmail.com
3. Interdisciplinary Research Center of Autoimmune Diseases, University of Piemonte Orientale, 28100 Novara, Italy
4. Endocrinology, Department of Translational Medicine, University of Piemonte Orientale, 28100 Novara, Italy
* Correspondence: flavia.prodam@med.uniupo.it; Tel.: +39-0321-660-693

Received: 9 August 2018; Accepted: 12 September 2018; Published: 18 September 2018

Abstract: The purposes of this study were to evaluate the differences in Mediterranean diet and its components among primary and secondary school children and adolescents living in northern Italy, and the associations with the weight status. Adherence was assessed by the KIDMED (Mediterranean Diet Quality Index) questionnaire on 669 subjects (6–16 years) attending five schools of Novara. The adherence was poor in 16.7%, average in 63.7%, and high in 19.6% of the students. Poor adherence was more frequent in primary than in secondary schools (20.7% vs. 13.7%, $p < 0.04$). Some unhealthy behaviors were more prevalent in younger children. Children of other ethnic origins had a mixed behavior, choosing both traditional healthy and unhealthy foods. Besides male gender and primary school, in Italian children, the risk of overweight was directly associated with eating at fast-food restaurants (OR: 1.890, CI 95% 1.002–3.563), and inversely with consumption of vegetables more than once a day (OR: 0.588, CI 95% 0.349–0.991), and olive oil at home (OR: 0.382, CI 95% 0.176–0.826). In children of other ethnic origins, this risk was associated with skipping breakfast (OR: 16.046, CI 95% 1.933–133.266), or consuming commercial baked good or pastries for breakfast (OR: 10.255, CI 95% 1.052–99.927). The overall KIDMED score correlated with height (β: 0.108; $p < 0.005$). Poor food quality is replacing the Mediterranean dietary pattern in children and adolescents, in particular among younger children. Because the risk of overweight was associated with different components of the Mediterranean diet depending on ethnic origins, tailored nutritional programs remain a need.

Keywords: Mediterranean diet; questionnaire; children; adolescents; obesity

1. Introduction

The Mediterranean diet (MD) is considered a model of a healthy diet, in particular after the publication of the first results derived by the PREDIMED study that demonstrated a reduction of cardiovascular mortality in subjects adherent to this dietary pattern [1]. MD has been associated with lower prevalence and/or incidence of several diseases, among others, type 2 diabetes, hypertension, cardiovascular diseases, and certain cancers that are all associated to overweight [2–5]. This is likely due to its composition rich in vegetables, fruits, legumes, whole cereals, as well as many sources of fiber and antioxidants, including fish, nuts, and extra-virgin olive oil. Moreover, the intake of sweets and trans fatty acids is low.

Although MD is beneficial, with the urbanization of people living in the Mediterranean area, in particular children and adolescents are deviating to a "Western diet" more rich in saturated fat, refined grains, simple carbohydrates and processed foods [6]. This phenomenon has been named nutrition transition and is one of the players implicated in the high prevalence of overweight and obesity in countries supposed to adopt a traditional MD [5,7]. A large meta-analysis of randomized controlled trials on MD reported a little but significant decrease in weight (-1.75 kg) and BMI (-0.57 kg/m^2) in those adherents to MD [8]. Although intriguing results have been obtained in trials, the dissociation between higher obesity prevalence in Mediterranean countries and lower prevalence of many of its comorbidities in subjects adherent to a MD pattern is still an issue, in particular in pediatrics.

Studies investigating nutrition habits are needed to plan tailored strategies of interventions to educate on a healthy diet. In 2004, Serra-Majem et al. developed the KIDMED (Mediterranean Diet Quality Index for children and adolescents) score, a nutritional index validated in several languages that evaluates the adherence to MD and the quality of diet in children and adolescents [9]. Although it is simple to use in the clinical practice as well as in other epidemiological settings, only a few studies have been explored the adherence to the MD and to the risk of obesity in the young school population in Italy [10–13]. Most have been conducted in the southern part of Italy [14,15], where the obesity rate is higher than in other areas of the country [16], thus the generalizability has to be further demonstrated. The most extensive study using a modified version of the KIDMED score portrayed a school population of 1740 8–9-year-old children living in north Italy (Friuli, Venezia, Giulia and Liguria) and was conducted in 2009. The authors showed that only the 5.0% of the cohort was classified as high adherent to the MD, with the best rate (6.0%) in the north [17].

Although the benefits of the MD pattern can be considered as a synergistic interaction among all its components, a few studies reported protective or detrimental effects related to specific foods in adults with differences in prospective cohort or randomized controlled studies [5]. Vegetable intake was negatively associated, whereas higher intake of sweets, sugar-sweetened beverages, and fast foods was associated with obesity in a study on MD adherence conducted among adolescents living in Sicily [14]. No other Italian data have been published.

Based on the above, data on MD adherence are insufficient in children living in northern Italy. The first purpose of this study was to evaluate the differences in Mediterranean diet and its components among primary and secondary school children and adolescents living in Novara, a city of northern Italy characterized by an urban community employed in both agriculture and industry. The second purpose was to evaluated the associations of MD adherence and its components with the weight status.

2. Subjects and Methods

2.1. Population and Anthropometric Examination

This was a cross-sectional study conducted in April and May 2017. The study is a part of a cross-sectional study on pediatric obesity approved by the Ethical Committee of the Maggiore della Carità Hospital (CE 95/12).

We included 3 primary and 2 secondary schools of Novara. In 2017, the population of Novara was estimated at 104,183, with 18,634 people $\leq$14 years old. The average annual income per capita for the population is estimated around 16,132 Euro [18]. Before starting the enrollment, schools of Novara were classified according to socio-economic status based on estimates of the district's socio-economic status in which they were located. We contacted all the schools by phone; to be selected they needed not to have developed a specific structured education program on MD in the year of recruitment.

Eight schools respected all the inclusion criteria and were balanced for socio-economic status. Three of them refused to participate in the survey because no scholastic days were available. For all enrolled schools, all students attending all years were invited to participate with a letter carefully explaining the purpose of the study both to them and to their parents, and written informed consent was obtained. In addition, the children and adolescents provided their verbal assent on the day of the questionnaire. To be included in the analysis, participants should write and read fluently Italian.

In each school, data collection was performed by two pediatric nurses, one nutritionist, two physicians and a member of the department of the school policies who was responsible for the program. Questionnaires were completed during school hours in the classroom in the presence of a teacher, the nutritionist and at least one nurse and one physician. The staff helped with the questionnaire interpretation if needed. Questionnaires were anonymous. Students were requested to report their sex and date of birth. Nurses and physicians also performed the auxological examination after the completion of the questionnaire which returned at that moment. Anthropometric data were reported on the questionnaire form. Some days after the testing session a closing visit with a lesson on the MD and the MD food pyramid was conducted by the study staff.

Anthropometric measurements were performed in duplicate for each subject, wearing light indoor clothing and without shoes. Weight was measured to the nearest 100 g with a spring scale tested daily for accuracy and calibrated against a set of standard weights (Salus, Inc., Gaggiano, Milano, Italy). Height was measured with a standard laboratory stadiometer to the nearest 0.5 cm during maximal expiration. BMI was calculated as the ratio between weight (kg) and squared height (m^2). BMI-SDS was calculated according to the LMS methods on the Italian charts [19]. Subjects were also stratified according to BMI categories (underweight, normal weight, overweight, obesity and morbid obesity) of the International Obesity Task Force [20].

Ethnicity was defined as the country of origin of the mother, in case of the different origin of both parents.

2.2. Evaluation of Adherence to the MD

We used the Italian version KIDMED index [21], a questionnaire of 16 dichotomous (positive/negative) items appropriate for youngsters. The answers with a positive connotation in relation to the MD are assigned a value of +1 (12 items), and those with a negative connotation, a value of −1 (4 items). The items explore the consumption of fruits, vegetables, fish, pasta/rice, cereals, yoghurt/cheese/dairy products, nuts, commercial baked and processed foods, breakfast habits and the frequency of skipping breakfast, fast-food frequency, sweet consumption, and olive oil during meals at home.

The overall score can range from −4 to 12. Total KIDMED scores were classified as follows: ≤3 reflects a poor adherence (very low diet quality), 4–7 an average adherence (improvement needed to adjust intake to MD patterns), and ≥8 a good adherence to the MD (optimal diet quality).

2.3. Statistical Analysis

Continuous data are expressed as mean, standard deviation (SD) and CI 95%. Prevalence of KIDMED, weight categories, and "yes" answers at each questionnaire item are reported as a percentage. The sample size was calculated according to the mean prevalence of low MD adherence according to the literature [8] with 95% confidence interval and an accuracy of ±4.0% of the average value of the adherence. A sample of 585 individuals was estimated as sufficient. Because the prevalence of obesity was relatively low, overweight and obese categories were considered together in the final analysis. Data were also stratified between primary and secondary schools. Socio-demographic level was defined according to that of the district area where the school was located. Kolmogorov–Smirnov test was used to test normality of variables' distribution. Student's independent t-test and Mann–Whitney U-test were used for normally and not normally distributed continuous variables, respectively. Two-tailed chi-square or Fisher exact test was used to evaluate differences in categorical variables, as appropriate.

Univariate and multivariate logistic regression was used to assess the association of weight status with the odds ratio (OR, 95% CI) of gender, school level, ethnicity, MD adherence, or KIDMED items, as well as of MD adherence with gender, school level, ethnicity, and weight status. Because of several ethnic origins, ethnicity was categorized for statistical analyses as Italian and non-Italian. KIDMED items inserted in the models were those significant in the univariate analysis. Goodness-of-fit was evaluated by using the Hosmer and Lemeshow test; all the models were accepted because the χ^2 was not significant. Interactions among variables (gender, school level, and ethnicity) were also explored; when p was >0.05 data in multinomial logistic analysis were only presented together. The KIDMED score and anthropometric parameters were also tested as continuous variables through linear regression stepwise analyses and the results are represented as standardized β coefficients. The level of statistical significance for analysis was set at $p < 0.05$. Statistical analysis was performed with SPSS for Windows version 17.0 (SPSS Inc., Chicago, IL, USA).

3. Results

3.1. Characteristics of the Population

The study was carried out in 669 subjects (324 males and 345 females) aged 11.2 (2.2) (CI 95% 11.0–11.4) years. All families and children gave their consent to participate in the study. Everybody completed the questionnaire and accepted the clinical visit. The analysis excluded six out of 705 subjects (0.9%) because they did not read and write fluently in Italian. All questionnaires were complete. The primary and secondary school samples were composed by 290 (138 males, 152 females) and 379 (186 males, 193 females) subjects, respectively. Six hundred twelve subjects (91.5%) were Italian. The remaining 57 subjects were born to parents from other ethnic origins. The majority of the subjects had a normal weight (n = 558; 83.4%); only 94 (14.1%) and 17 (2.5%) of them were overweight or obese, respectively. The prevalence of overweight plus obesity was higher in primary than in secondary schools (23.4% vs. 11.3%, χ^2: 17.384, $p < 0.0001$), in males than females (21.3% vs. 12.2%, χ^2: 10.047, $p < 0.0001$), and in subjects of other ethnic origins than those Italian (28.1% vs. 15.5%, χ^2: 5.932, $p < 0.001$).

Sex, type of school, and ethnicity in the three-predictor model of OWB were all significant (model χ^2: 31.971, $p < 0.001$) without interactions, accounting for 7.9% of the total variance (Nagelkerke R^2), and the correct prediction rate was about 83.4%. In particular, the risk to be OWB was associated with male gender (OR: 2.024, CI 95% 1.322–3.099, $p < 0.0001$), primary school (OR: 2.387, CI 95% 1.562–3.648, $p < 0.0001$), and other ethnic origins (OR: 1.947, CI 95% 1.031–3.676, $p < 0.03$) in the corrected model. Table 1 represents demographic characteristics.

Table 1. Anthropometric characteristics of the 669 subjects, by school level.

	All	Primary School	Secondary School	p
Gender				
M	324 (48.4%)	138 (47.5%)	186 (49.0%)	0.755
F	345 (51.6%)	152 (52.5%)	193 (51.0%)	
Age (years)	11.2 (2.2) (11.0–11.4)	9.0 (1.3) (8.8–9.2)	12.9 (1.1) (12.8–13.1)	0.0001
Ethnicity				
Italian	612 (91.5%)	258 (89.0%)	354 (93.4%)	
Eastern European	22 (3.3%)	7 (2.4%)	15 (4.0%)	0.03
African	25 (3.7%)	22 (7.6%)	3 (0.8%)	
Asian	4 (0.6%)	1 (0.3%)	3 (0.8%)	
South American	6 (0.9%)	2 (0.7%)	4 (1.0%)	
Height (cm)	147.9 (15.6) (146.8–149.2)	134.6 (10.3) (133.4–135.8)	158.2 (10.5) (157.1–159.3)	0.0001

Table 1. Cont.

	All	Primary School	Secondary School	p
Weight (Kg)	40.4 (12.6) (39.5 41.4)	31.3 (7.6) (30.5 32.3)	47.4 (11.2) (46.3–48.5)	0.0001
BMISDS	−0.476 (1.028) (−0.554, −0.398)	−0.309 (1.076) (−0.433, −0.185)	−0.604 (0.972) (−0.703, −0.507)	0.0001
BMI category Normal-weight Overweight Obese	558 (83.4%) 94 (14.1%) 17 (2.5%)	222 (76.5%) 57 (19.7%) 11 (3.8%)	336 (88.6%) 37 (9.8%) 6 (1.6%)	0.0001

Data are expressed as mean ± SD, CI 95%, absolute numbers and percentages. Differences among categorical variables were tested by Chi-square test. Associations between variables were tested by Student's independent t-test (BMISDS), or Mann–Whitney U-test (age, height, and weight). Abbreviations: F, female; M, male. BMI was stratified according to the IOTF criteria.

3.2. KIDMED

The adherence to the MD (scores ≤ 3) was poor in 16.7%, average (scores 4–7) in 63.7%, and high (scores ≥ 8) in 19.6% of the students. The overall score ranged from −1 to 11. The peak score was 6 (17.0%).

The prevalence rate of the three categories of adherence was similar between males and females, normal-weight (NW) and overweight/obese (OWB) subjects. The prevalence rate of poor adherence to the MD was significantly higher in primary than in secondary schools (20.7% vs. 13.7%, $p < 0.04$), with an equal rate of high adherence (19% vs. 20.1%). The four-predictor model of MD adherence (χ^2: 8.000, $p < 0.04$) showed that only primary school was associated to a high risk of low MD adherence (OR: 1.618, CI 95% 1.068–2.452, $p < 0.01$), accounting for 2.1% of the total variance (Nagelkerke R^2), and the correct prediction rate was about 83.3%. Table 2 shows the distribution of the levels of adherence among subgroups.

Table 2. Distribution of the adherence to the MD of the study population and relative odd ratios among subcategories.

	KIDMED Score	p	KIDMED Score Low	KIDMED Score Medium	KIDMED Score High	p	Adj OR (CI 95%) of High Adherence
School Primary	5.4 (2.3) (5.1 5.7)	0.094	60 (20.7%)	175 (60.3%)	55 (19.0%)	0.04	1
Secondary	5.6 (2.1) (5.5–5.9)		52 (13.7%)	251 (66.2%)	76 (20.1%)		1.618 (1.068–2.452)
Weight NW	5.6 (2.1) (5.4–5.8)	0.364	91 (16.3%)	359 (64.3%)	108 (19.4%)	0.610	1
OWB	5.6 (2.4) (4.9–5.9)		21 (18.9%)	67 (60.4%)	23 (20.7%)		0.868 (0.504–1.494)
Gender M	5.6 (2.1) (5.5–5.9)	0.062	47 (14.5%)	209 (64.5%)	68 (21.0%)	0.062	1
F	5.4 (2.2) (5.2–5.7)		65 (18.8%)	217 (62.9%)	63 (18.3%)		0.725 (0.478–1.098)
Ethnicity Italian	5.5 (2.1) (5.4–5.8)	0.092	103 (16.8%)	389 (63.6%)	120 (19.6%)	0.672	1
Others	5.5 (2.2) (5.0–6.1)		9 (15.8%)	37 (64.9%)	11 (19.3%)		0.850 (0.400–1.494)
All	5.5 (2.1) (5.4–5.7)	//	112 (16.7%)	426 (63.7%)	131 (19.6%)	//	//

KIDMED score as continuous variables is expressed as mean (SD) and CI 95%. Adjusted Odd Ratios (OR) were calculated by binary logistic regression analysis with low adherence as reference category in dependent variable, and school level, gender, weight status, and ethnicity as independent variables. Medium and high adherences were considered together. The ORs were referred to secondary school, female gender, OWB, and other ethnic origin. Abbreviations: F, female; M, male; NW, normal-weight; OWB, overweight + obese. //: not calculable.

The risk of OWB previously described was not modified by the introduction in the model of the MD adherence either as category or as continuous variable.

The overall KIDMED score did not correlate with weight, BMI, and BMI SDS. Diversely, it correlated with height (β: 0.108; B: 0.015, CI 95% 0.005–0.026 $p < 0.005$) also when corrected for gender, age or school level, and ethnicity.

3.3. KIDMED Items

We analyzed the prevalence of "yes" answers in several subcategories.

Subjects with the lowest adherence to the MD answered "yes" less frequently in the positive questions, and more frequently in the negative ones ($p < 0.0001$) than those with the highest adherence to the MD. A similar distribution of answers was only reported on the daily intake of candy and sweets (Table A1).

In primary schools, children ate fewer vegetables once a day (χ^2: 5.413, $p < 0.01$), fewer pulses once a week (χ^2: 4.459, $p < 0.02$), and skipped breakfast (χ^2: 5.375, $p < 0.01$). They also consumed more frequently pasta or rice almost every day (χ^2: 4.4672, $p < 0.01$), ate at fast-food restaurants (χ^2: 6.585, $p < 0.007$), consumed commercial baked good or pastries for breakfast (χ^2: 17.034, $p < 0.0001$) or took sweets and candy several times every day (χ^2: 18.610, $p < 0.0001$) than in secondary schools.

OWB consumed less olive oil (χ^2: 4.704, $p < 0.02$), and more frequently ate at fast-food restaurants (χ^2: 11.748, $p < 0.001$), skipped breakfast (χ^2: 3.556, $p < 0.04$) or consumed commercial baked good or pastries for breakfast (χ^2: 6.717, $p < 0.006$) than NW. Interestingly, OWB consumed more frequently vegetables once a day (χ^2: 4.762, $p < 0.01$) or more than once a day (χ^2: 4.000, $p < 0.03$) than NW.

Males skipped breakfast less (χ^2: 3.187, $p < 0.04$) and consumed fish more regularly several times per week (χ^2: 8.172, $p < 0.003$), but more frequently also ate at fast-food restaurants (χ^2: 4.230, $p < 0.02$), and consumed commercial baked good or pastries for breakfast (χ^2: 2.984, $p < 0.04$) than females.

Children of other ethnic origins consumed more fish (χ^2: 6.460, $p < 0.008$), cereals or grain for breakfast (χ^2: 3.705, $p < 0.03$), two yoghurts and/or some cheese (χ^2: 6.083, $p < 0.01$) but more frequently also ate at fast-food restaurants (χ^2: 5.505, $p < 0.02$), skipped breakfast (χ^2: 6.621, $p < 0.01$), consumed commercial baked good or pastries for breakfast (χ^2: 4.238, $p < 0.05$), or took sweets and candy several times every day (χ^2: 6.847, $p < 0.008$) than those Italian.

Table 3 shows the distribution of subjects with respect to each item among subgroups.

In the crude analysis, the risk of OWB was associated with eating at fast-food restaurants (OR: 1.845, CI 95% 1.056–3.223, $p < 0.03$), frequent daily consumption of sweet and candies (OR: 1.946, CI 95% 1.238–3.059, $p < 0.004$), and in primary schools also with olive oil consumption at home (OR: 0.362, CI 95% 0.133–0.984, $p < 0.04$).

In the model weighted for all the items founded significant in the descriptive analysis, the risk of OWB (χ^2: 57.393, $p < 0.0001$) was associated with the male gender (OR: 2.008, CI 95% 1.285–3.163, $p < 0.002$), the primary school (OR: 2.412, CI 95% 1.533–3.795, $p < 0.0001$), eating raw or cooked vegetables once a day (OR: 0.610, CI 95% 0.376–0.990, $p < 0.04$), olive oil consumption at home (OR: 0.521, CI 95% 0.255–0.973, $p < 0.05$), and consumed commercial baked good or pastries for breakfast (OR: 1.534, CI 95% 1.001–2.426, $p < 0.05$). The model accounted for 13.9% of the total variance (Nagelkerke R^2), and the correct prediction rate was about 83.3%. We also split the analysis for the ethnicity due to the relative number of foreign children and significant interaction with some items. In Italian children, besides male gender and primary school, the risk of OWB (χ^2: 54.208, $p < 0.0001$) was associated inversely with eating raw or cooked vegetables more than once a day (OR: 0.588, CI 95% 0.349–0.991, $p < 0.04$), and olive oil consumption at home (OR: 0.382, CI 95% 0.176–0.826, $p < 0.01$), and directly with eating at fast-food restaurants (OR: 1.890, CI 95% 1.002–3.563, $p < 0.04$). The model accounted for 14.2% of the total variance, and the correct prediction rate was about 84.2%. Diversely, in children of other ethnic origins, besides primary school, the risk of OWB (χ^2: 22.201, $p < 0.03$) was associated with skipping breakfast (OR: 16.046, CI 95% 1.933–133.266, $p < 0.01$), or consuming commercial baked goods or pastries for breakfast (OR: 10.255, CI 95% 1.052–99.927, $p < 0.03$). The model accounted for 46.4% of the total variance, and the correct prediction rate was about 80.7%.

Table 3. Distribution of "yes" answers by school level, weight status, gender, and ethnicity.

	School Level		Weight		Gender		Ethnicity	
	Primary School	Secondary School	NW	OWB	M	F	Italian	Other
Consumption of a fruit or a fruit juice every day [1]	215 (74.1%)	292 (77.0%)	426 (76.3%)	81 (73.0%)	253 (78.1%)	254 (73.6%)	462 (75.5%)	45 (78.9%)
Consumption of a second fruit every day [1]	141 (48.6%)	180 (47.5%)	264 (47.3%)	57 (51.4%)	153 (47.2%)	168 (48.7%)	291 (47.5%)	30 (52.6%)
Consumption of raw or cooked vegetables 1 time a day [1]	**146 (50.3%)**	**225 (59.4%)**	**299 (50.3%)**	**72 (64.9%)**	**181 (55.9%)**	**190 (55.1%)**	**335 (54.7%)**	**36 (63.2%)**
Consumption of raw or cooked vegetables >1 time a day [1]	79 (27.2%)	121 (31.9%)	158 (28.3%)	42 (37.8%)	101 (31.2%)	99 (28.7%)	185 (30.2%)	15 (26.3%)
Consumption of fish regularly (at least 2–3 times a week) [1]	138 (47.6%)	177 (46.7%)	256 (45.9%)	59 (53.2%)	**171 (52.8%)**	**144 (41.7%)**	**279 (45.6%)**	**36 (63.2%)**
Eating >1 time per week to a fast-food (hamburger) restaurant [2]	**57 (19.7%)**	**47 (12.4%)**	**75 (13.4%)**	**29 (26.1%)**	**60 (18.5%)**	**44 (12.8%)**	**89 (14.5%)**	**15 (26.3%)**
Consumption of beans >1 time per week [1]	**150 (51.7%)**	**227 (56.7%)**	313 (56.1%)	64 (57.7%)	189 (50.1%)	188 (49.9%)	347 (56.7%)	30 (52.6%)
Consumption of pasta or rice almost every day (≥5 times a week) [1]	**251 (86.6%)**	**304 (80.2%)**	466 (83.5%)	89 (80.2%)	267 (82.4%)	288 (83.5%)	510 (83.3%)	45 (78.9%)
Consumption of cereals or grains (bread, etc.) for breakfast [1]	166 (57.2%)	223 (58.8%)	328 (58.8%)	61 (55.0%)	197 (60.8%)	192 (55.7%)	**349 (57.0%)**	**40 (70.2%)**
Consumption of nuts regularly (at least 2–3 times per week) [1]	75 (25.9%)	92 (24.3%)	134 (24.0%)	33 (29.7%)	80 (24.7%)	87 (25.2%)	149 (24.3%)	18 (31.6%)
Consumption of olive oil at home [1]	264 (91.0%)	354 (93.4%)	**521 (93.4%)**	**97 (87.4%)**	300 (92.6%)	318 (92.2%)	567 (92.6%)	51 (89.5%)
Skipping breakfast [2]	**43 (14.8%)**	**83 (21.9%)**	**98 (17.6%)**	**28 (25.2%)**	**52 (16.0%)**	**74 (21.4%)**	**108 (17.6%)**	**18 (31.6%)**
Consumption of a dairy product for breakfast (yoghurts, milk, etc.) [1]	225 (77.6%)	275 (72.6%)	422 (75.6%)	78 (70.3%)	248 (76.5%)	252 (73.0%)	459 (75.0%)	41 (71.9%)
Consumption of commercially baked goods or pastries for breakfast [2]	**182 (62.8%)**	**117 (46.7%)**	**287 (51.4%)**	**72 (64.9%)**	**185 (57.1%)**	**174 (50.4%)**	**321 (52.5%)**	**38 (66.7%)**
Consumption of 2 yoghurts and/or cheese (40 g) daily [1]	114 (39.3%)	170 (44.9%)	236 (42.3%)	48 (43.2%)	144 (44.4%)	140 (40.6%)	**251 (41.0%)**	**33 (57.9%)**
Consumption of sweets or candy several times every day [2]	**154 (53.1%)**	**138 (36.4%)**	287 (51.4%)	72 (64.9%)	190 (58.6%)	187 (54.2%)	**258 (42.2%)**	**34 (59.6%)**

Numbers and percentages are referred to "yes" answers. The denominators are those described in Table 1. [1] Items with a positive answer (+1). [2] Items with a negative score (−1). Bold numbers are those significant in the univariate logistic regression. Abbreviations. F, female; M, male; NW, normal-weight; OWB, overweight + obese.

4. Discussion

Data on adherence to MD have been explored above all on Greek and Spanish pediatric populations. Italian data are relatively few and mainly referred to children aged 8–9 years, or adolescents living in the southern part of the country. We demonstrated that schoolchildren and adolescents, in particular primary school or overweight/obese students, are more likely to have dietary behaviors close to a Western dietary pattern. Moreover, pediatric subjects of other ethnic origins have mixed behaviors, as happens in the nutrition transition. Some specific unhealthy food choices are more prevalent, such as eating at fast-food restaurants, skipping breakfasts, consumption of commercially baked goods or pastries for breakfast, and of sweets several times every day. The risk of overweight/obesity was not associated with the overall adherence to MD, but with specific food habits different depending on ethnicity.

Firstly, we observed that the prevalence of overweight and obesity (17.6%) in our cohort was quite lower than that reported by the GBD 2015 Obesity Collaborators on children and adolescents younger than 20 years [22], the IDEFICS study on children aged 2–10 years [23], and the WHO European Childhood Obesity Surveillance Initiative on primary schoolchildren [24]. This result is likely due to the different age range in our school cohort (6–15 years), beyond a geographical reason being well known that the highest rate of overweight and obesity is in the southern part of Italy. Accordingly, the last Piedmont data derived by the "OKkio alla SALUTE" project on children aged 8–9 years are comparable with the prevalence (24.0% vs. 23.4%) observed in our primary schoolchildren and with a higher risk to be obese in males [16,25]. Moreover, we recorded a higher prevalence of overweight and obesity in children and adolescents of other ethnic origins than in Italian students. This finding is in agreement with data demonstrating that the prevalence of overweight and obesity has a negative gradient with social position and income across Europe [23].

Secondly, the overall prevalence of good adherence to the MD is less than 20%. Good adherence varies in the literature from 4.3% in Greek 10–12-year-old adolescents to 53.9% in Spanish children. Most of the studies conducted in southern European countries and recently reviewed reported that about half of pediatric individuals have an average adherence, while nearly half may have poor adherence [10,11]. Our data reflect those derived by the majority of the European studies [11]. Regarding Italy, our results are similar from the Calabrian Sierras Community Study (CSCS) which investigated a population attending primary and secondary schools in a 14-town southern Italian community [26]. We also observed a lower prevalence of good adherence in students attending primary than secondary school, suggesting that younger children are more subjected to unhealthy choices. In fact, the attendance at a primary school is the only significant risk factor related to a poor MD adherence. This result is in contrast with the majority of the data that reported a negative trend in MD adherence with age [10,11]. Unfortunately, the CSCS study did not stratify the data for the school level [27]. On the other hand, the prevalence in our secondary school sample is similar to that reported by other studies on adolescents living in southern Italy [14,25,27]. It has to be considered that other socio-demographic factors such as parents' education and income are inconsistently associated across European countries due to different demographic and education changes [11]. Although we included only those schools where no prevention programs on the diets were performed in the last year, the enlargement of the study by including all the schools of Novara, accurate data on the socio-economic level, and parental weight could explain if an unexpected selection bias occurred.

Gender and overweight were not associated with the adherence to the MD. Although some studies suggest that in Western societies women tend to have better dietary habits than men [28], and MD has been associated to the prevention of obesity in adults [29], our results are in line with available European data in children recently systematically reviewed [10,11,30]. These findings suggest again that both obesity and social differentiation are complex events. Overeating, lack of physical activity, low sleep quality, and the family environment should be considered. On the other hand, the differences by gender, weight, and ethnicity on the items of the KIDMED index we recorded could help in explaining the phenomenon.

Our study reported a generally better quality of the diet among those children and adolescents more adherent to the MD than those with low adherence, except for the daily intake of sweets that was somewhat common. Moreover, we observed that younger children presented more unhealthy food choices than adolescents. This result is in line with a higher rate of poor adherence to the MD in the primary schoolchildren, as discussed above. The lower intake of vegetables and pulses resembles results obtained by the ZOOM8 study in 2009 and the last report of the "OKkio alla SALUTE" study in 2016 [16,31]. A negative association between MD adherence and snacks, sweets, commercial goods, and fast-foods has frequently been reported in other European pediatric populations [10,11,16]. It is interesting that primary schoolchildren consumed a more Westernized diet, skipping breakfast, eating several times per week at fast-food restaurants, consuming commercial baked goods, and sweets. This phenomenon could be boosted by geographical reasons, being our study conducted in an urban area [25]. In line with this hypothesis, we recorded a mixed dietary behavior in children and adolescents of other ethnic origins. In fact, the latter maintained a higher intake of more traditional foods, such as fish, cereals or grain for breakfast, and yoghurts and/or some cheese, suggesting more home-made foods in their family environment. On the other hand, contemporarily, they frequently ate at fast-food restaurants, skipped breakfast, consumed commercial baked goods for breakfast, or sweets and candy several times every day. These findings well picture the nutrition transition described in European countries including those of the Mediterranean area [7,11]. Overeating, eating anything or disliked foods, and eating at friends' home were all identified as strategies to cope with food insecurity [32]. Frequent consumption of fast food/junk calorie dense foods have been reported in several developing countries [33], and these behaviors could be replicated when low-income families move abroad, and less control over the youngest generations occurs for several reasons [11].

As previously described, the adherence to the MD did not predict the weight status. Moreover, in the literature, there is inconsistency also in the evidence about the role of specific food groups [34]. However, we recorded some associations with single KIDMED items. First, the risk of being OWB was related to eating at fast-food restaurants and daily intake of commercial baked goods or pastries for breakfast. This result is in agreement with two systematic reviews, one reporting the role of ultra-processed foods and the other that of sugar-sweetened drinks and sweets snacking with increased obesity risk also in the pediatric populations [35,36]. Direct associations between fast food availability and obesity in lower-income children have been described [37]. The adherence to MD depends on many foods with specific and synergistic activities on metabolism. It is likely that dense energy foods rich in simple carbohydrates and saturated fats have a major role in the development of obesity, in particular in younger children.

Moreover, food habits associated with the risk of OWB are different depending on ethnic backgrounds. The higher risk of OWB in those of other ethnic origins related to unhealthy choices for breakfast with skipping it or consuming commercial sweets and pastries suggests that the urbanization of life may lead to a more stressful lifestyle also in migrant people with less time spent on cooking, more time out of home, and dinner as the principal meal consumed with the family. All these factors could influence the food choices of the youngest children.

Interestingly, OWB subjects consumed less olive oil at home, and the risk of OWB was significantly and inversely associated with the intake of olive oil. The fact that the olive oil intake is associated with BMI is still debated. A study in children observed that the likelihood to increase their BMI was less in those who consumed only olive oil than in those who consumed other oils [38]. A recent review did not observe an increase in weight with an enriched-olive oil diet [39], although the Food4Me study recently recorded a direct correlation with the increase in weight in adults [34]. However, these last data are a little bit ambiguous reporting at the same time an inverse relationship with the intake of monounsaturated fats.

Furthermore, OWB children and adolescents consumed more frequently vegetables than NW ones. This finding could be contrasting with their other food habits. However, the risk of OWB was inversely associated with the intake of vegetables more than once a day. In addition, in the ZOOM study, OWB subjects consumed more vegetables than NW children [30], suggesting that the answers to these items hide an overeating behavior that overcomes the protective effects of healthy dietary choices [40].

Finally, we observed a direct association between the KIDMED score and height. To our knowledge, this result has not been reported by other studies on the adherence to the MD, because they have been focused on BMI, waist or waist-to-height without considering height alone [10,11], with the exception of one study limited to nine-year-old children [41]. Since children with a medium/high adherence to the MD have a more balanced diet in terms of nutrients and functional foods [10], these habits can explain our data. In particular, a diet poor in micronutrients and high-quality proteins from milk products, pork meat, and fish has been shown to negatively influence stature [42–44]. The reanalysis of data derived by HELENA and IDEFICS cohorts could confirm our findings.

This study has some limitations. First, it was a cross-sectional study design. Therefore, it is a limited set to establish causal relationships between MD and health outcome, and then conclusions are indications for further prospective and experimental investigations. Second, we only used the KIDMED score, without integrating it with a food frequency questionnaire. Adherence indexes, such as KIDMED score, have been validated and used in epidemiological surveys, but their reliability and reproducibility in assessing diet quality in the single subject have not been demonstrated yet [10,11]. Indeed, data on diet composition related to KIDMED score can be only inferred from related limited literature. We cannot exclude that some nutrients are main players more than food habits we reported. On the other hand, we used the most used index of adherence in pediatric literature [10,11], and the precise and driven administration to our cohort, in particular to younger children, supports the accuracy of our data. In fact, some authors suggest that the variability of adherence to MD across studies also results from the different administration methodologies [10]. Third, data on physical activity and sleep quality are lacking. Sedentary behaviors have been demonstrated to be correlated with the risk of OWB and low adherence to MD [10,11], and, then, co-linearity with some variable could exist. Fourth, specific data on the socio-economic level were not obtained, and schools were only stratified according to the socio-economic level of the district area they were located, and an unexpected selection bias could have occurred. Indeed, more accurate investigations of these variables, including also parental education, could have a role and improve the prediction of the OWB risk. On the other hand, this study could give a significant contribution to research since recent data on northern Italy are lacking and it could be compared with similar studies conducted in the Southern part of Italy, as well as in other urban European areas. We presented data divided for school level, gender and ethnicity and this will help in making more effective reviews on the topic. In particular, we focused on how different food habits influence the risk of OWB depending on ethnicity. These data are crucial for further investigations and description of the nutrition transition phenomenon with urbanization. Moreover, weight and height were not self-reported, and this increased the accuracy of the relationship between weight status and MD adherence.

In general, our study confirms that both children and adolescents have a poor MD adherence in an urban area of northern Italy, in line with other Italian and European data [10,11]. Furthermore, the mixed food behaviors occurring in individuals of different ethnic origins suggests that tailored prevention programs are needed to mitigate in this category of people the nutrition transition resulting from urbanization and changes of lifestyle habits of their families. These programs are urgent in hopes of preserving traditional healthy food habits. Moreover, the risk of OWB seems directly and indirectly associated more with specific food categories in pediatrics. These results should be confirmed but suggest that we have to increase nutrition knowledge in children and parents, as well as nutrition researchers should work hard.

5. Conclusions

In conclusion, we observed a relatively low high adherence to the MD in children and adolescents, in particular in those attending primary schools. Skipping breakfast, eating at fast-food restaurants, intake of processed foods and sweets are the main unhealthy choices, in particular in those OWB or of other ethnic origins. Differences in adherence to the MD and food intake between primary and secondary school, NW and OWB subjects and ethnic groups should be taken into account. Strategies tailored explicitly to subgroups are needed. Prevention campaigns should be conducted to improve food quality and drive to consume home-made healthy foods. The phenomenon of the nutrition transition should be accurately investigated, in particular in younger children and those in low-income brackets.

Author Contributions: Conceptualization, F.P. and S.B.; Methodology, F.A., R.R., D.C., and F.P.; Software, R.R. and F.C.; Validation, A.S., Formal Analysis, F.A., F.C., and F.P.; Investigation, F.A., R.R., A.S., D.C., F.C., and R.D.B. Data Curation, R.D.B; Writing—Original Draft Preparation, F.A. and F.P.; Writing—Review and Editing, S.B.; Supervision, S.B. and F.P.; and Funding Acquisition, F.P.

Funding: This research received no external funding.

Acknowledgments: The authors thanks all the children and their parents. The study was supported by the Department of Health Sciences, University of Piemonte Orientale. The funder had no role in the study design, data collection and analysis.

Conflicts of Interest: The authors declare no conflict of interest.

Appendix

Table A1. Comparison of the each KIDMED item in children with the lowest (score ≤ 3) and the highest adherence (score ≥8) to the Mediterranean diet and worst lifestyle.

	KIDMED Score Low (N = 112)	KIDMED Score High (N = 131)	p
Consumption of a fruit or a fruit juice every day [1]	45.5%	83.1%	0.0001
Consumption of a second fruit every day [1]	17.0%	87.0%	0.0001
Consumption of raw or cooked vegetables 1 time a day [1]	17.9%	87.0%	0.0001
Consumption of raw or cooked vegetables >1 time a day [1]	9.8%	64.1%	0.0001
Consumption of fish regularly (at least 2–3 times a week) [1]	16.1%	73.3%	0.0001
Eating >1 time per week to a fast-food (hamburger) restaurant [2]	37.5%	9.2%	0.0001
Consumption of beans >1 time per week [1]	24.1%	84.7%	0.0001
Consumption of pasta or rice almost every day (≥5 times a week) [1]	66.1%	88.5%	0.0001
Consumption of cereals or grains (bread, etc.) for breakfast [1]	23.2%	85.5%	0.0001
Consumption of nuts regularly (at least 2–3 times per week) [1]	14.3%	48.9%	0.0001
Consumption of olive oil at home [1]	77.7%	100.0%	0.0001
Skipping breakfast [2]	37.5%	5.3%	0.0001
Consumption of a dairy product for breakfast (yoghurts, milk, etc.) [1]	42.9%	95.4%	0.0001
Consumption of commercially baked goods or pastries for breakfast [2]	66.1%	37.4%	0.0001
Consumption of 2 yoghurts and/or cheese (40 g) daily [1]	32.1%	56.5%	0.0001
Consumption of sweets or candy several times every day [2]	50.0%	40.5%	0.087

[1] Items with a positive answer (+1). [2] Items with a negative score (−1). Data are represented as percentages. The data were analyzed by univariate logistic regression.

References

1. Estruch, R.; Ros, E. Primary Prevention of Cardiovascular Disease with a Mediterranean Diet Supplemented with Extra-Virgin Olive Oil or Nuts. *N. Engl. J. Med.* **2018**, *378*, e34. [CrossRef] [PubMed]

2. Esposito, K.; Maiorino, M.I. A Journey into a Mediterranean Diet and Type 2 Diabetes: A Systematic Review with Meta-Analysis. *BMJ Open* **2015**, *5*, e008222. [CrossRef] [PubMed]
3. Mattioli, A.V.; Palmiero, P. Mediterranean Diet Impact on Cardiovascular Diseases: A Narrative Review. *J. Cardiovasc. Med.* **2017**, *18*, 925–935. [CrossRef] [PubMed]
4. Schwingshackl, L.; Schwedhelm, C. Adherence to Mediterranean Diet and Risk of Cancer: An Update Systematic Review and Meta-Analysis. *Nutrients* **2017**, *9*, 1063. [CrossRef] [PubMed]
5. Grosso, G.; Marventano, S. A comprehensive meta-analysis on evidence of Mediterranean diet and cardiovascular disease: Are individual components equal? *Crit. Rev. Food Sci. Nutr.* **2017**, *57*, 3218–3232. [CrossRef] [PubMed]
6. Tsakiraki, M.; Grammatikopoulou, M.G. Nutrition transition and health status of Cretan women: Evidence from two generations. *Public Health Nutr.* **2011**, *14*, 793–800. [CrossRef] [PubMed]
7. Belahsen, R. Nutrition transition and food sustainability. *Proc. Nutr. Soc.* **2014**, *73*, 385–388. [CrossRef] [PubMed]
8. Esposito, K.; Kastorini, C.M. Mediterranean diet and weight loss: Meta-analysis of randomized controlled trials. *Metab. Syndr. Relat. Disord.* **2011**, *9*, 1–12. [CrossRef] [PubMed]
9. Serra-Majem, L.; Ribas, L. Food, youth and the Mediterranean diet in Spain. Development of KIDMED, Mediterranean Diet Quality Index in children and adolescents. *Public Health Nutr.* **2004**, *7*, 931–935. [CrossRef] [PubMed]
10. Idelson, P.I.; Scalfi, L. Adherence to the Mediterranean Diet in children and adolescents: A systematic review. *Nutr. Metab. Cardiovasc. Dis.* **2017**, *27*, 283–299. [CrossRef] [PubMed]
11. Grosso, G.; Galvano, F. Mediterranean diet adherence in children and adolescents in southern European countries. *NFS J.* **2017**, *3*, 16–19. [CrossRef]
12. Rosi, A.; Calestani, M.V. Weight Status Is Related with Gender and Sleep Duration but Not with Dietary Habits and Physical Activity in Primary School Italian Children. *Nutrients* **2017**, *9*, 579. [CrossRef] [PubMed]
13. Corte, C.D.; Mosca, A. Good adherence to the Mediterranean diet reduces the risk for NASH and diabetes in pediatric patients with obesity: The results of an Italian Study. *Nutrition* **2017**, *39*, 8–14. [CrossRef] [PubMed]
14. Mistretta, A.; Marventano, S. Mediterranean diet adherence and body composition among Southern Italian adolescents. *Obes. Res. Clin. Pract.* **2017**, *11*, 215–226. [CrossRef] [PubMed]
15. Buscemi, S.; Marventano, S. Role of anthropometric factors, self-perception, and diet on weight misperception among young adolescents: A cross-sectional study. *Eat. Weight Disord.* **2018**, *23*, 107–115. [CrossRef] [PubMed]
16. Spinelli, A.; Nardone, P. Centro Nazionale per la prevenzione delle malattie e la promozione della salute. OKkio alla Salute: I dati nazionali 2016. Available online: http://www.epicentro.iss.it|okkioallasalute (accessed on 30 July 2018).
17. Roccaldo, R.; Censi, L. Adherence to the Mediterranean diet in Italian school children (The ZOOM8 Study). *Int. J. Food Sci. Nutr.* **2014**, *65*, 621–628. [CrossRef] [PubMed]
18. Sede territoriale per il Piemonte e la Valle d'Aosta. Available online: https://www.istat.it/it/piemonte (accessed on 30 July 2018).
19. Cacciari, E.; Milani, S. Italian cross-sectional growth charts for height, weight and BMI (2 to 20 yr). *J. Endocrinol. Investig.* **2006**, *29*, 581–593. [CrossRef] [PubMed]
20. Cole, T.J.; Lobstein, T. Extended international (IOTF) body mass index cut-offs for thinness, overweight and obesity. *Pediatr. Obes.* **2012**, *7*, 284–294. [CrossRef] [PubMed]
21. Studio ZOOM8: L'alimentazione e l'attività fisica dei bambini della scuola primaria. Available online: https://www.researchgate.net/publication/259967194_Studio_ZOOM8_l%27alimentazione_e_l%27attivita_fisica_dei_bambini_della_scuola_primaria (accessed on 30 July 2018).
22. GBD 2015 Obesity Collaborators. Health Effects of Overweight and Obesity in 195 Countries over 25 Years. *N. Engl. J. Med.* **2017**, *377*, 13–27. [CrossRef] [PubMed]
23. Ahrens, W.; Pigeot, I. Prevalence of overweight and obesity in European children below the age of 10. *Int. J. Obes.* **2014**, *38*, S99. [CrossRef] [PubMed]
24. Childhood Obesity Surveillance Initiative—Euro Who Int. PDF File Childhood Obesity Surveillance Initiative COSI FACTSHEET Childhood Obesity Surveillance Initiative HIGHLIGHTS 2015-17 Preliminary Data. Available online: www.euro.who.int/__data/.../372426/wh14-cosi-factsheets-eng.pdf?ua=1 (accessed on 30 July 2018).

25. Grosso, G.; Marventano, S. Factors associated with adherence to the Mediterranean diet among adolescents living in Sicily, Southern Italy. *Nutrients* **2013**, *5*, 4908–4923. [CrossRef] [PubMed]
26. Martino, F.; Puddu, P.E. Mediterranean diet and physical activity impact on metabolic syndrome among children and adolescents from Southern Italy: Contribution from the Calabrian Sierras Community Study (CSCS). *Int. J. Cardiol.* **2016**, *225*, 284–288. [CrossRef] [PubMed]
27. Santomauro, F.; Lorini, C. Adherence to Mediterranean diet in a sample of Tuscan adolescents. *Nutrition* **2014**, *30*, 1379–1383. [CrossRef] [PubMed]
28. Lee, H.; Kang, M. Gender analysis in the development and validation of FFQ: A systematic review. *Br. J. Nutr.* **2016**, *115*, 666–671. [CrossRef] [PubMed]
29. Grosso, G.; Mistretta, A. Mediterranean diet and cardiovascular risk factors: A systematic review. *Crit. Rev. Food Sci. Nutr.* **2014**, *54*, 593–610. [CrossRef] [PubMed]
30. Agostinis-Sobrinho, C.; Santos, R. Optimal Adherence to a Mediterranean Diet May Not Overcome the Deleterious Effects of Low Physical Fitness on Cardiovascular Disease Risk in Adolescents: A Cross-Sectional Pooled Analysis. *Nutrients* **2018**, *10*, E815. [CrossRef] [PubMed]
31. Martone, D.; Roccaldo, R. Food consumption and nutrient intake in Italian school children: Results of the ZOOM8 study. *Int. J. Food Sci. Nutr.* **2013**, *64*, 700–705. [CrossRef] [PubMed]
32. Smith, C.; Richards, R. Dietary intake, overweight status, and perceptions of food insecurity among homeless Minnesotan youth. *Am. J. Hum. Biol.* **2008**, *20*, 550–563. [CrossRef] [PubMed]
33. Mistry, S.K.; Puthussery, S. Risk factors of overweight and obesity in childhood and adolescence in South Asian countries: A systematic review of the evidence. *Public Health* **2015**, *129*, 200–209. [CrossRef] [PubMed]
34. Celis-Morales, C.; Livingstone, K.M. Correlates of overall and central obesity in adults from seven European countries: Findings from the Food4Me Study. *Eur. J. Clin. Nutr.* **2018**, *72*, 207–219. [CrossRef] [PubMed]
35. Malik, V.S.; Pan, A. Sugar-sweetened beverages and weight gain in children and adults: A systematic review and meta-analysis. *Am. J. Clin. Nutr.* **2013**, *98*, 1084–1102. [CrossRef] [PubMed]
36. Poti, J.M.; Braga, B. Ultra-processed Food Intake and Obesity: What Really Matters for Health-Processing or Nutrient Content? *Curr. Obes. Rep.* **2017**, *6*, 420–431. [CrossRef] [PubMed]
37. Cobb, L.K.; Appel, L.J. The relationship of the local food environment with obesity: A systematic review of methods, study quality, and results. *Obesity (Silver Spring)* **2015**, *23*, 1331–1344. [CrossRef] [PubMed]
38. Haro-Mora, J.J.; García-Escobar, E. Children whose diet contained olive oil had a lower likelihood of increasing their body mass index Z-score over 1 year. *Eur. J. Endocrinol.* **2011**, *165*, 435–439. [CrossRef] [PubMed]
39. Buckland, G.; Gonzalez, C.A. The role of olive oil in disease prevention: A focus on the recent epidemiological evidence from cohort studies and dietary intervention trials. *Br. J. Nutr.* **2015**, *113*, S94–S101. [CrossRef] [PubMed]
40. Dubois, L.; Farmer, A.P. Preschool children's eating behaviours are related to dietary adequacy and body weight. *Eur. J. Clin. Nutr.* **2007**, *61*, 846–855. [CrossRef] [PubMed]
41. Jennings, A.; Welch, A. Diet quality is independently associated with weight status in children aged 9–10 years. *J. Nutr.* **2011**, *141*, 453–459. [CrossRef] [PubMed]
42. Rubio-López, N.; Llopis-González, A. Dietary Calcium Intake and Adherence to the Mediterranean Diet in Spanish Children: The ANIVA Study. *Int. J. Environ. Res. Public Health* **2017**, *14*, E637. [CrossRef] [PubMed]
43. Wang, H.; Tian, X. Growth disparity of motherless children might be attributed to a deficient intake of high-quality nutrients. *Nutr. Res.* **2016**, *36*, 1370–1378. [CrossRef] [PubMed]
44. Bawaked, R.A.; Schröder, H. Association of diet quality with dietary inflammatory potential in youth. *Food Nutr. Res.* **2017**, *61*, 1328961. [CrossRef] [PubMed]

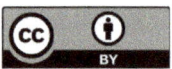

© 2018 by the authors. Licensee MDPI, Basel, Switzerland. This article is an open access article distributed under the terms and conditions of the Creative Commons Attribution (CC BY) license (http://creativecommons.org/licenses/by/4.0/).

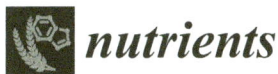

Article

Differences in Mediterranean Diet Adherence between Cyclists and Triathletes in a Sample of Spanish Athletes

José Joaquín Muros [1] and Mikel Zabala [2,*]

1. Department of Didactics of Musical, Plastic and Corporal Expression, University of Granada, 18071 Granada, Spain; jjmuros@ugr.es
2. Department of Physical Education, University of Granada, 18071 Granada, Spain
* Correspondence: mikelz@ugr.es; Tel.: +34-958-246-350

Received: 11 September 2018; Accepted: 8 October 2018; Published: 11 October 2018

Abstract: Adherence to the Mediterranean diet (MD) has rapidly declined in Mediterranean countries due to the increasing introduction of the Western diet. The aim of this study was to describe adherence to the MD within a sample of athletes from Spain. A second aim was to predict adherence to various components of the MD according to region, sex, and sport discipline. A cross-sectional study was conducted with a sample of 4037 (34.14 ± 9.28 years old) cyclists and triathletes (men: 90.1%). Participants self-reported their sex, date of birth, the number of years they had been practicing their sport, height, weight, sport discipline (cyclist, triathlon), and region. Mediterranean Diet Adherence Screener (MEDAS) was used to determine level of adherence to the MD. Women reported a higher MEDAS score and body mass index (BMI) ($p < 0.000$) than men. Cyclists reported a lower MEDAS score (7.44, SD 2.12 vs. 7.85, SD 2.08), and older age (37.72, SD 9.67 vs. 34.54, SD 8.58) and BMI (23.74, SD 2.69) vs. 22.85, SD 2.28) than triathletes. The study showed that a large proportion of the surveyed athletic population were not meeting the MD guidelines, with particularly low consumption amongst men and cyclists. There were no regional effects. Nutritional guidelines for athletes should be individual rather than general and follow specifications identified by the present research.

Keywords: Mediterranean diet; athletes; Spain

1. Introduction

The Mediterranean diet (MD) is rich in vegetables, fruit, legumes, nuts, and cereals, with olive oil as the staple dietary fat. The typical MD includes moderate to high intake of fish, moderate intake of dairy products, and low consumption of meat products [1]. Adherence to the MD has been proven to have health benefits for adults, such as protection against cardiovascular disease [2], type 2 diabetes [3], and metabolic syndrome, and improving blood pressure, waist circumference, high-density lipoprotein cholesterol, triacylglycerol, and glucose concentration [4].

Despite these health benefits, adherence to the MD has been rapidly declining in Mediterranean countries [5] including Spain [6]. These countries are replacing the MD with a Western diet, which is rich in animal products, refined carbohydrates, and fat and lacking in consumption of fruit and vegetables.

The benefits of physical exercise for health are well recognised [7]. An increase in physical activity has a significant role in the prevention of diseases such as cardiovascular disease, obesity, diabetes mellitus, cancer, depression, Alzheimer disease, arthritis, and osteoporosis [8]. Studies have shown an association between high levels of physical activity and Mediterranean diet adherence [6–9]. Trends since the late 1990s also show adherence to be consistently higher in southern regions [10], partly due to the warmer climate and closer proximity to the Mediterranean Sea [11]. However, no study has conducted this analysis for athletes who participate specifically in cycling or triathlons. It is currently unknown if cyclists and triathletes demonstrate different dietary practices with relation to MD adherence.

The aim of this study was to describe adherence to the MD within a sample of physically active adults who regularly engage in cycling or triathlons from all regions of Spain. We hypothesised that there would likely be differences in the nutritional habits between participants who engaged in cycling and those who engaged in triathlons. Although both sports are endurance sports, triathlon is considered to be a new sport compared with cycling and motivations for practice are likely to be different. A second aim was to predict adherence to various components of the MD according to region, sex, and discipline.

2. Materials and Methods

2.1. Design

This study used a cross-sectional design with a convenience sample. The demographic characteristics and the Mediterranean Diet Adherence Screener (MEDAS) were introduced into the application Google Drive® (Alphabet, Mountain View, CA, USA). The final questionnaire and instructions were sent by e-mail to the Royal Spanish Cycling Federation and to the Spanish Triathlon Federation, who forwarded them to all of their associated members. To be eligible for inclusion, participants had to be over 18 years old and have previously provided permission to their Federation to send e-mails to them. Research was conducted in 2016.

We adhered to the ethical principles of the Declaration of Helsinki for medical research. Ethical approval was granted by the Ethics Committee of the University of Granada, Spain (approval code: 883).

2.2. Subjects

A sample of 4037 (36.14 ± 9.28 years old) cyclists and triathletes (male: 90.1%) from across Spain (Table 1) was used for this study. There were 75,871 cyclists (male: 95%) federated in Spain during 2016 of which 2037 (male: 95.5%) satisfactorily completed the questionnaire and 27,760 triathletes (male: 82.3%) federated in Spain during 2016 of which 2000 (male: 84.5%) satisfactorily completed the questionnaire.

Table 1. Characteristics of study sample.

Characteristic	MEDAS Points (SD)	Male N (%)	Cyclists N (%)	Age Years (SD)	BMI kg/m² (SD)	Time Practicing Years (SD)
Overall (n = 4037)	7.64 (2.11)	3636 (90.07)	2037 (50.46)	36.14 (9.28)	23.30 (2.54)	9.31 (9.18)
North (n = 2340)	7.63 (2.09)	2108 (90.08)	1156 (49.40)	36.53 (9.63)	23.22 (2.53)	9.75 (9.61)
Aragon (n = 199)	7.59 (1.83)	184 (92.46)	125 (62.81)	37.13 (9.30)	23.25 (2.41)	9.86 (8.71)
Asturias (n = 160)	7.43 (1.88)	150 (93.75)	117 (73.13)	34.89 (10.10)	23.45 (2.74)	11.44 (9.64)
Balearic Islands (n = 112)	7.39 (2.00)	104 (92.86)	50 (44.64)	36.45 (9.14)	23.45 (2.22)	8.08 (8.53)
Basque Country (n = 265)	7.83 (1.90)	241 (90.94)	119 (44.91)	36.31 (9.29)	23.24 (2.41)	10.55 (9.80)
Cantabria (n = 135)	7.22 (2.09)	130 (96.30)	133 (98.52)	37.71 (8.33)	23.99 (2.33)	11.71 (10.31)
Castile and Leon (n = 268)	7.80 (2.24)	248 (92.54)	173 (64.55)	36.65 (10.32)	23.24 (2.52)	11.91 (10.58)
Catalonia (n = 476)	7.76 (2.03)	393 (82.56)	160 (33.61)	37.06 (9.84)	23.10 (2.41)	8.53 (9.57)
Community of Madrid (n = 452)	7.60 (2.18)	404 (89.38)	166 (36.73)	37.17 (9.51)	23.14 (2.81)	8.84 (9.39)
Galicia (n = 203)	7.38 (2.24)	185 (91.13)	86 (42.36)	34.08 (9.19)	22.93 (2.56)	8.74 (8.61)
La Rioja (n = 13)	7.62 (1.61)	11 (84.62)	0 (0.00)	36.08 (6.56)	23.02 (2.88)	3.54 (3.97)
Navarre (n = 61)	7.97 (1.91)	58 (95.08)	27 (44.26)	36.18 (11.10)	22.79 (1.97)	11.46 (10.07)
South (n = 1693)	7.66 (2.12)	1528 (90.25)	881 (52.04)	35.61 (8.76)	23.40 (2.55)	8.70 (8.51)
Andalusia (n = 971)	7.61 (2.18)	906 (93.31)	680 (70.03)	36.39 (8.83)	23.61 (2.66)	9.76 (8.86)
Canary Islands (n = 137)	7.30 (2.11)	125 (91.24)	55 (40.15)	35.44 (8.34)	23.46 (2.69)	8.24 (7.76)
Castile-La Mancha (n = 58)	7.90 (1.92)	50 (86.21)	5 (8.62)	31.98 (7.63)	23.04 (2.61)	4.34 (4.09)
Ceuta (n = 2)	9.00 (0.00)	2 (100.0)	0 (0.00)	41.50 (6.36)	22.49 (0.89)	15.50 (10.61)
Melilla (n = 11)	6.82 (1.94)	10 (90.91)	8 (72.73)	37.00 (6.45)	25.47 (3.08)	6.82 (7.47)
Extremadura (n = 132)	7.33 (2.15)	120 (90.91)	96 (72.73)	36.18 (9.98)	23.42 (2.48)	10.55 (9.06)
Region of Murcia (n = 105)	7.76 (1.94)	93 (88.57)	34 (32.38)	33.85 (8.40)	22.93 (2.24)	8.46 (8.86)
Valencian Country (n = 277)	8.12 (1.95)	222 (80.14)	3 (1.08)	33.98 (8.01)	22.81 (2.01)	5.35 (6.50)
p-value	0.466	0.736	0.088	0.001	0.042	0.008
Men (n = 3636)	7.59		1946 (53.52)	36.60 (9.15)	23.54 (2.46)	9.66 (9.31)
Women (n = 401)	8.15		91 (22.69)	31.96 (9.40)	21.08 (2.16)	6.13 (7.17)
p-value	0.000		0.000	0.000	0.000	0.000
Cyclists (n = 2037)	7.44 (2.12)	1946 (95.53)		37.72 (9.67)	23.74 (2.69)	12.98 (10.03)
Triathletes (n = 2000)	7.85 (2.08)	1690 (84.50)		34.54 (8.58)	22.85 (2.28)	5.56 (6.31)
p-value	0.000	0.000		0.000	0.000	0.000

MEDAS: Mediterranean Diet Adherence Screener; BMI: Body mass index.

2.3. Variables

Participants were asked to self-report their sex, data of birth, years practicing their sport, marital status, height, weight, sport discipline (cyclist, triathlon), and region (North: Aragon, Asturias, Balearic Islands, Basque Country, Cantabria, Castile and Leon, Catalonia, Community of Madrid, Galicia, La Rioja, or Navarre; South: Andalusia, Canary Islands, Castile-La Mancha, Ceuta, Melilla, Extremadura, Region of Murcia, and Valencian Country). Body mass index (BMI) was calculated as weight divided by height squared (kg/m^2). For ease of interpretation, categorical variables of sex (men and women), sport discipline (cyclists and triathlon), and region (north and south) were dichotomised. A total of 11% of the participants lived alone. Regarding marital status, 46.4% were single, 49.8% married, and 3.7% divorced.

MEDAS [12] was used to determine the level of adherence to the MD. This questionnaire consists of 14 items related to Mediterranean dietary patterns, 12 questions on food consumption frequency, and 2 questions on food intake habits, according to characteristics of the Spanish Mediterranean diet. Each question was scored 0 or 1 producing a derived score ranging from 0 to 14. One point was given for using olive oil as the principal source of fat for cooking and one for preferring white meat over red meat. One point was given for consumptions of: four or more tablespoon of olive oil per day; two or more servings of vegetables per day; three or more pieces of fruit per day; less than one serving of red meat, burgers, or sausages per day; less than one serving of butter, margarine, or cream per day; less than one carbonated and/or sugar-sweetened beverage per day; seven or more cups (100 mL) of wine per week; three or more servings of pulses per week; three or more servings of fish/seafood per week; less than two commercial pastries such as cookies or cakes per week; three or more servings of nuts per week; and two or more servings per week of boiled vegetables, pasta, rice, or other dishes with sauce, tomatoes, garlic, onion, or leeks sautéed in olive oil. The higher the score, the greater the adherence to the MD. Two MEDAS items were not included in the binary logistic regression model due to the lack of variation in responses, with more than 95% reporting using olive oil as the principal source of fat and less than 5% reporting meeting recommendations for consumption of wine. Although MEDAS was designed to evaluate elderly people, it is also suitable for assessing MD adherence in younger adults and adults [13].

2.4. Statistical Analysis

The mean for all quantitative variables is presented alongside the standard deviation. Normality of the data was tested using the Kolmogorov-Smirnov test with Lilliefort's correction and homoscedasticity was assessed using the Levene test. After verifying that the variables were non-normally distributed, the data were analysed using the U Mann-Whitney test for two-group comparison. Categorical variables are presented according to their frequency distribution and associations between them were determined using the Chi-square test.

Three binary logistic regression models were used to predict the probability of observations of the 12 items of the MEDAS according to sex, sport discipline, and region: Model 1: region (north and south) was entered as the predictor variable, representing a basic model adjusted for years practicing the relevant sport, BMI, sex, and sport discipline; Model 2: sport discipline was entered as the predictor variable, which was a basic model adjusted for years practicing the relevant sport, BMI, sex and region; and Model 3: sex was entered as the predictor variable, which was a basic model adjusted for years practicing the relevant sport, BMI, sport discipline, and region. Model fit was assessed using Nagelkerke R^2. The model demonstrated acceptable fit to data: Model 1 R^2: 0.269, Model 2 R^2: 0.336, and Model 3 R^2: 0.310. Data were analysed using the IBM-SPSS version 22.0 statistical programme for Windows (Armonk, NY, USA: IBM Corp.). The level of significance was set at 0.05.

3. Results

Data for MEDAS overall score, age, BMI, and time practicing the relevant sport for all study participants according to region, sex, and sport discipline are shown in Table 1. There were no significant differences according to region (north vs. south) in terms of MEDAS overall score, sex, and sport discipline. Northern participants were significantly older ($p < 0.01$), with lower BMI ($p < 0.05$), and reported more time practicing their relevant sport ($p < 0.001$). There were significant differences according to sex in relation to MEDAS overall score, age, BMI, and time practicing the relevant sport ($p < 0.000$). Women reported a higher MEDAS score and BMI, and lower age and time practicing their relevant sports. According to discipline, cyclists reported a lower MEDAS score and higher age, BMI, and time practicing their sport ($p < 0.000$).

Binary logistic regression analysis was conducted in order to predict adherence to various components of the MD as described by the different items on the MD questionnaire (Table 2). Participants who lived in the north were less likely than those living in the south to report meeting guidelines for the weekly consumption of olive oil (odds ratio (OR) = 0.75, 95% confidence interval (CI) = 0.64, 0.87); red meat, burgers, or sausages (OR = 0.75, 95% CI = 0.64, 0.87); nuts (OR = 0.86, 95% CI = 0.76, 0.99); and boiled vegetables, pasta, rice, or other dishes with tomato sauce, garlic, onion, or leeks sautéed in olive oil (OR = 0.85, 95% CI = 0.73, 0.99). Participants living in the north were more likely to meet recommendations for consumption of butter, margarine, or cream (OR = 1.48, 95% CI = 1.25, 1.75) and carbonated and/or sugar-sweetened beverages (OR = 1.44, 95% CI = 1.25, 1.65). They were also more likely to report preferring white meat over red meat (OR = 0.66, 95% CI = 0.55, 0.78). According to sport discipline, cyclists were less likely than triathletes to meet recommendations for consumption of fruit (OR = 0.74, 95% CI = 0.63, 0.88), carbonated and/or sugar-sweetened beverages (OR = 0.74, 95% CI = 0.63, 0.88), and nuts (OR = 0.67, 95% CI = 0.57, 0.79). Cyclists were more likely than triathletes to meet recommendations for boiled vegetables, pasta, rice, or other dishes with tomato sauce, garlic, onion, or leeks sautéed in olive oil (OR = 1.23, 95% CI = 1.01, 1.49). Model 3 considered sex as a predictor. Women were less likely than men to meet recommendations for consumption of pulses (OR = 0.68, 95% CI = 0.51, 0.90), nuts (OR = 0.78, 95% CI = 0.61, 0.99), and boiled vegetables, pasta, rice, or other dishes with tomato sauce, garlic, onion, or leeks sautéed in olive oil (OR = 0.53, 95% CI = 0.42, 0.69). Women were more likely to meet recommendation for consumption of vegetables per day (OR = 2.22, 95% CI = 1.72, 2.85) and red meat, burgers, or sausages per day (OR = 1.44, 95% CI = 1.11, 1.86).

Table 2. Binary logistic regression for the different aspects of the Mediterranean diet.

Variables	Model 1			Model 2			Model 3		
	OR	CI (95%)	p Value	OR	CI (95%)	p Value	OR	CI (95%)	p Value
Do you consume ≥4 tablespoon of olive oil per day?	0.75	0.64–0.87	0.000	1.20	0.99–1.45	0.061	1.14	0.85–1.53	0.374
Do you consume ≥2 servings of vegetables per day?	0.92	0.80–1.05	0.215	0.91	0.76–1.08	0.283	2.22	1.72–2.85	0.000
Do you consume ≥3 pieces of fruit per day?	1.07	0.94–1.23	0.300	0.74	0.63–0.88	0.000	0.91	0.70–1.17	0.458
Do you consume <1 serving of red meat, hamburger, or sausages per day?	0.75	0.64–0.87	0.000	1.06	0.88–1.28	0.532	1.44	1.11–1.86	0.006
Do you consume <1 serving of butter, margarine, or cream per day?	1.48	1.25–1.75	0.000	1.06	0.87–1.31	0.558	0.99	0.72–1.38	0.963
Do you consume <1 carbonated and/or sugar-sweetened beverages per day?	1.44	1.25–1.65	0.000	0.74	0.63–0.88	0.001	1.31	0.99–1.73	0.059
Do you consume ≥3 serving of pulses per week?	1.06	0.92–1.23	0.429	1.11	0.93–1.33	0.252	0.68	0.51–0.90	0.008
Do you consume ≥3 serving of fish/seafood per week?	1.12	0.97–1.29	0.125	0.88	0.74–1.05	0.157	1.07	0.83–1.37	0.597
Do you consume <2 commercial pastry such as cookies or cake per week?	0.93	0.81–1.06	0.280	1.06	0.90–1.25	0.500	1.19	0.93–1.54	0.174
Do you consume ≥3 serving of nuts per week?	0.86	0.76–0.99	0.030	0.67	0.57–0.79	0.000	0.78	0.61–0.99	0.047
Do you prefer to eat chicken, turkey, or rabbit instead of beef, pork, hamburgers, or sausages?	0.66	0.55–0.78	0.000	0.92	0.75–1.14	0.453	1.36	0.97–1.90	0.071
Do you consume ≥2 times per week boiled vegetables, pasta, rice, or other dishes with a sauce tomato, garlic, onion, or leeks sautéed in olive oil?	0.85	0.73–0.99	0.046	1.23	1.01–1.49	0.037	0.53	0.42–0.69	0.000

OR: Odds Ratio; CI: Confidence Interval.

4. Discussion

One of the main findings highlighted in this study was that a large proportion of the measured population did not meet MD guidelines. We also examined different individual aspects of the MD guidelines according to sex, sport discipline, and region.

The overall mean MEDAS score for the present sample of Spanish cyclists and triathletes was 7.64, higher than 6.34, which was reported in a representative sample of non-institutionalised Spanish adults aged 18 years old or older [6]. Although the overall MEDAS score was higher than that previously reported in a Spanish sample, it is still short of describing strict accordance to the MD ($\geq$9 points) [14]. Abandonment of MD habits have been previously reported in Mediterranean countries such as Spain [6], Greece [15], and Italy [16]. These countries are slowly replacing their traditional patterns of eating with Western dietary patterns rich in animal products, refined carbohydrates, and fat, and low consumption of fruit and vegetables. Levels of physical activity could explain differences in the overall MEDAS score of the present sample and that reported previously in another sample of non-institutionalised Spanish adults. Previous studies showed associations between high MD scores and high levels of daily physical activity, including in a sample of European adults [17] and a Spanish sample [18]. Another study found that cycling was associated with higher values of adherence to a MD, irrespective of training volume [19].

In the present study, there were no significant differences according to region (north vs. south) in terms of overall MEDAS score. The present findings contradict those previously reported by Abellán Alemán et al. [20], which showed that South-eastern Spain had the lowest score for adherence to the MD due to low consumption of fish and plant products. A study by Bach-Faig et al. [10] reported MD adherence over 20 years to be significantly higher in some southern Mediterranean regions of Spain, such as Andalusia. Teenagers from the southern region of Italy also showed the highest regional adherence for their country [21]. The different samples examined in these studies could explain the differences reported, as the present study was conducted with a sample of athletes and a physically active lifestyle was previously associated with a greater adherence to the MD independent of region [18,22]. Other potential confounders, such as socio-economic and educational status, should also be considered, as previous studies demonstrated that individuals with low socioeconomic and educational levels report low consumption of fish, fruit, and fresh vegetables [23,24]. In our study, those participants who were living in the northern regions were less likely than those living in the south to report meeting guidelines for the weekly consumption of olive oil. Although more than 95% of participants in both regions used olive oil as the principal source of fat for cooking, 78.5% participants who were living in the south consumed four or more tablespoons of olive oil per day in comparison to 74.1% of the participants who lived in the north. Also, participants who lived in the south consumed more boiled vegetables, pasta, rice, or other dishes with tomato sauce, garlic, onion, or leeks sautéed in olive oil. This can be explained by the finding that southern participants used more olive oil as oil for cooking. Participants who lived in the north were less likely than those living in the south to report meeting guidelines for red meat consumption. This corroborates previous results that showed that people living in the lower northern areas of Spain consumed more red meat and dairy products [20]. However, participants who lived in the south were also less likely to meet the recommendation for consumption of carbonated and or sugar-sweetened beverages. A number of factors could explain these findings. It is possible than the warmer climate contributes to a greater consumption of these beverages.

Women received a higher MEDAS score than men. A systematic review within Greek and Cypriot populations did not find statistically significant differences according to sex [25]. Contrasting results were found in a sample from Catalonia [26] and in a representative sample of Spanish adults in which women had lower adherence to the MD than men. This difference was mostly due to a lower consumption of wine amongst women with differences disappearing when wine was excluded from MD calculations [6]. Differences in the present research could also be related to the nutritional habits and knowledge of the included athletes. A comparison study with collegiate athletes previously showed that male athletes consume fast food or restaurant meals more frequently and have higher and more frequent weekly alcohol intake during the competitive season than women [27]. Female Australian elite athletes also reported a better diet quality than male athletes in addition to better nutrition knowledge [28]. A previous systematic review also reported that athletes' knowledge was equal to or better than non-athletes and that this knowledge was greater in women than in men [29]. Regarding specific components of the MD, women were more likely than men to meet the recommendations for daily consumption of vegetables (59.1% vs. 36.1%) and red meat (34.9% vs. 23.2%). Similar results were found by de Boer et al. [30] who concluded that differences could be driven by greater health consideration and awareness of climate change amongst women. Recommendations for consumption of pulses and fish should be given special consideration as the percentage of athletes following this MD recommendation in the present study was very small (less than 30% for pulses and less than 40% for fish), regardless of sex. Our results correspond with results reported for the general population of Spain, which suggest 22% meet the recommendation for pulses and only 30.2% consume three to four portions of fish/seafood per week [20].

With regards to discipline, triathletes had a higher MEDAS scored than cyclists. No previous studies reported adherence to the MD in a sample of triathletes and only two studies reported adherence to the MD in cyclists. One of these reported higher adherence to the MD amongst cyclists than amongst inactive adults [19]. Similar results were found in the second study, in which young male cyclists reported higher adherence to the MD than a matched group of non-cyclists [31]. In the present study, triathletes were more likely to meet the recommendation for consumption of fruit, nuts, and carbonated and or sugar-sweetened beverages than cyclists. This could be related to motives for participating in different endurance sports. Many cyclists were motivated by competition, whereas triathletes tended to be motivated by fitness, health benefits, and weight loss [32].

Regarding the recommendation for wine consumption, our results found that less than 5% of all surveyed athletes followed this guideline independent of sex, age, region, or discipline. Several factors could explain these findings. Firstly, alcohol is included on the list of prohibited substances and methods for athletes, meaning that they only occasionally consume alcohol [33]. The proportion of athletes that never consumed alcohol was higher than in a regular population and teetotal individuals would not be encouraged to commence drinking [34]. Despite the benefits of red wine on heart and kidney protection from ischemia-reperfusion injury [35], the recommendation concerning wine within this type of population should be optional and always with meals.

Two main recommendations emerge from the present findings. Firstly, although nutritional policies in Mediterranean countries have focused on the preservation of MD, nutritional intervention evidently requires comprehensive and specific messages about the different components of this diet. Specific recommendations should be elaborated for endurance sport athletes and specific recommendations for other sports should also be studied.

Limitations of the present study include its cross-sectional design, which precludes drawing conclusions on the direction of associations and inhibits the investigation of causal relationships. Adherence to a Mediterranean diet was measured using a validated questionnaire. The questionnaire has inherent limitations of precision due to reliance on self-reported data and the choice of research method, which precludes independent verification. However, the risk of error was minimized by ensuring anonymity of responses. The use of self-reporting to assess a number of variables increases the possibility of measurement error. However, MEDAS has previously demonstrated high validity and reliability in similar populations. The questionnaire was validated alongside the established food frequency questionnaire (FFQ), producing an average MEDAS score estimate of 105% of the FFQ score estimate suggesting that it is a valid instrument for rapid estimation of adherence to the MD. Weight and height were self-reported as opposed to directly measured due to time, financial resources, and labor constraints. Although this method is less accurate than direct measurement, it has demonstrated good agreement and validity in healthy weight populations. It was not possible to evaluate the socioeconomic status (SES) of individuals in this study. Future studies should measure SES where possible.

5. Conclusions

To the best of our knowledge, this is one of few investigations that describe adherence to a Mediterranean diet in a sample of athletes, and this is the first to analyse differences between cyclists and triathletes in a sample of Spanish athletes. This study is also the first to describe different nutritional patterns according to region, sex, and sport discipline in a sample of athletes. Future interventions should focus on an increase in vegetables and a decrease in red meat and hamburgers or sausages as a source of protein, especially in men. Another important focus of nutritional interventions with athletes should be an increase in pulses and fish/seafood independent of sex, region, or discipline, an increase in the consumption of fruit, and decreased consumption of carbonated sugar-sweetened drinks amongst cyclists. The study showed that a large proportion of the surveyed athletic population were not meeting MD guidelines, with particularly low consumption amongst men and cyclists. The findings have important implications for the design of nutritional interventions for athletes across Spain. It is essential to provide nutritional guidelines to athletes that consider the present findings rather than just promoting the MD in general.

Author Contributions: J.J.M. and M.Z. conceived the hypothesis of the study, participated in data collection, analysed the data, wrote the paper and approved the final manuscript.

Funding: This research received no external funding.

Acknowledgments: The authors thank both Cycling and Triathlon Spanish national federations for their collaboration in the data collection, especially Javier Chavarren (Head of Education in the Spanish Triathlon Federation). The authors also thank Emily Knox for revising the English language.

Conflicts of Interest: The authors declare no conflict of interest.

References

1. Trichopoulou, A.; Costacou, T.; Barnia, C.; Trichopoulos, D. Adherence to a Mediterranean diet and survival in a Greek population. *N. Engl. J. Med.* **2003**, *348*, 2599–2608. [CrossRef] [PubMed]
2. Estruch, R.; Ros, E.; Salas-Salvadó, J.; Covas, M.I.; Corella, D.; Arós, F.; Gómez-Gracia, E.; Ruiz-Gutiérrez, V.; Fiol, M.; Lapetra, J.; et al. Primary prevention of cardiovascular disease with a Mediterranean diet. *N. Engl. J. Med.* **2013**, *368*, 1279–1290. [CrossRef] [PubMed]
3. Schwingshackl, L.; Missbach, B.; König, J.; Hoffmann, G. Adherence to a Mediterranean diet and risk of diabetes: A systematic review and meta-analysis. *Public Health Nutr.* **2015**, *18*, 1292–1299. [CrossRef] [PubMed]
4. Kastorini, C.M.; Milionis, H.J.; Esposito, K.; Giugliano, D.; Goudevenos, J.A.; Panagiotakos, D.B. The effect of Mediterranean diet on metabolic syndrome and its components: A meta-analysis of 50 studies and 534,906 individuals. *J. Am. Coll. Cardiol.* **2011**, *57*, 1299–1313. [CrossRef] [PubMed]
5. Vareiro, D.; Bach-Faig, A.; Quintana, B.R.; Bertomeu, I.; Buckland, G.; de Almeida, M.D.; Serra-Majem, L. Availability of Mediterranean and non-Mediterranean foods during the last four decades: Comparison of several geographical areas. *Public Health Nutr.* **2009**, *12*, 1667–1675. [CrossRef] [PubMed]
6. León-Munoz, L.M.; Guallar-Castillón, P.; Graciani, A.; López-García, E.; Mesas, A.E.; Aguilera, M.T.; Banegas, J.R.; Rodríguez-Artalejo, F. Adherence to the Mediterranean diet pattern has declined in Spanish adults. *J. Nutr.* **2012**, *142*, 1843–1850. [CrossRef] [PubMed]
7. Mansoubi, M.; Pearson, N.; Clemes, S.; Biddle, S.J.H. The relationship between sedentary behaviour and physical activity in adults: A systematic review. *Prev. Med.* **2014**, *69*, 28–35. [CrossRef] [PubMed]
8. Lobelo, F.; Rohm Young, D.; Sallis, R.; Garber, M.D.; Billinger, S.A.; Duperly, J.; Hutber, A.; Pate, R.R.; Thomas, R.J.; Widlansky, M.E.; et al. Routine assessment and promotion of physical activity in healthcare setting: A scientific statement from de American Heart Association. *Cirulation* **2018**, *17*, e495–e522. [CrossRef] [PubMed]

9. Patino-Alonso, M.C.; Recio-Rodríguez, J.I.; Belio, J.F.; Colominas-Garrido, R.; Lema-Bartolomé, J.; Arranz, A.G.; Agudo-Conde, C.; Gomez-Marcos, M.A.; García-Ortiz, L.; EVIDENT Group. Factors associated with adherence to the Mediterranean diet in the adult population. *J. Acad. Nutr. Diet.* **2014**, *114*, 583–589. [CrossRef] [PubMed]
10. Bach-Faig, A.; Fuentes-Bol, C.; Ramos, D.; Carrasco, J.L.; Roman, B.; Bertomeu, I.F.; Cristià, E.; Geleva, D.; Serra-Majem, L. The Mediterranean diet in Spain: Adherence trends during the past two decades using the Mediterranean Adequacy Index. *Public Health Nutr.* **2011**, *14*, 622–628. [CrossRef] [PubMed]
11. Arriscado, D.; Knox, E.; Zabala, M.; Zurita-Ortega, F.; Dalmau, J.M.; Muros, J.J. Different healthy habits between northern and southern Spanish school children. *J. Public Health* **2017**, *25*, 653–660. [CrossRef] [PubMed]
12. Schröder, H.; Fitó, M.; Estruch, R.; Martínez-González, M.A.; Corella, D.; Salas-Salvadó, J.; Lamuela-Raventós, R.; Ros, E.; Salaverría, I.; Fiol, M.; et al. A short screener is valid for assessing Mediterranean diet adherence among older Spanish men and women. *J. Nutr.* **2011**, *141*, 1140–1145. [CrossRef] [PubMed]
13. Bamia, C.; Martimianaki, G.; Kritikou, M.; Trichopoulou, A. Indexes for assessing adherence to a Mediterranean diet from data measured through brief questionnaires: Issues raised from the analysis of a Greek population study. *Curr. Dev. Nutr.* **2017**, *1*, 1–8. [CrossRef] [PubMed]
14. Sánchez-Taínta, A.; Estruch, R.; Bullo, M.; Corella, D.; Gomez-Gracia, E.; Fiol, M.; Algorta, J.; Covas, M.I.; Lapetra, J.; Zazpe, I.; et al. Adherence to a Mediterranean-type diet and reduced prevalence of clustered cardiovascular risk factors in a cohort of 3204 high-risk patients. *Eur. J. Cardiovasc. Prev. Rehabil.* **2008**, *15*, 589–593. [CrossRef] [PubMed]
15. Arvaniti, F.; Panagiotakos, D.B.; Pitsavos, C.; Zampelas, A.; Stefanadis, C. Dietary habits in a Greek sample of men and women: The ATTICA study. *Cent. Eur. J. Public Health* **2006**, *14*, 74–77. [CrossRef] [PubMed]
16. Sofi, F.; Vecchio, S.; Giuliani, G.; Marcucci, R.; Gori, A.M.; Fedi, S.; Casini, A.; Surrenti, C.; Abbate, R.; Gensini, G.F. Dietary habits, lifestyle and cardiovascular risk factors in a clinically healthy Italian population: The 'Florence' diet is not Mediterranean. *Eur. J. Clin. Nutr.* **2005**, *59*, 584–591. [CrossRef] [PubMed]
17. Fallaize, R.; Livingstone, K.M.; Celis-Morales, C.; Macready, A.L.; San-Cristobal, R.; Navas-Carretero, S.; Marsaux, C.F.; O'Donovan, C.B.; Kolossa, S.; Moschonis, G.; et al. Association between diet-quality scores, adiposity, total cholesterol and markers of nutritional status in European adults: Findings from the FoodMe study. *Nutrients* **2018**, *10*, 49. [CrossRef] [PubMed]
18. Bibiloni, M.D.M.; González, M.; Julibert, A.; Llompart, I.; Pons, A.; Tur, J.A. Ten-year trends (1999–2010) of adherence to the Mediterranean diet among the Balearic Islands' adult population. *Nutrients* **2017**, *9*, E749. [CrossRef] [PubMed]
19. Mayolas-Pi, C.; Munguia-Izquierdo, D.; Peñarrubia-Lozano, C.; Reverter-Masia, J.; Bueno-Antequera, J.; López-Laval, I.; Oviedo-Caro, M.Á.; Murillo-Lorente, V.; Murillo-Fuentes, A.; Paris-García, F.; et al. Adherence to the Mediterranean diet in inactive adults, indoor cycling practitioners and amateur cyclists. *Nutr. Hops.* **2017**, *35*, 131–139. [CrossRef]
20. Abellán Alemán, J.; Zafrilla Rentero, M.P.; Montoro-García, S.; Mulero, J.; Pérez Garrido, A.; Leal, M.; Guerrero, L.; Ramos, E.; Ruilope, L.M. Adherence to the "Mediterranean diet" in Spain and its relationship with cardiovascular risk (DIMERICA study). *Nutrients* **2016**, *8*, 680. [CrossRef] [PubMed]
21. Noale, M.; Nardi, M.; Limongi, F.; Siviero, P.; Caregaro, L.; Crepaldi, G.; Maggi, S.; Mediterranean Diet Foundation Study Group. Adolescents in southern regions of Italy adhere to the Mediterranean diet more than those in the northern regions. *Nutr. Res.* **2014**, *34*, 771–779. [CrossRef] [PubMed]
22. Moreno, L.A.; Sarría, A.; Popkin, B.M. The nutrition transition in Spain: A European Mediterranean country. *Eur. J. Clin. Nutr.* **2002**, *56*, 992–1003. [CrossRef] [PubMed]
23. Mertens, E.; Kuijsten, A.; Dofková, M.; Mistura, L.; D'Addezio, L.; Turrini, A.; Dubuisson, C.; Favret, S.; Havard, S.; Trolle, E.; et al. Geographic and socioeconomic diversity of food and nutrients intake: A comparison of four European countries. *Eur. J. Nutr.* **2018**. [CrossRef] [PubMed]
24. Darmon, N.; Drewnowski, A. Does social class predict diet quality? *Am. J. Clin. Nutr.* **2008**, *87*, 1107–1117. [CrossRef] [PubMed]
25. Kiriacou, A.; Evans, J.M.; Economides, N.; Kyriacou, A. Adherence to the Mediterranean diet by the Greek and Cypriot population: A systematic review. *Eur. J. Public Health* **2015**, *25*, 1012–1018. [CrossRef] [PubMed]

26. Bondia-Pons, I.; Serra-Majem, L.; Castellote, A.I.; López-Sabater, M.C. Compliance with the European and national nutritional objectives in a Mediterranean population. *Eur. J. Clin. Nutr.* **2007**, *61*, 1345–1351. [CrossRef] [PubMed]
27. Hull, M.V.; Jagim, A.R.; Oliver, J.M.; Greenwood, M.; Busteed, D.R.; Jones, M.T. Gender differences and access to a sport dietitian influence dietary habits or collegiate athletes. *J. Int. Soc. Sports Nutr.* **2016**, *13*, 38. [CrossRef] [PubMed]
28. Spronk, I.; Heaney, S.E.; Prvan, T.; O'Connor, H.T. Relationship between general nutrition knowledge and dietary quality in elite athletes. *Int. J. Sport Nutr. Exerc. Metab.* **2015**, *25*, 243–251. [CrossRef] [PubMed]
29. Heaney, S.; O'Connor, H.; Michael, S.; Gifford, J.; Naghton, G. Nutrition knowledge in athletes: A systematic review. *Int. J. Sport Nutr. Exerc. Metab.* **2011**, *21*, 248–261. [CrossRef] [PubMed]
30. de Boer, J.; Schosler, H.; Aiking, H. "Meatless days" or "less but better"? Exploring strategies to adapt Western meat consumption to health and sustainability challenges. *Appetite* **2014**, *76*, 120–128. [CrossRef] [PubMed]
31. Sánchez-Benito, J.L.; Sánchez-Soriano, E.; Ginart Suárez, J. Assessment of the Mediterranean diet adequacy index of a collective of young cyclists. *Nutr. Hosp.* **2009**, *24*, 77–86. [PubMed]
32. Dolan, S.H.; Houston, M.; Martin, S.B. Survey results of the training, nutrition, and mental preparation of triathletes: Practical implications of findings. *J. Sports Sci.* **2011**, *29*, 1019–1028. [CrossRef] [PubMed]
33. O'Brien, C.P.; Lyons, F. Alcohol and the athlete. *Sports Med.* **2000**, *29*, 295–300. [CrossRef] [PubMed]
34. George, E.S.; Kucianski, T.; Mayr, H.L.; Moschonis, G.; Tierney, A.C.; Itsiopoulos, C. A Mediterranenan diet model in Australia: Strategies for translating the traditional Mediterranean diet into a multicultural setting. *Nutrients* **2018**, *10*, 465. [CrossRef] [PubMed]
35. Ortega, R. Importance of functional foods in the Mediterranean diet. *Public Health Nutr.* **2006**, *9*, 1136–1140. [CrossRef] [PubMed]

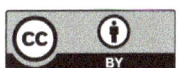

© 2018 by the authors. Licensee MDPI, Basel, Switzerland. This article is an open access article distributed under the terms and conditions of the Creative Commons Attribution (CC BY) license (http://creativecommons.org/licenses/by/4.0/).

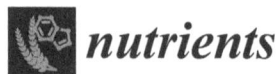

Review

Relationship between Mediterranean Dietary Polyphenol Intake and Obesity

Sara Castro-Barquero [1,2], Rosa M. Lamuela-Raventós [3,4], Mónica Doménech [1,2,4] and Ramon Estruch [1,2,4,5,*]

1. Institut d'Investigacions Biomèdiques August Pi i Sunyer (IDIBAPS), 08036 Barcelona, Spain; sacastro@clinic.cat (S.C.-B.); mdomen@clinic.cat (M.D.)
2. Department of Medicine, Faculty of Medicine and Health Sciences, University of Barcelona, 08036 Barcelona, Spain
3. Department of Nutrition, Food Science and Gastronomy, XaRTA, INSA-UB, School of Pharmacy and Food Science, University of Barcelona, 08028 Barcelona, Spain; lamuela@ub.edu
4. CIBEROBN Fisiopatología de la Obesidad y Nutrición, Instituto de Salud Carlos III, 28029 Madrid, Spain
5. Department of Internal Medicine Institut d'Investigacions Biomèdiques August Pi Sunyer (IDIBAPS), Hospital Clinic, University of Barcelona, 08036 Barcelona, Spain
* Correspondence: restruch@clinic.cat; Tel.: +34-93-227-54-00 (ext. 2276)

Received: 21 September 2018; Accepted: 14 October 2018; Published: 17 October 2018

Abstract: Obesity is a multifactorial and complex disease defined by excess of adipose mass and constitutes a serious health problem. Adipose tissue acts as an endocrine organ secreting a wide range of inflammatory adipocytokines, which leads to systemic inflammation, insulin resistance, and metabolic disorders. The traditional Mediterranean diet is characterized by a high phenolic-rich foods intake, including extra-virgin olive oil, nuts, red wine, vegetables, fruits, legumes, and whole-grain cereals. Evidence for polyphenols' effect on obesity and weight control in humans is inconsistent and the health effects of polyphenols depend on the amount consumed and their bioavailability. The mechanisms involved in weight loss in which polyphenols may have a role are: activating β-oxidation; a prebiotic effect for gut microbiota; inducing satiety; stimulating energy expenditure by inducing thermogenesis in brown adipose tissue; modulating adipose tissue inhibiting adipocyte differentiation; promoting adipocyte apoptosis and increasing lipolysis. Even though the intake of some specific polyphenols has been associated with body weight changes, there is still no evidence for the effects of total polyphenols or some polyphenol subclasses in humans on adiposity.

Keywords: dietary intake; catechins; resveratrol; olive oil; wine; BMI

---

1. Introduction

The global overweightness and obesity epidemic is increasing at an alarming rate and constitutes a serious global public health problem, affecting over 27.5% of the worldwide adult population and 47.1% of children [1]. Between 1980 and 2013, the worldwide prevalence of overweight and obese individuals increased from 857 million to 2.1 billion [1]. There is some evidence that the obesity epidemic is leveling off in some populations, although the prevalence of excess weight remains high in many countries of the world. The health consequences associated with obesity have been widely recognized: overall mortality, cardiovascular disease (CVD), hypertension, type 2 diabetes mellitus (T2DM), hyperlipidemia, stroke, cancer, osteoarthritis, chronic kidney disease, and gynecological problems, among others [2]. The medium-to-long-term consequences of obesity lead to rendering the health system unsustainable and, consequently, an urgent priority must be given to finding solutions for this issue that should be based on the best scientific evidence available.

Obesity is a multifactorial complex disease defined by excess of adipose mass, which occurs through adipocyte hypertrophy and hyperplasia [3]. The adipose tissue is an endocrine organ that secretes a wide variety of inflammatory adipocytokines, such as tumor necrosis factor alpha (TNF-α), interleukin-6 (IL-6), resistin, leptin, and adiponectin. Visceral adiposity is associated with a higher production of these inflammatory adipocytokines, leading to systemic inflammation, insulin resistance, and several obesity-related metabolic disorders [4]. This inflammation due to obesity can be reversed with weight loss, which causes a reduction in fat mass and proinflammatory adipokines. Moreover, the intake of foods rich in bioactive compounds such as omega-3 fatty acids and polyphenols have been described to decrease low-degree inflammation [3].

2. The Mediterranean Diet

The link between adherence to the traditional Mediterranean diet (MedDiet) and the risk of cardiovascular disease (CVD) are mediated by several mechanisms, including reduction in low-degree inflammation [5–7], high plasma concentration of adiponectin, improvement of endothelial function [8], diminution of oxidative stress [9], low concentration of atherogenic lipoproteins, and lower levels of oxidized low-density lipoprotein (LDL) particles [10]. The high-density lipoprotein (HDL) functionality was also improved by the MedDiet. Cholesterol efflux capacity, specifically the HDL esterification index and HDL antioxidant and anti-inflammatory capacity, and vasoprotective effects inducing nitric oxide synthesis by endothelial cells are increased [11]. Furthermore, there are other inflammatory biomarkers related to CVD and atherosclerotic process that may be modulated by lifestyle, such as C-reactive protein (CRP), IL-6, and homocysteine [7,12].

The MedDiet is characterized by a high intake of phenolic compounds, which are present in the main key foods of this dietary pattern: extra-virgin olive oil (EVOO), nuts, red wine, legumes, vegetables, fruits, and whole-grain cereals. Phenolic compounds, usually called polyphenols (Figure 1) [13], are important candidates responsible for the beneficial effects of the MedDiet. A continuous and prolonged polyphenol intake is related to blood pressure and adiposity lowering effects, improvements in lipid profile, and also anti-inflammatory effects, which all act as CVD protectors [14].

Mediterranean Diet and Weight Loss

Although the long-term health benefits of the MedDiet are well established, its efficacy for weight loss at ≥12 months in overweight or obese individuals remains controversial. A systematic review of five randomized clinical trials (RCTs) [15] studied the effect of the MedDiet on weight loss in overweight or obese individuals comparing MedDiet interventions with low-fat diets, a low-carbohydrate diet, and the American Diabetes Association (ADA) diet. In this review, the MedDiet showed greater weight loss than the low-fat diets (range of the mean values: −4.1 to −10.1 kg vs. −2.9 to −5.0 kg), but similar weight loss compared with the other two interventions (range of the mean values: −4.1 to −10.1 kg vs. −4.7 to −7.7 kg). Epidemiological evidence for the association between the adherence to a traditional MedDiet with reduction of body weight and waist circumference is unclear. In 2011, Esposito et al. published a meta-analysis of 16 RCTs, which shows that a greater adherence to the MedDiet causes more weight loss as compared with a control diet [5]. Moreover, in none of the 16 RCTs was MedDiet adherence correlated with weight gain. Many components of the MedDiet may favor weight loss due to the abundance of plant-based foods, which provide high dietary fiber intake with a low energy density and low glycemic load. However, the effect of the MedDiet on body weight was greater in association with an energy-restricted MedDiet plan (−3.88 kg) or physical activity improvements (−4.01 kg) [16].

Huo et al. studied the effect of a Mediterranean-style diet on T2DM patients in terms of glycemic control, weight loss, and cardiovascular risks factors. Body mass index (BMI) was decreased in participants who followed the MedDiet (mean difference, −0.29 kg/m^2; 95% CI, −0.46 to −0.12) compared with those in the control diets [16].

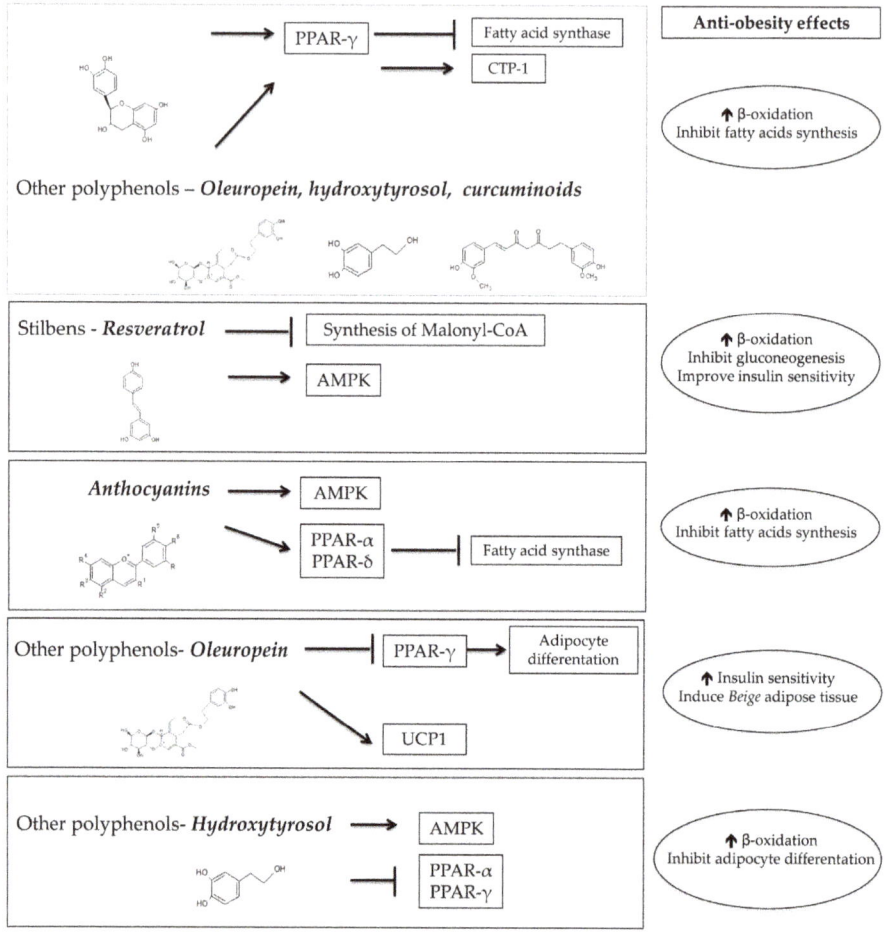

Figure 1. Molecular mechanisms of polyphenols involved in obesity. PPAR-γ: peroxisome proliferator-activated receptor gamma; CTP-1: tricarboxylate transport protein 1; AMPK: 5′-adenosine monophosphate-activated protein kinase; PPAR-α: peroxisome proliferator-activated receptor alpha; PPAR-δ: peroxisome proliferator-activated receptor delta; PPAR-γ: peroxisome proliferator-activated receptor gamma; → activation; ⊣ inhibition; and ↑ increase. ADC/ChemSketch (Advanced Chemistry Development, Inc., Toronto, ON, Canada) software was employed for chemical structures.

3. Dietary Polyphenol Intake

The effects of polyphenols depend on the amount and absorption of dietary polyphenols. Thus, to highlight the health benefits of polyphenols in humans, it is necessary to know the polyphenol content of the foods and the polyphenol subclasses' composition. Typically, polyphenol intake is currently evaluated using data extracted from food frequency questionnaires (FFQs). Recently, polyphenol intake has been measured using analysis of different biomarkers, mainly phase II enzyme-conjugated polyphenol metabolites, which are metabolites present in the bloodstream and urine and fecal samples. Unfortunately, there are thousands of potential biomarkers of polyphenol intake and there is no consensus yet [17]. On the other hand, Tresserra-Rimbau et al. studied the effect of dietary polyphenol intake on CVD, calculating the polyphenol consumption by matching FFQ data with the Phenol-Explorer database [14]. In this context, the effect of gut microbiota has to be considered, as it metabolizes part of the dietary polyphenols and its metabolism can modify their absorption, bioavailability, and biological activity. The interindividual variability in gut microbiota, which determines polyphenol absorption, can explain the variety of health effects in the mentioned studies.

Polyphenol Intake in the Mediterranean Countries

The intake of dietary polyphenols and the main food sources depends on the dietary pattern and the native foods of each region, as described in Table 1. In the case of Mediterranean countries, the European Prospective Investigation into Cancer (EPIC) Nutrition cohort described the differences among the polyphenol intake of the European regions, estimating individual polyphenols and subclasses [18]. The estimation of polyphenol intake was performed by 24-h dietary recall of 36,027 adults, and the phenolic compounds data was obtained using the Phenol-Explorer database. Interestingly, the Mediterranean countries (including Spain, Greece, Italy, and the south of France) showed the lowest intake of total polyphenols (around 1011 mg/day) compared with non-Mediterranean countries and the United Kingdom (around 1284 and 1521 mg/day, respectively) [18]. Nevertheless, the profile of polyphenol subclasses was very different: Mediterranean countries showed the highest intake of stilbenes and flavonoids (49–62% of total polyphenols), followed by phenolic acids (34–44%). In relation to the main food sources, polyphenols in Mediterranean countries come mainly from coffee, fruits (the main source of flavonoids, representing 45% of the intake), wine, and vegetables oils (representing 26% of lignans intake), whereas in the non-Mediterranean countries, polyphenols come from coffee, tea, and wine (40.9%, 17.4%, and 4.6% of total polyphenols, respectively) [18].

Another cohort from France, called SUpplémentation en VItamines et Minéraux AntioXydants (SU.VI.MAX), quantified the polyphenol intake by 24-h dietary records and the Phenol-Explorer database in 4942 subjects. The mean total polyphenol intake (TPI) was 1193 mg/day, with hydroxycinnamic acids being the highest consumed polyphenol subclass, followed by proanthocyanidins [19]. The main food sources of hydroxycinnamic acids were coffee, potatoes, and apples, whereas for proanthocyanidins, were fruits, cocoa products, and red wine.

An observational study focusing on the nutritional habits characterizing the Mediterranean lifestyle, performed in Sicily in southern Italy, named the Mediterranean healthy Eating, Aging, and Lifestyle study (MEAL), estimated the polyphenol intake of 2044 subjects by FFQs and the Phenol-Explorer database. The main objective of the study was to describe the polyphenol intake differentiating the subjects by their level of adherence to the MedDiet, as measured by the MEDI-LITE score [20]. Additionally, Godos et al. described the intake of polyphenol subclasses and the major food sources in the MEAL study population [21]. Total polyphenol intake was 664 mg/day, of which the main intakes by subclass were phenolic acids, followed by flavonoids (363 and 259 mg/day, respectively). Nuts were the main food source of polyphenols, accounting for around 28% of total polyphenol intake, followed by coffee, cherries, red wine, and tea. Despite the fact that the adherence to the Mediterranean diet was high, the intake of total polyphenols was lower than the other areas described. The study concluded that the most consumed subclasses were flavonoids among the individuals with the highest adherence to the MedDiet, with fruits, vegetables, and red wine being the main food contributors [22].

Table 1. Profile of the dietary polyphenol subclasses' intake among the Mediterranean countries.

Mediterranean Area	Polyphenol Subclass (% of TPI) [a]	Main Food Sources (% of TPI) [a]
Spain, Greece, Italy, and south of France [17]	Phenolic acids (49), flavonoids (45), other polyphenols (0.6), stilbenes, and lignans (<0.7)	Coffee (36), fruits (25), red wine (10)
France [18]	Phenolic acids (54), flavonoids (42)	Coffee (44), tea (7), apples (7), red wine (6)
Spain [23]	Flavonoids (54), phenolic acids (37), other polyphenols (8.7), stilbenes, and lignans (<0.3)	Coffee (18), oranges (16), apples (12), olives and olive oil (11), red wine (6)
Sicily (Italy) [20,21]	Phenolic acids (53), flavonoids (37), lignans (0.4), stilbenes (0.3)	Nuts (28), coffee (7), red wine (6), tea (5)

TPI; Total polyphenol intake. [a] Dietary polyphenol intake was determined by the Phenol-Explorer Database (http://phenol-explorer.eu/, accessed on July 2018) for all the areas described.

The PREDIMED cohort (PREvención con DIeta MEDiterránea), comprised of a Spanish population at high cardiovascular risk, studied the effect of dietary polyphenol intake and the incidence of cardiovascular events [14]. Tresserra-Rimbau et al. described the intake of polyphenol subclasses' intake and the major food sources of the PREDIMED study subjects also using FFQs and the Phenol-Explorer database. Similar to the Italian population, the main intakes by subclass were flavonoids (443 mg/day), followed by phenolic acids (304 mg/day) [23]. Fruits were the main total polyphenols contributor, accounting for around 44%. Within the flavonoids, flavanols were strongly related to CVD prevention (HR = 0.4 (0.23–0.72)) and were mostly consumed from red wine (32%) and apples (31%) [14]. This study concluded that a higher intake of flavanols was associated with a 60% reduction of cardiovascular event and mortality risk. Despite the fact that the main phenolic acids subclass consumed was hydroxycinnamic acids, the intake of hydroxybenzoic acids was related to a lower incidence of CVD (HR = 0.47 (0.26–0.86)). It should be pointed out that increased intake of lignans was also related to CVD prevention (HR = 0.51 (0.30–0.86)), even though their intake was lower than 1 mg/day.

The main key foods of the MedDiet in the PREDIMED cohort were EVOO and nuts. EVOO and olives provide around 11% of the total polyphenol intake. The phenolic profile of EVOO and olives is unique, with 98% of the polyphenols being inside the 'other phenolic acids' and 'other polyphenols' subclasses. Among these subclasses, oleuropein is associated with antidiabetes, antiatherosclerosis, and anti-inflammation properties [24]. This characteristic phenolic profile has resulted in health benefits, a claim which was recognized by the European Food Safety Authority (EFSA) [25].

4. Antiobesity Effects of Dietary Polyphenols

Evidence for polyphenols' effect on obesity and weight control in humans is inconsistent due to the heterogeneity among study design, study populations, intervention period, and polyphenol supplements. These potential effects are summarized in Table 2. Some intervention clinical trials with polyphenol-enriched foods, such as an apple juice, showed a significant reduction in body fat mass but not in body weight, BMI, or waist circumference [26]. However, a recent double-blinded, randomized, parallel clinical trial conducted in 17 type 1 obesity participants (BMI between 30.1 and 33.3 kg/m^2) with a polyphenol supplement of 370 mg of total polyphenols showed a significant reduction in body weight, BMI, and waist and hip circumference compared with a placebo group after 12 weeks of intervention [27]. Moreover, only a few studies have studied the relationship between TPI from diet and weight control. Guo et al. [28] analyzed the association between body weight and TPI using a urine biomarker in a high cardiovascular risk population in a long-term study. After five years of follow-up, they showed an inverse association between total polyphenol excretion (TEP) and BMI, body weight, and waist circumference [28].

Similarly, a study conducted in the Mediterranean area demonstrated that higher dietary intake of flavonoids is inversely associated with an excess of weight and obesity [29]. Studies conducted in non-Mediterranean areas have shown an effect of polyphenol intake on weight control, but other clinical trials did not find any relationship between polyphenol intake and weight loss or changes in body composition (CITA).

A longitudinal study from a Netherlands cohort that included 4280 participants aged 55–69 years over 14 years of follow-up showed an association between a higher flavonoids intake and a lower increase in body mass index (BMI) in women ($p < 0.05$) [30]. Within the flavonoids, catechins are related with benefits in anthropometric parameters and body composition. More evidence that includes some studies with green tea extracts rich in catechins, epigallocatechin gallate (EGCG), showed a significant reduction in body weight, waist circumference, body fat mass, and visceral and subcutaneous fat [31]. Based on a meta-analysis of 11 studies, Hursel et al. concluded that catechin or an EGCG–caffeine mixture contained in green tea had a minimal effect on weight loss and weight loss maintenance [31]. Therefore, the clinical significance of the small changes seen in the body composition parameters indicates that green tea has no significant effect on weight loss and weight loss maintenance [32].

Resveratrol, a phenolic compound found in grapes, red wine, and some berries, also has potential antiobesity effects by inhibiting adipocyte differentiation and decreasing proliferation, mediated by adipocyte apoptosis and decreasing lipogenesis, promoting lipolysis and β-oxidation [30]. However, evidence about the effect of resveratrol intake on weight loss and weight loss maintenance is limited and the effects only seem to be achieved through dietary supplementation. Tome-Carneiro et al. performed several randomized, parallel, dose–response, placebo-controlled studies with a grape supplement rich in resveratrol and other grape polyphenols [33,34]. The effects were statistically significant for CVD risk factors: reduction in LDL-cholesterol, oxidized LDL, and thrombogenic plasminogen activator inhibitor type 1 (PAI-1), and increase in adiponectin and anti-inflammatory cytokines; however, they were not significant for adiposity parameters. Thus, the antiobesity potential and the optimal dose of resveratrol remain to be studied.

Despite the fact that the spice turmeric is not a characteristic food of the MedDiet, curcumin, a yellow-colored polyphenol from the curcuminoids subclass, is known for its health benefits such as anti-inflammatory, anticarcinogenesis, antiobesity, antiangiogenesis, and antioxidant activities [35]. The antiobesity properties of curcumin are similar to resveratrol, through inhibiting adipocyte differentiation, lipogenesis, reducing proinflammatory cytokines' synthesis in the adipose tissue, and promoting β-oxidation [35]. Similar to resveratrol, clinical trials to investigate the antiobesity properties of curcumin are limited. Ramirez-Bosca reported improvements in serum lipid profile through an increase in HDL-cholesterol and Apo A, as well as a decrease in LDL-cholesterol, ApoB, and the ApoB/ApoA ratio [36] with a supplement dose of 10 mg of a curcumin extract daily over 30 days.

Evidence from in vitro and experimental models suggests the potential effects of polyphenols on obesity, obesity-related inflammation, and other metabolic disorders. These studies show significant reduction of body weight by increasing basal metabolic rate, increasing β-oxidation, lowering triglycerides synthesis, and improving insulin sensitivity. Obese individuals have been reported to be more dependent on glucose oxidation rather that fat oxidation [37]. The mechanisms involved in weight loss where polyphenols may have a role are: inducing satiety; stimulating energy expenditure by inducing thermogenesis in brown adipose tissue; modulating adipose tissue by inhibiting adipocyte differentiation and promoting adipocyte apoptosis; modulating lipolysis; and activating β-oxidation [38]. Relative to metabolic disorders, an in vitro study about the effect of white tea EGCG showed improvements in cellular glucose metabolism mediated by glucose transporters (GLUTs) and a potential hypocholesterolemic effect stimulating LDL receptor binding activity [39].

Gut Microbiota and Prebiotic Potential of Dietary Polyphenols

The gut microbiota is, nowadays, strongly associated with several complex diseases, especially when this microbiota is imbalanced, also known as dysbiosis. This dysbiosis may be disrupted by lifestyle, such as excessive sanitation, diet, sedentarism, antibiotics, and so forth. Related to the topic of this review, the microbiota has a role in the host's metabolism, energy extraction, fat deposition, inflammatory status, gut barrier integrity, and also satiety [40]. The roles of the molecules generated from bacterial fermentation are crucial to establishing the causal relevance of the gut microbiota and health benefits.

Short-chain fatty acids (SCFAs) are formed from the fermentation of oligosaccharides, proteins, and peptides [41], with the main SCFA products being acetate, propionate, and butyrate. The consumption of complex carbohydrates from fruits and vegetables is associated with higher microbial production of SCFAs [42]. The contribution of SCFA products against obesity has been linked to decreasing weight gain by preventing fat accumulation [43–45]. Fernandes et al. showed that obese subjects present higher SCFA products in stool samples than lean subjects because of the differences in their colonic fermentation [42]. The before-mentioned SCFA main products display different mechanisms to induce satiety: butyrate acts on intestinal cells, increasing GLP-1 production [46], and propionate increases intestinal gluconeogenesis [45], both pathways leading to improvements in glucose homeostasis and increasing satiety.

Besides the microbial products, the gut microbiota is crucial for the metabolism and degradation of some other compounds. Branched-chain amino acids (BCAAs) are elevated in obesity and T2DM, which are contributing to the development of obesity-related insulin resistance. A reduction in BCAA level is strongly correlated with improvements in insulin sensitivity, more so than weight loss [47]. Interestingly, the composition of the gut bacteria, specifically the invasion of *Bacteroides* spp., may improve the efficiency of BCAA degradation [48].

Nevertheless, the main tool to balance the gut microbiota is diet. This notion is promoting the use of prebiotics, which are mainly dietary components such as nondigestible carbohydrates. Other dietary compounds not absorbed by the small intestine, such as polyphenols, are accumulated in the large intestine, thus being exposed to the enzymatic activities of the gut microbiota [49]. In vitro studies suggested that polyphenols may act as prebiotics by enhancing the growth of beneficial bacteria such as *Lactobacillus* spp. and *Bifidobacterium* spp. [50]. Related to the SCFAs, polyphenols from plum were reported to decrease fecal SCFAs in obese rats and, consequently, prevent weight gain in association with the changes in the bacterial composition of the gut microbiota by increasing *Faecalibacterium* spp., *Lactobacillus* spp., and *Bacteroidetes* spp. proliferation [50]. The potential prebiotic effect of proanthocyanidin on *Akkermansia muciniphila* is well described by Anhê et al. [51]. The pathways through which proanthocyanidins can enhance *Akkermansia* proliferation are: increasing mucus secretion to the intestinal lumen by goblet cells; proanthocyanidins and other polyphenols may use free oxygen radicals in the intestinal lumen, creating an environment only favorable for strict aerobic species; antimicrobial effects of polyphenols may help to degrade competitive bacteria of *Akkermansia*.

Relative to proanthocyanidins, a dietary supplement of grape seed extract in six female pigs caused a change in the distribution of the microbiota, increasing *Lachnospiraceae*, unclassified *Clostridales*, *Lactobacillus*, and *Ruminococcacceae* [52]. The same experimental models used by Quifer-Rada et al. described the molecular mechanisms of the potential hypocholesterolemic effects of proanthocyanidins shown in human studies [53]. The grape seed extract increases biliary excretion and reduces micellar solubility, which translates to a higher excretion of cholesterol in feces [54].

Table 2. Potential health benefits on body weight by Mediterranean diet polyphenols.

Phenolic Compound	Potential Health Benefits	References
Total polyphenols	↓ Body weight, BMI, and waist and hip circumferences	[26]
Total polyphenols	Prebiotic effect ↑ *Lactobacillus* spp., *Bifidobacterium* spp., *Faecalibacterium* spp., and *Bacteroidetes* spp. proliferation	[49]
Total polyphenols	↓ SFCAs excretion	[49]
Flavonoids	↓ BMI	[27]
Epigallocatechin gallate (EGCG) and green tea extracts	↓ Body weight, fat mass, and visceral and subcutaneous fat	[31]
Proanthocyanidins	↑ Proliferation of the *Akkermansia muciniphila* spp.	[50]
Proanthocyanidins	↓ Total cholesterol levels ↑ Biliary excretion and micellar solubility	[52]
Resveratrol	↓ Adipocyte proliferation ↓ Lipogenesis ↑ Lipolysis and β-oxidation	[28]

[1] BMI: Body mass index; SFCAs: Short-chain fatty acids; ↓ significant decrease; and ↑ significant increase.

5. Mechanism Involved

Catechins, mainly green tea EGCC, promote β-oxidation by regulating the expression in adipose tissue of peroxisome proliferator-activated receptor gamma (PPAR-γ) and fatty acid synthase (FAS), while increasing the levels of CPT-1, a protein that facilitates the transport of fatty acids to the mitochondria, which is a limiting step for β-oxidation [54].

In the case of resveratrol, its involvement in regulating β-oxidation has been studied by increasing 5′-adenosine monophosphate-activated protein kinase (AMPK) activity through preventing the degradation of intracellular cyclic adenosine monophosphate (cAMP) [55]. The AMPK function is to regulate glucose transport and fatty acid metabolism. Therefore, its activation may lead to fatty acid oxidation and suppression of hepatic gluconeogenesis as well as improvements in insulin sensitivity. Other studies revealed that resveratrol could mediate the expression of PPAR-γ [56] or promote β-oxidation by inhibiting the synthesis of malonyl-CoA [57], which is a precursor and promoter of fatty acid synthesis.

Curcumin contains polyphenols, and there is substantial evidence about its effectiveness in stimulating β-oxidation, inhibiting fatty acid synthesis, and decreasing fat storage [38]. The molecular pathways are similar to EGCG in the upregulation of CPT-1, but also entail the reduction of lipid biosynthesis by the downregulation of fatty acid synthesis enzymes [58].

Within the flavonoids, anthocyanins have been reported as having a role as antiobesity agents. Anthocyanins are widely found in fruits, such as apples with peel, strawberries, blueberries, blackberries, and blood oranges. To induce fatty acid oxidation, the postulated pathways are the modulation of AMPK synthesis and regulation of the expression of genes participating in β-oxidation [59].

Regarding EVOO polyphenols, tyrosol derivates, such as oleuropein, are involved in energy metabolism and adiposity [60], reducing the expression of PPAR-γ, compromising adipocyte differentiation, and improving insulin sensitivity [61]. Another interesting mechanism studied by Oi-Kano et al. in experimental models showed an increase in uncoupling protein 1 (UCP1) expression, which translates to the formation of "beige" adipose tissue, leading to a decrease of visceral fat mass [62]. Hydroxytyrosol and its derivatives constitute around 90% of the total polyphenol content of EVOO [63]. In vitro studies reported that hydroxytyrosol downregulates the expression of PPAR-α and -γ, which is translated to a reduction in adipocyte size [64]. Additionally, an increase in AMPK and lipase (hormone-sensitive and phosphorylated lipase) was observed in adipocytes exposed to hydroxytyrosol [65]. Furthermore, these effects were not reported to have an impact on body weight and adiposity in humans [65].

There are several mechanisms of action involved and each polyphenol presents different pathways, as shown in Figure 1.

However, more randomized clinical trials are needed to verify if the ability of polyphenols to act as antioxidants and anti-inflammatory mediators, through suppressing the effects of oxidative stress and inflammation, can be translated to antiobesity effects.

6. Conclusions

The characteristic phenolic profile of the MedDiet differs from other dietary patterns, especially in the Mediterranean countries, where EVOO and olives are food sources that provide unique phenolic compounds with health benefits.

The health effects of polyphenols depend on the amount consumed and their bioavailability, which is low, and systemic concentrations of phenolic compounds may reach the millimolar range. As previously mentioned, the gut microbiota might be the most remarkable factor for the absorption and metabolism of dietary polyphenols. Moreover, bioavailability can be also modulated by the effects of culinary techniques, dietary patterns, or alteration of phase I/II metabolism by pharmacological or dietary agents.

However, the essential step towards the understanding of the protective effects of polyphenols against overweightness, unhealthy body composition, obesity-related inflammatory processes, and metabolic syndrome status is to estimate their consumption by dietary recalls (through 24-h dietary recall or FFQs) or other methods such as measurements of urine concentration of key polyphenols, in order to identify the compounds most likely to provide the greatest protection.

Even though the intake of some specific polyphenols has been associated with body weight improvements, there is still no evidence for the effects of total polyphenols or some polyphenol subclasses. Further randomized controlled trials are needed to confirm the promising protective effects of polyphenols on weight gain, obesity, and CVD. This research field might be useful for setting food and health counselling goals for overweightness and obesity, and additionally, to establish dietary recommendations for individuals and population groups and desired minimum levels of polyphenol intake.

Author Contributions: Conceptualization, R.E. and S.C.-B.; writing—original draft preparation, S.C.-B.; writing—review and editing, M.D. and R.M.L.-R.

Funding: This research received no external funding.

Conflicts of Interest: R.M.L.-R.: receiving lecture fees from Cerveceros de España, and receiving lecture fees and travel support from Adventia. R.E. reports serving on the board of and receiving lecture fees from the Research Foundation on Wine and Nutrition (FIVIN); serving on the boards of the Beer and Health Foundation and the European Foundation for Alcohol Research (ERAB); receiving lecture fees from Cerveceros de España and Sanofi-Aventis; and receiving grant support through his institution from Novartis. The other authors declare no conflict of interest.

References

1. Ng, M.; Fleming, T.; Robinson, M.; Thomson, B.; Graetz, N.; Margono, C.; Mullany, E.C.; Biryukov, S.; Abbafati, C.; Abera, S.F.; et al. Global, regional, and national prevalence of overweight and obesity in children and adults during 1980–2013: A systematic analysis for the Global Burden of Disease Study 2013. *Lancet* **2014**, *384*, 766–781. [CrossRef]
2. Williams, E.P.; Mesidor, M.; Winters, K.; Dubbert, P.M.; Wyatt, S.B. Overweight and obesity: Prevalence, Consequences and Causes of a Growing Public Health Problem. *Curr. Obes. Rep.* **2015**, *4*, 363–370. [CrossRef] [PubMed]
3. Siriwardhana, N.; Kalupahana, N.S.; Cekanova, M.; Lemieux, M.; Greer, B.; Moustaid-Moussa, N. Modulation of adipose tissue inflammation by bioactive food compounds. *J. Nutr. Biochem.* **2013**, *24*, 613–623. [CrossRef] [PubMed]

4. Kalupahana, N.S.; Moustaid-Moussa, N.; Claycombe, K.J. Immunity as a link between obesity and insulin resistance. *Mol. Asp. Med.* **2012**, *33*, 26–34. [CrossRef] [PubMed]
5. Esposito, K.; Kastorini, C.M.; Panagiotakos, D.B.; Giugliano, D. Mediterranean diet and weight loss: Meta-analysis of randomized controlled trials. *Metab. Syndr. Relat. Disord.* **2011**, *9*, 1–12. [CrossRef] [PubMed]
6. Mena, M.P.; Sacanella, E.; Vazquez-Agell, M.; Morales, M.; Fitó, M.; Escoda, R.; Serrano-Martínez, M.; Salas-Salvadó, J.; Benages, N.; Casas, R.; et al. Inhibition of circulating immune cell activation: A molecular antiinflamatory effect of the Mediterranean diet. *Am. J. Clin. Nutr.* **2009**, *89*, 248–256. [CrossRef] [PubMed]
7. Urpi-Sarda, M.; Casas, R.; Chiva-Blanch, G.; Romero-Mamamni, E.S.; Valderas-Martínez, P.; Arranz, S.; Andres-Lacueva, C.; Llorach, R.; Medina-Remón, A.; Lamuela-Raventos, R.M.; et al. Virgin olive oil and nuts as key foods of the Mediterranean diet effects on inflammatory biomarkers related to atherosclerosis. *Pharmacol. Res.* **2012**, *65*, 577–583. [CrossRef] [PubMed]
8. Marin, C.; Ramirez, R.; Delgado-Lista, J.; Yubero-Serrano, E.M.; Perez-Martinez, P.; Carracedo, J.; Garcia-Rios, A.; Rodriguez, F.; Gutierrez-Mariscal, F.M.; Gomez, P.; et al. Mediterranean diet reduces endothelial damage and improves the regenerative capacity of endothelium. *Am. J. Clin. Nutr.* **2011**, *93*, 267–274. [CrossRef] [PubMed]
9. Dai, J.; Jones, D.P.; Goldberg, J.; Ziegler, T.R.; Bostick, R.M.; Wilson, P.W.; Manatunga, A.K.; Shallenberger, L.; Jones, L.; Vaccarino, V. Association between adherence to the Mediterranean diet and oxidative stress. *Am. J. Clin. Nutr.* **2011**, *88*, 1364–1370.
10. Jones, J.L.; Fernandez, M.L.; McIntosh, M.S.; Najm, W.; Calle, M.C.; Kalynych, C.; Vukich, C.; Barona, J.; Ackermann, D.; Kim, J.E.; et al. A Mediterranean-style low-glycemic-load diet improves variables of metabolic syndrome in women, in addition of a phytochemical-rich medical food enhances benefits on lipoprotein metabolism. *J. Clin. Lipidol.* **2011**, *5*, 188–196. [CrossRef] [PubMed]
11. Hernáez, Á.; Castañer, O.; Elosua, R.; Pintó, X.; Estruch, R.; Salas-Salvadó, J.; Corella, D.; Arós, F.; Serra-Majem, L.; Fiol, M.; et al. Mediterranean Diet Improves High-Density Lipoprotein Function in High-Cardiovascular-Risk Individuals. *Circulation* **2017**, *135*, 633–643. [CrossRef] [PubMed]
12. Fitó, M.; Cladellas, M.; de la Torre, R.; Martí, J.; Muñoz, D.; Schröder, H.; Alcántara, M.; Pujadas-Bastardes, M.; Marrugat, J.; López-Sabater, M.C.; et al. Anti-inflammatory effect of virgin olive oil in stable coronary disease patients: A randomized, crossover, controlled trial. *Eur. J. Clin. Nutr.* **2008**, *62*, 570–574. [CrossRef] [PubMed]
13. Phenol-Explorer, An Online Comprehensive Database on Polyphenol Contents in Foods. 2010. Available online: http://www.phenol-explorer.eu (accessed on 21 September 2018).
14. Tresserra-Rimbau, A.; Rimm, E.B.; Medina-Remon, A.; Martinez-Gonzalez, M.A.; dela Torre, R.; Corella, D.; Salas-Salvador, J.; Gómez-Garcia, E.; Lapetra, J.; Arós, F.; et al. Inverse association between habitual polyphenol intake and incidence of cardiovascular events in the PREDIMED study. *Nutr. Metab. Cardiovasc. Dis.* **2014**, *24*, 639–647. [CrossRef] [PubMed]
15. Mancini, J.G.; Filion, K.B.; Atallah, R.; Eisenberg, M.J. Systematic Review of the Mediterranean Diet for Long-Term Weight Loss. *Am. J. Med.* **2016**, *129*, 407–415. [CrossRef] [PubMed]
16. Huo, R.; Du, T.; Xu, Y.; Xu, W.; Chen, X.; Sun, K.; Yu, X. Effects of Mediterranean-style diet on glycemic control, weight loss and cardiovascular risk factors among type 2 diabetes individuals: A meta-analysis. *Eur. J. Clin. Nutr.* **2015**, *69*, 1200–1208. [CrossRef] [PubMed]
17. Probst, Y.; Guan, V.; Kent, K. A systematic review of food composition tools used for determining dietary polyphenol intake in estimated intake studies. *Food Chem.* **2018**, *238*, 146–152. [CrossRef] [PubMed]
18. Zamora-Ros, R.; Knaze, V.; Rothwell, J.A.; Hémon, B.; Moskal, A.; Overvad, K.; Tjønneland, A.; Kyrø, C.; Fagherazzi, G.; Boutron-Ruault, M.C.; et al. Dietary polyphenol intake in Europe: The European Prospective Investigation into Cancer and Nutrition (EPIC) study. *Eur. J. Nutr.* **2016**, *55*, 1359–1375. [CrossRef] [PubMed]
19. Pérez-Jiménez, J.; Fezeu, L.; Touvier, M.; Arnault, N.; Manach, C.; Hercberg, S.; Galan, P.; Scalbert, A. Dietary intake of 337 polyphenols in French Adults. *Am. J. Clin. Nutr.* **2011**, *93*, 1220–1228. [CrossRef] [PubMed]
20. Sofi, F.; Dinu, M.; Pagliai, G.; Marcucci, R.; Casini, A. Validation of a literature-based adherence score to Mediterranean diet: The MEDI-LITE score. *Int. J. Food Sci. Nutr.* **2017**, *68*, 757–762. [CrossRef] [PubMed]
21. Godos, J.; Marventano, S.; Mistretta, A.; Galvano, F.; Grosso, G. Dietary sources of polyphenols om the Mediterranean healthy Eating, Aging and Lifestyle (MEAL) study cohort. *Int. J. Food. Sci. Nutr.* **2017**, *68*, 750–756. [CrossRef] [PubMed]

22. Godos, J.; Rapisarda, G.; Marventano, S.; Galvano, F.; Mistretta, A.; Grosso, G. Association between polyphenol intake and adherence to the Mediterranean diet in Sicily, soythern Italy. *NFS J.* **2017**, *8*, 1–7. [CrossRef]
23. Tresserra-Rimbau, A.; Medina-Remón, A.; Pérez-Jiménez, J.; Martínez-González, M.A.; Covas, M.I.; Corella, D.; Salas-Salvador, J.; Gómez-Gracia, E.; Lapetra, J.; Arós, F.; et al. Dietary intake and major food sources of polyphenols in a Spanish population at high cardiovascular risk: The PREDIMED study. *Nutr. Metab. Cardiovasc. Dis.* **2013**, *23*, 953–959. [CrossRef] [PubMed]
24. Covas, M.I.; Nyyssonen, K.; Poulsen, H.E.; Kaikkonen, J.; Zunft, H.J.; Kiesewetter, H.; Gaddi, A.; de la Torre, R.; Mursu, J.; Bäumler, H.; et al. The effect of polyphenols in olive oil on heart disease risk factors: A randomized trial. *Ann. Intern. Med.* **2006**, *145*, 333–341. [CrossRef] [PubMed]
25. EFSA Panel on Dietetic Products NaAN. Scientific Opinion on the substantiation of health claims related to polyphenols in olive and protection of LDL particles from oxidative damage (ID 1333, 1638, 1639, 1696, 2865), maintenance of normal blood HDLcholesterol concentrations (ID 1639), maintenance of normal blood pressure (ID 3781), "anti-inflammatory properties" (ID 1882), "contributes to the upper respiratory tract health" (ID 3468), "can help to maintain a normal function of gastrointestinal tract" (3779), and "contributes to body defences against external agents" (ID 3467) pursuant to Article 13(1) of Regulation (EC) No 1924/20061. *EFSA J.* **2011**, *9*, 2033.
26. Barth, S.W.; Koch, T.C.L.; Watzl, B.; Dietrich, H.; Will, F.; Bub, A. Moderate effects of apple juice consumption on obesity-related markers in obese men: Impact of diet-gene interaction on body fat content. *Eur. J. Nutr.* **2012**, *51*, 841–850. [CrossRef] [PubMed]
27. Cases, J.; Romain, C.; Dallas, C.; Gerbi, A.; Cloarec, M. Regular consumption of Fiit-ns, a polyphenol extract from fruit and vegetables frequently consumed within the Mediterranean diet, improves metabolic ageing of obese volunteers: A. randomized, double-blind, parallel trial. *Int. J. Food. Sci. Nutr.* **2015**, *66*, 120–125. [CrossRef] [PubMed]
28. Guo, X.; Tresserra-Rimbau, A.; Estruch, R.; Martinez-Gonzalez, M.A.; Medina-Remon, A.; Fitó, M.; Corella, D.; Salas-Salvadó, J.; Portillo, M.P.; Moreno, J.J.; et al. Polyphenol levels are inversely correlated with body weight and obesity in an elderly population after 5 years of follow up (The Randomised PREDIMED Study). *Nutrients* **2017**, *9*, 452. [CrossRef] [PubMed]
29. Marranzano, M.; Ray, S.; Godos, J.; Galvano, F. Association between dietary flavonoids intake and obesity in a cohort of adults living in the Mediterranean area. *Int. J. Food Sci. Nutr.* **2018**, *26*, 1–10. [CrossRef] [PubMed]
30. Wang, S.; Moustaid-Moussa, N.; Chen, L.; Mo, H.; Shastri, A.; Su, R.; Bapat, P.; Kwun, I.; Shen, C.L. Novel insights of dietary polyphenols and obesity. *J. Nutr. Biochem.* **2014**, *25*, 1–18. [CrossRef] [PubMed]
31. Hursel, R.; Viechtbauer, W.; Westerterp-Plantenga, M.S. The effects of green tea on weight loss and weight maintenance: A meta-analysis. *Int. J. Obes.* **2009**, *33*, 956–961. [CrossRef] [PubMed]
32. Jurgens, T.M.; Whelan, A.M.; Killian, L.; Doucette, S.; Kirk, S.; Foy, E. Green tea for weight loss and weight maintenance in overweight or obese adults. *Cochrane Database Syst. Rev.* **2012**, *12*, CD008650. [CrossRef] [PubMed]
33. Kim, S.; Jin, Y.; Choi, Y.; Park, T. Resveratrol exerts anti-obesity effects via mechanisms involving down-regulation of adipogenic and inflammatory processes in mice. *Biochem. Pharmacol.* **2011**, *81*, 1343–1351. [CrossRef] [PubMed]
34. Tome-Carneiro, J.; Gonzalvez, M.; Larrosa, M.; Garcia-Almagro, F.J.; Aviles-Plaza, F.; Parra, S.; Yáñez-Gascón, M.J.; Ruiz-Ros, J.A.; García-Conesa, M.T.; Tomás-Barberán, F.A.; et al. Consumption of a grape extract supplement containing resveratrol decreases oxidized LDL and ApoB in patients undergoing primary prevention of cardiovascular disease: A triple-blind, 6- month follow-up, placebo-controlled, randomized trial. *Mol. Nutr. Food Res.* **2013**, *56*, 810–821. [CrossRef] [PubMed]
35. Meydani, M.; Hasan, S.T. Dietary polyphenols and obesity. *Nutrients* **2010**, *2*, 737–751. [CrossRef] [PubMed]
36. Ramirez-Bosca, A.; Soler, A.; Carrion, M.A.; Diaz-Alperi, J.; Bernd, A.; Quintanilla, C.; Quintanilla Almagro, E.; Miguel, J. An hydroalcoholic extract of curcuma longa lowers the apo B./apo A. ratio. Implications for atherogenesis prevention. *Mech. Ageing Dev.* **2000**, *119*, 41–47. [CrossRef]
37. Cox, L.M.; Blaser, M.J. Pathways in microbe-induced obesity. *Cell Met.* **2013**, *17*, 883–894. [CrossRef] [PubMed]

38. Rupasinghe, H.P.V.; Sekhon-Loodu, S.; Mantso, T.; Panayiotidis, M.I. Phytochemicals in regulating fatty acids β-oxidation: Potential underlying mechanisms and their involvement in obesity and weight loss. *Pharmacol. Ther.* **2016**, *165*, 153–163. [CrossRef] [PubMed]
39. Tenore, G.C.; Stiuso, P.; Campiglia, P.; Novellino, E. In vitro hypoglycaemic and hypolipidemic potential of white tea polyphenols. *Food Chem.* **2013**, *141*, 2379–2384. [CrossRef] [PubMed]
40. Cummings, J.H.; Macfarlane, G.T. The control and consequences of bacterial fermentation in the human colon. *J. Appl. Bacteriol.* **1991**, *70*, 443–459. [CrossRef] [PubMed]
41. Hester, C.M.; Jala, V.R.; Langille, M.G.; Umar, S.; Greiner, K.A.; Haribabu, B. Fecal microbes, short chain fatty acids, and colorectal cancer across racial/ethnic groups. *World J. Gastroenterol.* **2015**, *21*, 2759–2769. [CrossRef] [PubMed]
42. Fernandes, J.; Su, W.; Rahat-Rozenbloom, S.; Wolever, T.M.; Comelli, E.M. Adiposity, gut microbiota and faecal short chain fatty acids are linked in adult humans. *Nutr. Diabetes* **2014**, *4*, e121. [CrossRef] [PubMed]
43. Den Besten, G.; Bleeker, A.; Gerding, A.; van Eunen, K.; Having, R.; van Dijk, T.H.; Oosterveer, M.H.; Jonker, J.W.; Groen, A.K.; Reijngoud, D.J.; et al. Short-chain fatty acids protect against high-fat diet-induced obesity via a PPARgamma-dependent switch from lipogenesis to fat oxidation. *Diabetes* **2015**, *64*, 2398–2408. [CrossRef] [PubMed]
44. De Vadder, F.; Kovatcheva-Datchary, P.; Goncalves, D.; Vinera, J.; Zitoun, C.; Duchampt, A.; Bäckhed, F.; Mithieux, G. Microbiota-generated metabolites promote metabolic benefits via gut-brain neural circuits. *Cell* **2014**, *156*, 84–96. [CrossRef] [PubMed]
45. Lin, H.V.; Frassetto, A.; Kowalik, E.J., Jr.; Nawrocki, AR.; Lu, M.M.; Kosinski, J.R.; Hubert, J.A.; Szeto, D.; Yao, X.; Forrest, G.; et al. Butyrate and propionate protect against diet-induced obesity and regulate gut hormones via free fatty acid receptor 3-independent mechanisms. *PLoS ONE* **2012**, *7*, e35240. [CrossRef] [PubMed]
46. Shah, S.H.; Crosslin, D.R.; Haynes, C.S.; Nelson, S.; Turer, C.B.; Stevens, R.D.; Muehlbauer, M.J.; Wenner, B.R.; Bain, J.R.; Laferrère, B.; et al. Branched-chain amino acid levels are associated with improvement in insulin resistance with weight loss. *Diabetologia* **2012**, *55*, 321–330. [CrossRef] [PubMed]
47. Ridaura, V.K.; Faith, J.J.; Rey, F.E.; Cheng, J.; Duncan, A.E.; Kau, A.L.; Griffin, N.W.; Lombard, V.; Henrissat, B.; Bain, J.R.; et al. Gut microbiota from twins discordant for obesity modulate metabolism in mice. *Science* **2013**, *341*, 1241214. [CrossRef] [PubMed]
48. Cardona, F.; Andrés-Lacueva, C.; Tulipani, S.; Tinahones, F.Q.; Queipo-Ortuño, M.I. Benefits of polyphenols on gut microbiota and implications in human health. *J. Nutr. Biochem.* **2013**, *24*, 1415–1422. [CrossRef] [PubMed]
49. Duda-Chodak, A.; Tarko, T.; Satora, P.; Sroka, P. Interaction of dietary compounds, especially polyphenols, with the intestinal microbiota: A review. *Eur. J. Nutr.* **2015**, *54*, 325–341. [CrossRef] [PubMed]
50. Noratto, G.D.; Garcia-Mazcorro, J.F.; Markel, M.; Martino, H.S.; Minamoto, Y.; Steiner, J.M.; Byrne, D.; Suchodolski, J.S.; Mertens-Talcott, S.U. Carbohydrate-free peach (Prunus persica) and plum (Prunus domestica) juice affects fecal microbial ecology in an obese animal model. *PLoS ONE* **2014**, *9*, e101723. [CrossRef] [PubMed]
51. Anhê, F.F.; Varin, T.V.; Le Barz, M.; Desjardins, Y.; Levy, E.; Roy, D.; Marette, A. Gut microbiota dysbiosis in obesity-linked metabolic diseases and prebiotic potential of polyphenol-rich extracts. *Curr. Obes. Rep.* **2015**, *4*, 389–400. [CrossRef] [PubMed]
52. Choy, Y.Y.; Quifer-Rada, P.; Holstege, D.M.; Frese, S.A.; Calvert, C.C.; Mills, D.A.; Lamuela-Raventós, R.M.; Waterhouse, A.L. Phenolic metabolites and substantial microbiome changes in pig feces by ingesting grape seed proanthocyanidins. *Food Funct.* **2014**, *5*, 2298–2308. [CrossRef] [PubMed]
53. Quifer-Rada, P.; Choy, Y.Y.; Calvert, C.C.; Waterhouse, A.L.; Lamuela-Raventós, R.M. Use of metabolomics and lipidomics to evaluate the hypocholestreolemic efffect of Proanthocyanidins from grape seed in a pig model. *Mol. Nutr. Food Res.* **2016**, *60*, 1–9. [CrossRef] [PubMed]
54. Lee, M.S.; Kim, C.T.; Kim, Y. Green tea (−)-epigallocatechin-3-gallate reduces body weight with regulation of multiple genes expression in adipose tissue of diet-induced obese mice. *Ann. Nutr. Metab.* **2009**, *54*, 151–157. [CrossRef] [PubMed]
55. Chung, J.H.; Manganiello, V.; Dyck, J.R. Resveratrol as a calorie restriction mimetic: Therapeutic implications. *Trends Cell Biol.* **2012**, *22*, 546554. [CrossRef] [PubMed]

56. Aguirre, L.; Fernandez-Quintela, A.; Arias, N.; Portillo, M.P. Resveratrol: Anti-obesity mechanisms of action. *Molecules* **2014**, *19*, 18632–18655. [CrossRef] [PubMed]
57. Skudelska, K.; Szkudelski, T. Resveratrol, obesity and diabetes. *Eur. J. Pharmacol.* **2010**, *635*, 1–8. [CrossRef] [PubMed]
58. Ejaz, A.; Wu, D.; Kwan, P.; Meydani, M. Curcumin inhibits adipogenesis in 3T3-L1 adipocytes and angiogenesis and obesity in C57/BL mice. *J. Nutr.* **2009**, *39*, 791–797. [CrossRef] [PubMed]
59. Wu, T.; Tang, Q.; Gao, Z.; Yu, Z.; Song, H.; Zheng, X.; Chen, W. Blueberry and mulberry juice prevent obesity development in C57BL/g mice. *PLoS ONE* **2013**. [CrossRef] [PubMed]
60. Vogel, P.; Machado, I.K.; Garavaglia, J.; Zani, V.T.; De Souza, D.; Morelo Dal Bosco, S. Polyphenols benefits of olive leaf (*Olea europaea* L.) to human health. *Nutr. Hosp.* **2015**, *31*, 1427–1433.
61. Casado-Díaz, A.; Anter, J.; Müller, S.; Winter, P.; Quesada-Gómez, J.M.; Dorado, G. Transcriptomic analyses of the anti-adipogenic effects of oleuropein in human mesenchymal stem cells. *Food Funct.* **2017**, *8*, 1254–1270. [CrossRef] [PubMed]
62. Oi-Kano, Y.; Iwasaki, Y.; Toshiyuki, N.; Watanabe, T.; Goto, T.; Kawada, T.; Watanabe, K.; Iwai, K. Oleuropein aglycone enhances UCP1 expression in brown adipose tissue in high-fat-diet-induced obese rats by activating β-adrenergic signaling. *J. Nutr. Biochem.* **2017**, *40*, 209–218. [CrossRef] [PubMed]
63. De la Torre-Carbot, K.; Chávez-Servín, J.L.; Jaúregui, O.; Castellote, A.I.; Lamuela-Raventós, R.M.; Fitó, M.; Covas, M.-I.; Muñoz-Aguayo, D.; López-Sabater, M.C. Presence of virgin olive oil phenolic metabolites in human low density lipoprotein fraction: Determination by high-performance liquid chromatography-electrospray ionization tandem mass spectrometry. *Anal. Chim. Acta* **2007**, *583*, 402–410. [CrossRef] [PubMed]
64. Peyrol, J.; Riva, C.; Amiot, M.J. Hydroxytyrosol in the Prevention of Metabolic Syndrome and Related Disorders. *Nutrients* **2017**, *9*, 306. [CrossRef] [PubMed]
65. Hao, J.; Shen, W.; Yu, G.; Jia, H.; Li, X.; Feng, Z.; Wang, Y.; Weber, P.; Wertz, K.; Sharman, E.; et al. Hydroxytyrosol promotes mitochondrial biogenesis and mitochondrial function in 3T3-L1 adipocytes. *J. Nutr. Biochem.* **2010**, *21*, 634–644. [CrossRef] [PubMed]

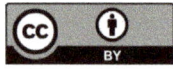

© 2018 by the authors. Licensee MDPI, Basel, Switzerland. This article is an open access article distributed under the terms and conditions of the Creative Commons Attribution (CC BY) license (http://creativecommons.org/licenses/by/4.0/).

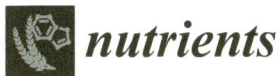

Article

Exploring the Perceived Barriers to Following a Mediterranean Style Diet in Childbearing Age: A Qualitative Study

Harriet Kretowicz, Vanora Hundley and Fotini Tsofliou *

Department of Human Science and Public Health, Centre for Midwifery, Maternal and Perinatal Health, Faculty of Health and Social Sciences, Bournemouth University, Bournemouth BH1 3LT, UK; s4933331@bournemouth.ac.uk (H.K.); vhundley@bournemouth.ac.uk (V.H.)
* Correspondence: ftsofliou@bournemouth.ac.uk; Tel.: +44-1202-961583

Received: 29 September 2018; Accepted: 2 November 2018; Published: 6 November 2018

Abstract: A considerable amount of research has focused on interventions in pregnancy to promote health in current and future generations. This has yielded inconsistent results and focus has turned towards improving health in the preconception period. Promotion of healthy dietary patterns similar to a Mediterranean diet in the preconception years has been suggested as a dietary strategy to prevent maternal obesity and optimize offspring health. However, it is uncertain whether adoption is acceptable in women of childbearing age. This qualitative study aims to investigate the perceived barriers to following a Mediterranean diet in women of childbearing age. Semi-structured focus groups were used to generate deep insights to be used to guide the development of a future intervention. Nulliparous women aged between 20 and 47 years were recruited ($n = 20$). Six focus groups were digitally audio recorded and transcribed verbatim by the researcher. Thematic analysis was used to analyze data, which occurred in parallel with data collection to ascertain when data saturation was reached. Five core themes were identified: Mediterranean diet features, perceived benefits, existing dietary behavior and knowledge, practical factors, and information source. The present study highlights that a Mediterranean diet is acceptable to childbearing-aged women, and the insights generated will be helpful in developing an intervention to promote Mediterranean diet adoption.

Keywords: Mediterranean diet; barriers; dietary change; childbearing age

1. Introduction

It is well established that the health of an expectant mother can significantly influence the health and wellbeing of the developing baby [1,2]. Nutrition is a major factor in optimizing health, and the impact of maternal nutrition on offspring has gained considerable attention in recent years. The ground for a focus on maternal nutrition are threefold: first, a large body of evidence from epigenetics suggests maternal nutrition can affect the body composition and metabolic health of the developing baby, at birth and in later life [3,4]; second, maternal obesity and excessive gestational weight gain are associated with a number of adverse pregnancy complications, including miscarriage [5], still birth [6], preeclampsia and hypertensive disorders [7], gestational diabetes mellitus (GDM) [8,9], emergency caesarean section [10], macrosomia [11], and preterm delivery [12] amongst others, and rates have doubled in the past two decades [13]; and finally, nutrition is a largely modifiable factor with an underestimated potential to provide significant improvement to both the short and long term health of mother and baby, and a reduction in pregnancy complications.

Several interventions have been developed with the aim of improving nutrition in pregnancy to minimize complications, improve offspring and maternal health, and to limit gestational weight gain [14]. However, while some trials have shown positive trends in eating behavior among obese pregnant women [15,16], a lack of beneficial clinical outcomes and an average reduction in gestational weight gain by a mere 0.7 kg [14] has made it difficult to draw firm conclusions about the efficacy of pregnancy interventions [17]. It is likely that intervention in pregnancy may be necessary to mitigate problems associated with poor maternal nutrition, but additional interventions are needed to optimize health and nutrition and prevent obesity prior to conception.

Promoting health and optimizing nutrition prior to pregnancy is supported by research that has found diet quality and health long before conception can also influence the health of future offspring and pregnancy outcomes [18–21]. However recent evidence suggests that women across the span of childbearing age from late adolescence up to 49 years [22] are not nutritionally prepared for pregnancy, with 9 in 10 eating fewer than five fruit and vegetable portions a day, consuming 50 g of free sugars daily on average, consuming only 17 g of fiber daily on average, and nearly 6 in 10 with folate levels below the clinical threshold [23]. In addition, it is unlikely that pregnancy is planned for years prior to conception and is often unexpected, allowing for sub-optimum nutrition status of the mother [23]. This, together with evidence suggesting that the gestation period may be too short to demonstrate significant behavior changes and the mixed results of clinical efficacy of interventions in pregnancy, suggests a need and potential benefit for interventions in the childbearing age population in general, and there is an emerging consensus that this strategy should be pursued [17]. In order to optimize the nutritional health in women prior to pregnancy, a supportive, evidence-based, and pragmatic method of nutrition and health promotion must be decided upon. Research into pre-pregnancy dietary patterns and health has consistently shown a dietary pattern which is high in vegetables, fruits, wholegrains, lean proteins, and fish, and low in red and processed meats and refined sugary foods is associated with positive health outcomes for both mother and offspring, and therefore should be adopted [19].

The Mediterranean diet (MD) is such a dietary pattern, and is characterized by high consumption of vegetables, fruits, legumes, extra virgin olive oil as the principal fat source, a moderate consumption of fish, lean protein, and dairy, and low consumption of processed foods and sweets [24]. The MD has been shown to prevent diseases associated with chronic inflammation, including coronary heart disease and stroke, type 2 diabetes, cognitive diseases, and obesity [25]. In addition, research has also demonstrated numerous benefits to the preconception and pregnancy periods, such as a reduced risk of hypertensive disorders [26], reduced risk of GDM [27], improvement in glucose tolerance [28], reduced gestational weight gain [29], reduction in depressive symptoms and risk of postnatal depression [30], and improved offspring homocysteine and lipoprotein levels [31].

It is therefore possible that following an MD pattern may have the potential to boost the overall health in women of childbearing age, whilst reducing the risk of complications during pregnancy and optimizing the health of mother and baby, if or when pregnancy should arise in the future. Yet, there are concerns relating to the feasibility of promoting the MD to young women in the U.K. and other non-Mediterranean populations and the acceptability to individuals currently consuming a Western diet [32,33], as there is evidence suggesting that low adherence to an MD is common in younger generations, with a decline in adherence even in Mediterranean countries [34,35]. However, prior research has shown the diet pattern to have high palatability, adherence, and transferability, even in non-Mediterranean countries [36–39]. To the best of our knowledge, there is no existing research that investigates the feasibility of promoting a Mediterranean dietary pattern to women of childbearing age. In order to utilize the Mediterranean diet as a way of promoting health and wellbeing and create the most effective, informative, and appealing intervention, it is necessary to develop a deep and thorough understanding of the possible barriers to following this dietary pattern and the ways to overcome them in this population of women.

The primary aim of the study was to explore barriers and enablers to following a Mediterranean style diet in women of childbearing age in the U.K.

2. Methods

A qualitative design was utilized. Semi-structured focus groups were chosen to gain a detailed insight into perceived barriers and enablers to following a Mediterranean style diet. This method was chosen because participants were able to give their own thoughts and build on the views of others, thus generating broad and in-depth discussions [40]. This method has been used in a wide range of health research, including to assess attitudes relating to lifestyle change [41], to identify health needs in specific populations [42], to investigate the feasibility and acceptability of behavioral interventions [43], and to also explore experiences of health interventions [44], as it is essential that a thorough understanding of the target population is gained [45].

The study utilized a convenience sample of university students and employed women identified through a snowballing approach [46]. Women aged 18–49 years old, who were U.K. residents, nulliparous, had low to medium MD adherence, and did not study or have an occupation directly related to nutrition were eligible to participate in the study. Participants were recruited via posters, social media, email, and in person. The research was undertaken between May and June 2017 and was approved by the Bournemouth University Research Ethics Committee.

Thirty-eight participants were initially recruited for the study. Three participants were ineligible due to parity and residency status. A further 15 participants withdrew prior to participation, leaving 20 in total, engaging in six focus groups.

Prior to focus group participation, participants were sent a document containing detailed information about the study and a link to a two-part online questionnaire which was used to confirm eligibility. Part one related to general information age, socioeconomic status, and parity, and required participants to self-report their height and weight. Participant characteristics are summarized in Table 1.

Table 1. Participants' Characteristics.

Demographic Data	Mean (SD)
Age (years), $n = 20$	26.8 (9.4)
BMI (kg/m^2)	23 (4)
	n
Employment Status	
University Student	13
Employed Non-Student	7
	n
Ethnicity	
White British	18
White Other	2
Median Mediterranean Diet Score (0–14)	5

Part two assessed MD adherence using the validated 14-item PREvencion con DIetaMEDiterranea (PREDIMED) score (MDPS) [47]. The range of possible scores for MDPS is 0–14, and those who had a high adherence (≥ 10) would not be eligible for participation as they were not considered to be inclusive in the target population. Figure 1 shows the distribution of participants' scores for MDPS. Overall mean MDPS was 5.6 ± 1.3; none of the twenty participants demonstrated high MD adherence, so all were included in the focus groups.

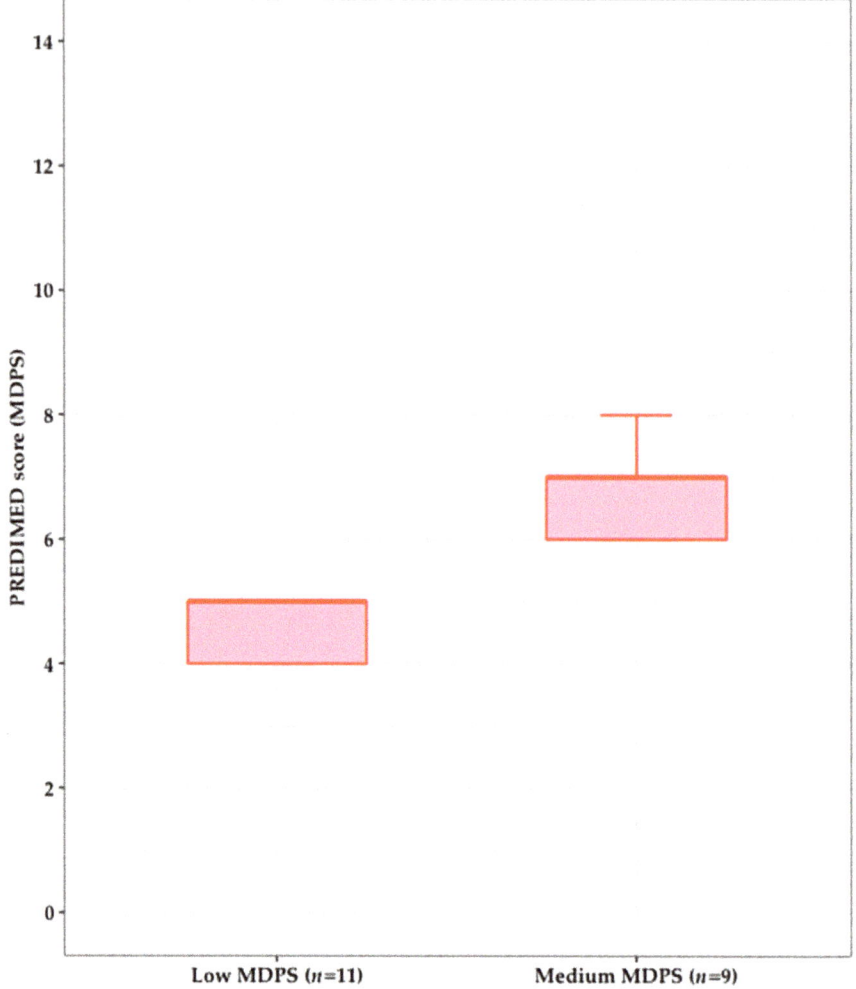

Figure 1. Participants' adherence to the MD assessed using the PREDIMED score (MDPS). In the boxplot showing the distribution of PREDIMED score (MDPS), eleven participants scored low on MDPS (≤5) (median 5, range 4–5), and nine participants had scores in medium tertile (median 7, range 6–8). The dark red horizontal line is the median.

The focus groups were led by a facilitator and conducted in a private room. The focus group procedure was explained and participants were reminded of the audio recording and their right to withdraw.

Participants were sent an MD information sheet, including an MD pyramid demonstrating the types and quantities of food and drink recommended in the diet patter, as well as information relating to the health benefits, based on current evidence. This allowed participants to familiarize themselves with the content of the dietary pattern and provided basic information in preparation for the focus groups. This information was also available for reference throughout the focus group process. Open-ended questions were used to guide discussions.

A semi-structured focus group guide was used with open-ended questions and probes allowing for the exploration of possible barriers to following an MD, with indicative topics including awareness of MD, motivations and eating behaviors, practicalities and social perception, and source preferences (Appendix A). Participants were given the opportunity to add or raise any additional points before concluding the focus groups, and on completion participants received a £5 gift voucher.

The digital audiotapes were transcribed verbatim by the facilitator (H.K.) after each focus group. Data collection and analysis co-occurred to asses when data collection could be concluded once emerging themes had reached saturation. This is a process whereby no new themes are generated from the data and there is repetition in emerging ideas. Focus group transcripts were analyzed using the process of inductive thematic analysis, as described by Braun and Clarke [48]. After the initial analysis, a second researcher (F.T.) reviewed the transcripts and independently coded for themes. Any discrepancies were resolved through discussion and additional review of the transcripts.

3. Results

The study identified five core themes encompassing perceived barriers and enabling factors to following a MD and include: MD features, perceived benefits, existing dietary behavior and knowledge, practical factors, and information source. Themes are illustrated with representative verbatim quotations from participants, represented numerically to protect anonymity, followed by participant age (e.g., (P. (n)/age (years))).

3.1. Mediterranean Diet Features

Several participants reported barriers and enablers relating to features of a MD. Two main subthemes were identified as the components of the MD and its perceived qualities. Participants indicated that a reduction in meat and an increase in plant-based foods would be difficult ("*I eat a lot of red meat, that's what I would find hard, making it more plant-based*" (P. 03/21)), and suggested the components of the diet were unappealing ("*it just looks quite bland . . . the lack of meat and like lentils and stuff, it's a bit off-putting, a bit lacklustre*" (P. 14/23)). Participants also believed that the low inclusion of sweet treats would also pose a barrier: "*not eating processed or refined stuff, or stuff high in sugar, I think I would really, really struggle with that*" (P. 18/21).

The perceived qualities of an MD were identified and considered to be enabling by many participants and included the non-restrictive nature of the diet: "*It's quite diverse, and there's quite a lot of different things you can eat, and normally you're quite restricted but it seems like most food groups are involved in the diet*" (P. 13/20). The description of the MD as a "diet" was seen to imply a negative quality to the diet, due to participants' existing experience and understanding of the term. The term "diet" elicited ideas of restriction, and many participants found its use off-putting in this context ("*when you say diet, you think of restrictions*" (P. 20/23)), and not conducive to the ethos of the MD: "*The word diet makes you automatically think losing weight, but I think whether it's a change in wording or you call it the Mediterranean lifestyle, because it is about physical activity, socializing, and rest and everything, and take the focus away from food . . . it's the diet word I think that puts people off, it's a lot of restriction isn't it*" (P. 14/23).

3.2. Perceived Benefits

Participants verbalized several motivations to following a healthy diet and subthemes of appearance, disease prevention, and psychological benefits were identified. Appearance was a commonly identified motivator, particularly in participants under 30 years of age, and it was suggested that benefits of a healthy diet for physical appearance were prioritized over health: "*I think of image and fitness, I probably should be but I don't feel like things like heart disease and stroke, I don't think about that at the moment, I think more about fitness and what I am going to look like in a bikini*" (P. 17/25).

It was therefore suggested that to enable adoption of an MD in this group that appearance benefits should be promoted rather than health benefits: "*It might even have to go down the route of 'you will have nice hair if you have this meal' or 'you will have good skin' and again focusing more on the looks, rather* than what it should be about with the whole, actual health and heart disease and stroke and things like that" (P. 20/23).

In addition to appearance being a primary motivating benefit to following a healthy diet, a significant motivating factor was the identification of disease prevention ("*I want to prevent things before they're at risk, you think I don't want diabetes so I'm going to change this, what I'm eating, I don't want to have heart disease when I'm older so I am going to think about this when I am eating*" (P. 17/25)), and psychological health ("*For me, when I am eating properly I'm less stressed ... it's more my mental health that I do it for*" (P. 20/23)).

Whilst promoting an MD for the benefits of disease prevention was considered enabling, promoting it in this group of women as a method of optimizing the health of their future offspring was considered off-putting, with participants suggesting that such a focus places too much responsibility on women: "*I'm going to take quite a strong feminist view here, this is promoting it completely at women ... to put all the emphasis on the mother eating healthily and the mother eating this diet for the sake of a baby seems an uncomfortable way of framing it for me*" (P. 06/42).

It also makes assumptions about the female role: "You feel kind of like a baby making machine, if they're like 'you need to do this because it will be good for your pregnancy' and just not highlight other things and be like actually this is really good for your health in the long term" (P. 05/22).

3.3. Existing Dietary Behavior and Knowledge

A common theme of existing dietary behavior and knowledge arose. Within this, dietary habits, nutritional awareness, and familial influences were identified.

Dietary habits were either a barrier or enabler depending on individual circumstance and habit: "*I know in other circumstances where people are brought up where take-aways are a regular occurrence, and I think to change from that to this sort of diet would be very difficult*" (P. 12/21); "*I think people who eat quite a normal diet, or healthy diet anyway, would be more likely to make changes*" (P. 09/42).

Existing dietary information was perceived as a significant barrier to following an MD, with participants expressing confusion with available dietary information and a difficulty in knowing which advice to follow: "*It sounds like you get a lot of benefits from the same diets and it gets really quite confusing, whenever I look up what's good for you and what's not there are cross cuts all over the place, so I never actually know what sort of diet is good for you*" (P. 12/21).

In addition, conflicting dietary health messages were considered off-putting, and it was indicated that this was a barrier to following any forms of dietary advice in general: "*There are so many different things out there, so many different diets that's a benefit and there's another bit of research that goes against it, and for everything they say is good, there is something else saying it's bad, so I don't really tend to pay too much attention*" (P. 14/23).

An absence of nutrition education was indicated as a barrier to following a MD, with the belief of a lack of taught cooking in childhood was a considerable barrier for following a healthy diet as an adult: "*People don't have home economics or cooking at school now do they? That's quite frightening isn't it, so then you learn from your mother and if your mother doesn't cook or your grandmother never cooks, you're never going to cook*" (P. 04/47).

Specific to an MD, re-education around dietary oils was also highlighted, as current perceptions of dietary fats were suggested as a barrier: "*I think more knowledge around olive oil, because people look at oil and think, 'Oh God, that's going to make me fat' so more education about why it's good and what makes it good*" (P. 04/47).

The impact of the influence of family members was verbalized as a possible barrier to following an MD. Some participants indicated that non-compliance from a partner would prevent personal adherence to the diet: "*I would love to cook with them [lentils and pulses] actually, I really would, but I would need to work on my other half, because he thinks a meal without meat is not a meal*" (P. 04/47); "*I think it's important to have the same kind of behavior towards food, because if you're around someone that has a negative relationship with food, you would be more likely to*" (P. 20/23).

Related to this, the upbringing and family values and practices around food was highlighted to be an enabler to following a Mediterranean style diet in this group of women: *"I think also because I have grown up with a healthy diet I enjoy that kind of stuff, I naturally think to put vegetables with my dinner, it's just how I've been brought up"* (P. 19/21).

3.4. Practical Factors

Practical factors relating to following a MD were highlighted as possible barriers. Within this, cooking skills, time and convenience, seasonal influence, and affordability were identified.

Participants indicated that cooking skills would be necessary to follow an MD: *"This diet is all about non-processed, it's all about the cooking"* (P. 06/42). This was not necessarily considered a problem in this group of women, but was suggested as a barrier for others: *"If I didn't cook and looked at this I would think I would just have to eat salad all the time"* (P. 04/47). However, it was also discussed that the content did not appear to in fact require more culinary ability that any other food preparation: *"I don't think it would be that different food prep from any other diet"* (P. 14/23).

Time and convenience were significant barriers for most participants, with preparation and cooking of fresh food perceived as time consuming and effortful, and therefore was not always possible due to busy lifestyles: *"I will finish work and go to the gym, so when I get home I just want to eat something that is quick"* (P. 07/33). Participants explained that if healthy food required too much time to prepare, then sometimes convenience food would be chosen instead: *"I know that if I was following a diet where every evening you had half an hour or an hour preparation, then some evenings I know I would just come home and order pizza instead"* (P. 13/20).

Seasonal influence and climate differences were suggested to have an impact on the ability to follow an MD, and participants believed that a Mediterranean climate facilitated following a MD (*"This has a big chunk of regular exercise, physical activity, socializing and rest ... the weather has a big effect on that, you can socialize more outside, you can do more things outside all year around"* (P. 01/24)) and unpredictable climate was implicated in food choice (*"You might not want to eat like that in the winter, you would want a lot more warm recipes"* (P. 13/20)). Coupled with this, the seasonal availability of produce was also considered problematic: *"When it comes to fresh diets, it's really dependent on the seasons, and it will change in the winter, it might be really hard and really expensive to get things then"* (P. 13/20).

Affordability of an MD was found to be both a barrier and enabler (*"Fruits and veg and quality meat is actually really quite expensive"* (P. 12/21)); however, the reduction in meat and increase in plant-based foods was conversely considered positively by some (*"I think fruit and vegetables can be expensive, but I think in this diet you are cutting out red meat which is also really expensive, like steak and stuff, that's expensive, so on the whole it would balance out"* (P. 03/21)) but it was suggested that the variety in the content of an MD made it possible to tailor adoption to individual affordability: *"I don't think it has to be expensive, eating healthy, as people think, because frozen vegetables have just as much nutritional value as fresh I think, and things like lentils and beans and pulses are very cheap"* (P. 09/42).

3.5. Information Source

Participants discussed their preferences for sources of diet and health information and source type and resource features were identified. Information was often sought from multiple sources, including the internet, traditional media such as magazines, social media, word of mouth, and books, however, the use of the internet was largely the main identified source of information, either as a primary source (*"I will always go online and find everything"* (P. 10/21)), or to seek validation of information gained elsewhere (*"I go by quite a lot of word of mouth, or I read a newspaper or magazine, then I will go on the internet and have a look"* (P. 13/20)). The internet was also considered an enabler due to the immediacy of access and the amount of information available: *"I think it is probably easier now than it ever has been before because it's so easy to find stuff online, from recipes to 'other ways to get more olive oil into your diet' or whatever, there's never been a better time to do this"* (P. 09/42). Conversely however, participants also expressed distrust about existing information and preferred reputable and evidence-based sources:

"it would have to be available from a reputable source . . . somewhere that is not 'The Sun' or 'Mail Online'" (P. 15/21).

Certain features were considered particularly appealing, and participants expressed a preference for blogs due to their interactivity and relatability (*"I think a blog is good . . . you feel like you're reading something you can relate to"* (P. 02/24)), as well as the inclusion of recipe ideas: *"things like recipe ideas or knowing how easy it is, or how easy it is to get ingredients would be helpful"* (P. 07/33).

4. Discussion

Although the feasibility and acceptability of the MD has been explored in older people and those in middle age [37,38,49,50], to date there has been no research that has investigated the feasibility of promoting an MD to women of childbearing age, with only evidence from cross-sectional studies in adolescent girls and women in early adulthood suggesting poor adherence to diet patterns similar to the MD [51,52]. Promoting a healthy diet in women of childbearing age can have a significant impact on both maternal and child health; however, the present study demonstrates that whilst an MD may be generally well received, adherence would require several obstacles to be overcome. Our findings suggest that in order to achieve behavioral change there would need to be reframing of ideas about diet, removal of barriers to change, and motivational buy-in.

One of the key points to address is how to reframe the diet in terms of language and benefits to make it more appealing. Participants' understanding and experience of the term "diet" came with negative connotations, including restriction and dissatisfaction. The description of an MD as a "diet" is therefore potentially off-putting, especially to those who have previously undertaken restrictive dietary practices. Linked with this notion is the perception that eating Mediterranean style foods is non-restrictive, with the inclusion of all food groups described as a significant enabling factor. Previous research on the use of language and terminology in health promotion messages has shown that language choice when promoting healthy eating is of critical importance [53], and therefore promotion of a MD as a "lifestyle" which emphasizes the lack of strict restriction is likely to be more appealing to this population of women.

Although a MD was considered non-restrictive where the reduction of red meat and increase in legumes was considered by participants to be particularly challenging, which has been previously reported [33,39,49,54]. Indeed, whilst implementing MD content in non-Mediterranean countries might prove challenging, there are simple practical approaches that can be offered to individuals who wish to adopt an MD in favor of a Western diet [32,33]. Participants suggested that education around cooking more plant-based meals and the provision of recipes would help address the limitations of content changes, such as increasing the consumption of legumes while substituting red or processed meat. Several practical barriers were highlighted in the study including time, knowledge, and finances. As found in other research on MD adoption and healthy eating [38,55], a lack of time to prepare food and the perceived cost implications of purchasing healthy food were highlighted as barriers [38,55–57]. To overcome these factors, it was suggested that a range of recipes with varying time requirements be provided, alongside cost reducing methods in order to change the perception that a healthy diet is expensive. Examples included providing information on cost per serving, leftover ideas to reduce wastage, and options for using frozen, tinned, and dried fruit, vegetables, and legumes, which are typically inexpensive. It may also be beneficial to highlight that the cost of consuming a healthy diet with increased fruit and vegetables may be offset by a reduction in meat products, as has also been shown in previous research [58].

Climate was highlighted as a possible barrier to healthy food choice, with participants specifying the belief that eating a healthy diet was easier in warmer climates and seasons, with "comforting" recipes being preferred in colder weather. This is consistent with previous research on climate and seasonal variation in dietary intake, which has shown variations in fruit and vegetable consumption across seasons [59–61] although research in this area is limited and there are conflicting results as to whether variations of significance exist [62]. Climate was also indicated in part as a financial barrier, with participants indicating that fresh produce would only be seasonally available and therefore be expensive to purchase imported goods. It was suggested that this could be overcome relatively simply by providing recipes containing seasonal produce. However, a larger scale intervention with governmental support may be necessary to increase consumption of fruit and vegetables in the population in general [33]. Some countries have successfully socially engineered fruit and vegetable availability, including the North Karelia project in Finland where the Ministry of Commerce and the Ministry of Agriculture promoted domestic berry and vegetable products and encouraged farmers to switch to growing these [63]. Such population-based interventions are expensive and complex to implement, but could be necessary to overcome this barrier [33].

Aside from barriers of practicalities, a lack of external support from partners and family members was considered a barrier and the sharing of behaviors and attitudes towards diet was considered key in the facilitation of healthy lifestyle. The perceived need for partner or familial support is in accordance with other dietary intervention research that has found social support to be an important factor in successful dietary adherence [64–66], and therefore targeting promotion and both men and women may encourage adherence.

Whilst the provision of recipes and dietary information may be helpful in overcoming some of the practical barriers highlighted, the provision of information alone is often insufficient to change behavior [53] Motivation is identified as a key component in health behavior change in theoretical models [67–70], and the perceived benefits of a healthy diet were motivations that emerged as a key theme. Appearance benefits were found to be a significant motivator, which supports previous research that suggests weight management and appearance benefits should be prioritized when promoting a healthy diet to young women [71]. It is possible that promoting an MD for appearance benefits may encourage adherence as well as conveying health benefits to this group of women.

Enabling factors of following an MD mostly centered around disease prevention, as has previously been shown in studies investigating MD adoption in non-Mediterranean countries [32]. Emphasis on the protective effects of the MD against non-communicable diseases (NCD) and for mental health benefits [72,73] would likely be beneficial in its promotion. Interestingly, although the health benefits of an MD were enabling factors, the reported benefits in preconception and pregnancy [26–31,74–76] were considered less important. Most participants indicated that the possibility of pregnancy was too far in the future to contemplate following a dietary pattern for benefits, and diet would not even be a concern in some participants unless there was difficulty in conception. Previous literature has shown that the proximity of goals can be influential in behavior change with proximal goals seen as more influential on behavior change than distant outcomes [77–79]. The present findings could therefore suggest that pregnancy-related benefits could be perceived as a short-term health goal, only relevant for those who are planning pregnancy. However, it is interesting to note that participants were able to conceptualize and accept that following a healthy eating pattern in the present would likely convey both short-term health benefits and NCD prevention in later life.

Whilst promotion of the diet for pregnancy benefits were perceived as irrelevant by some, they were also perceived negatively by other women, with the expression of the belief that promoting a diet at young women for pregnancy and offspring benefits places an emphasis on the reproductive role of women. This is contrary to previous research, which has found a reduced risk of health issues in pregnancy to be an enabling factor to healthy eating in young people [80]. Encouragement of preconception healthy is a priority, but it is important that pregnancy benefits are not over-emphasized to generate the perception that the MD is only applicable to those planning pregnancy.

In terms of information source of diet and health information, a range of sources were highlighted and most participants expressed a preference for use of the internet. Recipes, blogs and interactivity, photographs, and simple and clear evidence-based information were preferred, similar to features previously identified in other studies investigating acceptability of a MD [39]. The development of a future intervention promoting the MD should include these elements to assist in overcoming some of the identified barriers.

5. Strengths and Limitations

A thorough search of existing literature yielded no prior research investigating the perceived barriers to following an MD in women of childbearing age in the U.K., making this study the first of its kind. The qualitative methodology used enabled a deep and thorough understanding, which is recommended to aid the development of effective interventions [81] and will be used in the development of an MD-based intervention for the purposes of the promotion of optimum health in this group of women. Both university students and employed women were recruited for the study to promote heterogeneity amongst participants and to invoke a wide range of insights, and a broad age range was recruited to ensure adequate representation of the childbearing period. Inclusion of participants with only low to moderate adherence to the MD is also a significant strength to the study, as these women are the target population for a future intervention.

The limitations of the study relate to the relatively small sample size. There has been considerable discussion about the ideal size of a sample for qualitative research and, while differing views exist, a sample of 20 is usually considered adequate [82]. In addition, saturation of data was achieved in this group. The sample of women recruited for this study were well-educated, with all women educated to age 18 at a minimum and those who were not university students were employed in professional roles. This is, therefore, not representative of the wider population, and it is possible that individuals with other educational or socioeconomic backgrounds may have generated different data. In addition, even though adherence to an MD was low to moderate in all participants, all women believed that they currently followed a healthy lifestyle in general, suggesting a level of selection bias with an existing level of interest and motivation in healthy living. It is therefore possible that individuals with poor dietary habits will have generated different data to the participants in this study, and further investigation of barriers to following an MD in a broader sample of women would be warranted. Future research with different populations would be useful to identify whether barriers and facilitators differ in lower socioeconomic groups and other cultural contexts.

6. Conclusions

The nutrition of women of childbearing age has received considerable attention due to its modifiable nature. It has been suggested that the promotion of behavior change to follow dietary patterns similar to an MD is important because of the wide-ranging health benefits. It is necessary, however, to understand the possible barriers to following such a diet in women of childbearing age. This study identified five core themes including barriers and enablers, which should be addressed in the development of an intervention to effectively promote an encourage adherence to an MD. Based on these themes, five key points should be considered in the development of an intervention: (1) a reconsideration of language used to describe an MD and a focus on the qualities of the MD, such as its non-restrictive nature and inclusion of all food groups would likely be encouraging; (2) chronic disease prevention and long-term health benefits should be emphasized, along with the principle that a healthy diet will likely convey appearance related benefits should be highlighted to encourage adherence in this group; (3) the emphasis on benefits in pregnancy should be reserved specifically for those individuals planning pregnancy, as overemphasis could be off-putting; (4) emphasis should be placed on altering the perception that an MD is expensive and time consuming; and (5) the development of an intervention should have a strong and clear evidence base to support recommendations and elements of interactivity.

The insights gained from this formative research will be useful to assist in the development of a novel MD intervention for trial in a broad sample of women of childbearing age for the promotion of health prior to pregnancy.

Author Contributions: F.T. (corresponding author) conceived the idea, designed the study and analyzed the data. H.K. recruited participants, completed the interviews, and analyzed the data as part of an MSc program under the supervision of F.T. and V.H. All authors wrote the paper, for which H.K. prepared the first draft. All authors read and approved the final manuscript.

Funding: This research received no external funding and was conducted as part of an MSc program.

Acknowledgments: The authors would like to thank all volunteers for their participation as well as Orouba Almilaji for her assistance in the graphical display of PREDIMED score.

Conflicts of Interest: The authors declare no conflict of interest.

Appendix A. Focus Group Guide Which Was Used to Inform the Focus Groups

Guide Questions & Probes
Tell me what you previously knew about the Mediterranean diet.
How is it different to other diets you are aware of?
How do you think the known benefits would affect you and people like you?
If you were thinking about getting pregnant, when do you think you would start thinking about diet?
How do you think the known health benefits in pregnancy would affect you and people like you?
How would it affect you if this information was more widely available?
What are your thoughts about framing this diet specifically at young women?
What are your current motivations for following a healthy lifestyle?
How do you feel about the food in the Mediterranean diet in comparison to your usual diet?
Tell me what you feel about following this diet in your current lifestyle.
What are your thoughts about preparing the food in this diet?
Tell me what you think about the cost of this diet.
Tell me about how you normally find and access information on diet and lifestyle.
Tell me about features of resources that you find particularly helpful or unhelpful.

References

1. Barker, D.J. Maternal nutrition, fetal nutrition, and disease in later life. *Nutrition* **1997**, *13*, 807–813. [CrossRef]
2. Barker, M.; Dombrowski, S.U.; Colbourn, T.; Fall, C.H.D.; Kriznik, N.M.; Lawrence, W.T.; Norris, S.A.; Ngaiza, G.; Patel, D.; Skordis-Worrall, J.; et al. Intervention strategies to improve nutrition and health behaviors before conception. *Lancet* **2018**, *391*, 1853–1864. [CrossRef]
3. Blumfield, M.L. Update on the role of maternal diet in pregnancy and the programming of infant body composition. *Nutr. Bull.* **2015**, *40*, 286–290. [CrossRef]
4. Crume, T.L.; Brinton, J.T.; Shapiro, A.; Kaar, J.; Glueck, D.H.; Siega-Riz, A.; Dabeles, D. Maternal dietary intake during pregnancy and offspring body composition: The Healthy Start Study. *Am. J. Obstet. Gynecol.* **2016**, *609*, e1–e8. [CrossRef] [PubMed]
5. Marchi, J.; Berg, M.; Dencker, A.; Olander, E.K.; Begley, C. Risks associated with obesity in pregnancy, for the mother and baby: A systematic review of reviews. *Obes. Rev.* **2015**, *16*, 621–638. [CrossRef] [PubMed]
6. Chu, S.Y.; Kim, S.Y.; Lau, J.; Schmid, C.H.; Dietz, P.M.; Callaghan, W.M.; Curtis, K.M. Maternal obesity and risk of stillbirth: A meta-analysis. *Am. J. Obstet. Gynecol.* **2007**, *197*, 223–228. [CrossRef] [PubMed]
7. O'Brien, T.E.; Ray, J.G.; Chan, W. Maternal body mass index and the risk of preeclampsia: A systematic overview. *Epidemiology* **2003**, *14*, 368–374. [CrossRef] [PubMed]
8. Torloni, M.R.; Betran, A.P.; Horta, B.L.; Nakamura, M.U.; Atallah, A.N.; Moron, A.F.; Valente, O. Prepregnancy BMI and the risk of gestational diabetes: A systematic review of the literature with meta-analysis. *Obes. Rev.* **2009**, *10*, 194–203. [CrossRef] [PubMed]
9. Poston, L.; Bell, R.; Croker, H.; Flynn, A.C.; Godfrey, K.M.; Goff, L.; Hayes, L.; Khazaezadeh, N.; Nelson, S.M.; Oteng-Ntim, E.; et al. Effect of a behavioral intervention in obese pregnant women (the UPBEAT study): A multicenter, randomized controlled trial. *Lancet Diabetes Endocrinol.* **2015**, *3*, 767–777. [CrossRef]
10. Poobalan, A.S.; Aucott, L.S.; Gurung, T.; Smith, W.C.; Bhattacharya, S. Obesity as an independent risk factor for elective and emergency caesarean delivery in nulliparous women—Systematic review and meta-analysis of cohort studies. *Obes. Rev.* **2009**, *10*, 28–35. [CrossRef] [PubMed]
11. Gaudet, L.; Ferraro, Z.M.; Wen, S.W.; Walker, M. Maternal obesity and occurrence of fetal macrosomia: A systematic review and meta-analysis. *Biomed. Res. Int.* **2014**, *2014*. [CrossRef] [PubMed]
12. Smith, G.C.S.; Shah, I.; Pell, J.P.; Crossley, J.A.; Dobbie, R. Maternal obesity in early pregnancy and risk of spontaneous and elective preterm deliveries: A retrospective cohort study. *Public Health* **2007**, *97*, 157–162. [CrossRef]

13. Heslehurst, N.; Rankin, J.; Wilkinson, J.R.; Summerbell, C.D. A national representative study of maternal obesity in England, UK: Trends in incidence and inequalities in 619323 births, 1989–2007. *Int. J. Obes (Lond)*. **2010**, *34*, 420–428. [CrossRef] [PubMed]
14. International Weight Management in Pregnancy (i-WIP) Collaborative Group. Effect of diet and physical activity based interventions in pregnancy on gestational weight gain and pregnancy outcomes: Meta-analysis of individual participant data from randomized trials. *BMJ* **2017**, *19*. [CrossRef]
15. Dodd, J.M.; Newman, A.; Moran, L.J.; Deussen, A.R.; Grivell, R.M.; Moran, L.J.; Crowther, C.A.; Turnbull, D.; McPhee, A.J.; Wittert, G.; et al. The effect of antenatal dietary and lifestyle advice for women who are overweight or obese on emotional well-being: The LIMIT randomized trial. *Acta. Obstet. Gynecol. Scand.* **2015**, *99*, 309–318. [CrossRef] [PubMed]
16. Poston, L.; Caleyachetty, R.; Cnattingius, S.; Corvalan, C.; Uauy, R.; Herring, S.; Gillman, M.W. Preconceptional and maternal obesity: Epidemiology and health consequences. *Lancet Diabetes Endocrinol.* **2016**, *4*, 1025–1236. [CrossRef]
17. Hanson, M.; Barker, M.; Dodd, J.M.; Kumanyika, S.; Norris, S.; Steegers, E.; Stephenson, J.; Thangaratinam, S.; Yang, H. Interventions to prevent maternal obesity before conception, during pregnancy, and post-partum. *Lancet Diabetes Endocrinol.* **2017**, *5*, 65–76. [CrossRef]
18. Catalano, P.M.; Farrell, K.; Thomas, A.; Huston-Presley, L.; Mencin, P.; de Mouzon, S.H.; Amini, S.B. Perinatal risk factors for childhood obesity and metabolic dysregulation. *Am. J. Clin. Nutr.* **2009**, *90*, 1303–1313. [CrossRef] [PubMed]
19. Tobias, D.K.; Zhang, C.; Chavarro, J.; Bowers, K.; Rich-Edwards, J.; Rosner, B.; Mozaffarian, D.; Hu, F.B. Prepregnancy adherence to dietary patterns and lower risk of diabetes mellitus. *Am. J. Clin. Nutr.* **2012**, *96*, 289–295. [CrossRef] [PubMed]
20. Schoenaker, D.A.J.M.; Soedamah-Muthu, S.S.; Callaway, L.K.; Mishra, G.D. Pre-pregnancy dietary patterns and the risk of gestational diabetes mellitus: Results from an Australian population-based prospective cohort study. *Diabetologia* **2015**, *58*, 2726–2735. [CrossRef] [PubMed]
21. Grieger, J.A.; Grzeskowiak, L.E.; Clifton, V.L. Preconception dietary patterns in human pregnancies are associated with preterm delivery. *J. Nutr.* **2014**, *144*, 1075–1080. [CrossRef] [PubMed]
22. Parker, J.; Branum, A.; Axelrad, D.; Cohen, J. Adjusting national health and nutrition examination survey sample weights for women of childbearing age. *Vital Health Stat.* **2013**, *157*, 1–20.
23. Stephenson, J.; Heslehurst, N.; Hall, J.; Schoenaker, D.A.J.M.; Hutchinson, J.; Cade, J.E.; Poston, L.; Barrett, G.; Crozier, S.; Barker, M.; et al. Before the beginning: Nutrition and lifestyle in the preconception period and its importance for future health. *Lancet* **2018**, *391*, 1830–1841. [CrossRef]
24. Bach-Faig, A.; Berry, E.M.; Lairon, D.; Reguant, J.; Trichopoulou, A. Mediterranean diet pyramid today. Science and cultural updates. *Public Health Nutr.* **2011**, *14*, 2274–2284. [CrossRef] [PubMed]
25. Gotsis, E.; Anagnostis, P.; Mariolis, A.; Vlachou, A.; Katsiki, N.; Karagiannis, A. Health benefits of the Mediterranean diet: An update of research over the last 5 years. *Angiology* **2015**, *66*, 304–318. [CrossRef] [PubMed]
26. Schoenaker, D.A.J.M.; Soedamah-Muthu, S.S.; Callway, L.K.; Mishra, G. Pre-pregnancy dietary patterns and the risk of developing hypertensive disorders of pregnancy: Results from the Australian Longitudinal Study on Women's Health. *Am. J. Clin. Nutr.* **2015**, *102*, 94–101. [CrossRef] [PubMed]
27. Izadi, V.; Tehrani, H.; Haghighatdoost, F.; Dehghan, A.; Surkan, P.J.; Azadbakht, L. Adherence to the DASH and Mediterranean diets is associated with decreased risk for gestational diabetes mellitus. *Nutrition* **2016**, *32*, 1092–1096. [CrossRef] [PubMed]
28. Karamanos, B.; Thanopoulou, A.; Anastasiou, E.; Assaad-Khalil, S.; Albache, N.; Bachaoui, M.; Slama, C.B.; Ghomari, E.L.; Jotic, A.; Lalic, N.; et al. Relation of the Mediterranean diet with the incidence of gestational diabetes. *Eur. J. Clin. Nutr.* **2014**, *68*, 8–13. [CrossRef] [PubMed]
29. Silva-del Valle, M.A.; Sanchez-Villegas, A.; Serra-Majem, L. Association between the adherence to the Mediterranean diet and overweight and obesity in pregnant women in Gran Crania. *Nutr. Hosp.* **2013**, *28*, 654–659. [PubMed]
30. Chatzi, L.; Melaki, V.; Sarri, K.; Apostolaki, I.; Roumeliotaki, T.; Ibarluzea, J.; Tardon, A.; Amiano, P.; Lertxundi, A.; Iniguez, C.; et al. Dietary patterns during pregnancy and the risk of postpartum depression: The mother-child 'Rhea' cohort in Crete, Greece. *Public Health Nutr.* **2011**, *14*, 1663–1670. [CrossRef] [PubMed]

31. Gesteiro, E.; Bastida, S.; Rodriguez Bernal, B.; Sanchez-Muniz, F.J. Adherence to Mediterranean diet during pregnancy and serum lipid, lipoprotein and homocysteine concentrations at birth. *Eur. J. Nutr.* **2015**, *54*, 1191–1199. [CrossRef] [PubMed]
32. Martinez-Gonzalez, M.; Hershey, M.S.; Zazpe, I.; Trichopoulous, A. transferability of the Mediterranean diet to non-Mediterranean countries. What is and what is not the Mediterranean diet. *Nutrients* **2017**, *9*, 1126. [CrossRef] [PubMed]
33. Murphy, K.J.; Parletta, N. Implementing a Mediterranean-style diet outside the Mediterranean region. *Curr. Atheroscler. Rep.* **2018**, *20*. [CrossRef] [PubMed]
34. Grosso, G.; Galvano, F. Mediterranean diet adherence in children and adolescents in southern European countries. *NFS J.* **2016**, *3*, 13–19. [CrossRef]
35. Iaccarino Idelson, P.; Scalfi, L.; Valerio, G. Adherence to the Mediterranean diet in children and adolescents: A systematic review. *Nutr. Metab. Cardiovasc. Dis.* **2017**, *27*, 283–299. [CrossRef] [PubMed]
36. McManus, K.; Antinoro, L.; Sacks, F. A randomized controlled trial of a moderate-fat, low-energy diet compared with low fat, low energy diet for weight loss in overweight adults. *Int. J. Obes. (Lond.)* **2001**, *25*, 1503–1511. [CrossRef] [PubMed]
37. Lara, J.; McCrum, L.; Mathers, J.C. Association of Mediterranean diet and other health behaviors with barriers to healthy eating and perceived health among British adults of retirement age. *Maturitas* **2014**, *79*, 292–298. [CrossRef] [PubMed]
38. Papadaki, A.; Wood, L.; Sebire, S.J.; Jago, R. Adherence to the Mediterranean diet among employees in South West England: Formative research to inform a web-based, work-place nutrition intervention. *Prev. Med. Rep.* **2015**, *2*, 223–228. [CrossRef] [PubMed]
39. Cubillos, L.; Estrada del Campo, Y.; Harbi, K.; Keyserling, T.; Samuel-Hodge, C.; Reuland, D.S. Feasibility and acceptability of a clinic-based Mediterranean style diet intervention to reduce cardiovascular risk for Hispanic Americans with type 2 diabetes. *Diabetes Educ.* **2017**, *43*, 286–296. [CrossRef] [PubMed]
40. Wong, L.P. Focus group discussion: A tool for health and medical research. *Singap. Med. J.* **2008**, *49*, 256–261.
41. Glantz, S.A.; Jamieson, P. Attitudes towards second hand smoke, smoking, and quitting among young people. *Paediatrics* **2000**, *106*, E82. [CrossRef]
42. Brotman, S.; Ryan, B.; Cormier, R. The health and social service needs of gay and lesbian elders and their families in Canada. *Gerontologist* **2003**, *43*, 192–202. [CrossRef] [PubMed]
43. Ayala, G.X.; Elder, J. Qualitative methods to ensure acceptability of behavioral and social interventions to the target population. *J. Public Health Dent.* **2011**, *71*, S69–S79. [CrossRef] [PubMed]
44. Paul, G.; Keogh, K.; D'Eath, M.; Smith, S.M. Implementing a peer-support intervention for people with type 2 diabetes: A qualitative study. *Fam. Pract.* **2013**, *30*, 595–603. [CrossRef] [PubMed]
45. Ayala, G.X.; Elder, J.P.; Campbell, N.R.; Engelberg, M.; Olson, S.; Morena, C.; Serrano, V. Nutrition communication for a Latino community: Formative research foundations. *Fam. Community Health* **2001**, *24*, 72–87. [CrossRef] [PubMed]
46. Naderifar, M.; Goli, H.; Ghaljaie, F. Snowball sampling: A purposeful method of sampling in qualitative research. *Strides Dev. Med. Educ.* **2017**, *14*, E67670. [CrossRef]
47. Martinez-Gonzalez, M.A.; Garcia-Arellano, A.; Toledo, E.; Salas-Salvado, J.; Buil-Cosiales, P.; Corella, D.; Covas, M.I.; Schroder, H.; Aros, F.; Gomez-Gracia, E.; et al. A 14-item Mediterranean diet assessment tool and obesity indexes among high-risk subjects: The PREDiMED trial. *PLoS ONE* **2012**, *7*, E43134. [CrossRef] [PubMed]
48. Braun, V.; Clarke, V. Using thematic analysis in psychology. *Qual. Res. Psychol.* **2006**, *3*, 77–101. [CrossRef]
49. Erwin, C.M.; McEvoy, C.T.; Moore, S.E.; Prior, L.; Lawton, J.; Kee, F.; Cupples, M.E.; Young, I.S.; Appleton, K.; McKinley, M.C.; et al. A qualitative analysis exploring preferred methods of peer support to encourage adherence to a Mediterranean diet in a Northern European population at high risk of cardiovascular disease. *BMC Public Health* **2018**, *18*, 213. [CrossRef] [PubMed]
50. Lara, J.; Turbett, E.; Mckevic, A.; Rudgard, K.; Hearth, H.; Mathers, J.C. The Mediterranean diet among British older adults: Its understanding, acceptability, and the feasibility of a randomized brief intervention with two levels of dietary advice. *Maturitas* **2015**, *82*, 387–393. [CrossRef] [PubMed]
51. Boghossian, N.S.; Yeung, E.H.; Mumford, S.L.; Zhang, C.; Gaskins, A.J.; Wactawski-Wende, J.; Schisterman, E.F.; BioCycle Study Group. Adherence to the Mediterranean diet and body fat distribution in reproductive aged women. *Eur. J. Clin. Nutr.* **2013**, *67*, 289–294. [CrossRef] [PubMed]

52. Novak, D.; Stefan, L.; Prosoli, R.; Emeljanovas, A.; Mieziene, B.; Milanovic, I.; Radisavljevic-Janic, S. Mediterranean diet and its correlates among adolescents in Non-Mediterranean European Countires: A population-based study. *Nutrients* **2017**, *9*, 177. [CrossRef] [PubMed]
53. Buckton, C.H.; Lean, M.E.J.; Combet, E. 'Language is the source of misunderstandings'—Impact of terminology on public perceptions of health promotion messages. *BMC Public Health* **2015**, *15*, 579. [CrossRef] [PubMed]
54. Papadaki, A.; Thanasoulias, A.; Pound, R.; Sebire, S.J.; Jago, R. Employees' expectations of internet-based, workplace interventions promoting the Mediterranean diet: A qualitative study. *J. Nutr. Educ. Behav.* **2016**, *48*, 706–715. [CrossRef] [PubMed]
55. Middleton, G.; Keegan, R.; Smith, M.F.; Alkhatib, A.; Klonizakis, M. Implementing a Mediterranean diet intervention into a RCT: Lessons learned from a Non-Mediterranean Based Country. *J. Nutr. Health Aging* **2015**, *19*, 1019–1022. [CrossRef] [PubMed]
56. Morris, M.A.; Hulme, C.; Clarke, G.P.; Edwards, K.L.; Cade, J.E. What is the cost of a healthy diet? Using diet data from the UK Women's Cohort Study. *J. Epidemiol. Community Health.* **2014**, *68*, 1043–1049. [CrossRef] [PubMed]
57. Hartmann, C.; Dohle, S.; Siegrist, M. Importance of cooking skills for balanced food choices. *Appetite* **2013**, *65*, 125–131. [CrossRef] [PubMed]
58. Tong, T.Y.N.; Imamura, F.; Monsivais, P.; Brage, S.; Griffin, S.J.; Wareham, N.J.; Forouhi, N.G. Dietary cost associated with adherence to the Mediterranean diet, and its variation by socio-economic factors in the UK Fenland Study. *Br. J. Nutr.* **2018**, *119*, 685–694. [CrossRef] [PubMed]
59. Ziegler, R.G.; Wilcox, H.B.; Mason, T.J.; Bill, J.S.; Virgo, P.W. Seasonal variation in intake of carotenoids and vegetables and fruits among white men in New Jersey. *Am J Clin Nutr.* **1987**, *45*, 107–114. [CrossRef] [PubMed]
60. Cox, B.; Whichelow, M.J.; Prevost, A.T. Seasonal consumption of salad vegetables and fresh fruit in relation to the development of cardiovascular disease and cancer. *Public Health Nutr.* **2000**, *3*, 19–29. [CrossRef] [PubMed]
61. Capita, R.; Alonso-Calleja, C. Differences in reported winter and summer dietary intakes in young adults in Spain. *Int. J. Food Sci. Nutr.* **2005**, *56*, 431–443. [CrossRef] [PubMed]
62. Bernstein, S.; Zambell, K.; Amar, M.J.; Arango, C.; Kelley, R.C.; Miszewski, S.G.; Tryon, S.; Courville, A.B. Dietary intake patterns are consistent across seasons in a cohort of healthy Adults in a Metropolitan population. *J. Acad. Nutr. Diet.* **2016**, *116*, 38–45. [CrossRef] [PubMed]
63. Puska, P.; Stahl, T. Health in all policies—The Finnish initiative: Background, principles, and current issues. *Annu. Rev. Public Health* **2010**, *31*, 315–328. [CrossRef] [PubMed]
64. Kelsey, K.S.; Kirkley, B.G.; DeVellis, R.F.; Earp, J.A.; Ammerman, A.S.; Keyserling, T.C.; Shannon, J.; Simpson, R.J. Social support as a predictor of dietary change in a low-income population. *Health Educ. Res.* **1996**, *11*, 383–395. [CrossRef]
65. Scholz, U.; Hornung, R.; Ochsner, S.; Knoll, N. Does social support really help to eat a low-fat diet? Main effects and gender differences of received social support within the health action process approach. *Appl. Psychol. Health Well Being* **2013**, *5*, 270–290. [CrossRef] [PubMed]
66. Hammarstrom, A.; Fjellman Wiklund, A.; Lindahl, B.; Larsson, C.; Ahlgren, C. Experiences of barriers and facilators to weight-loss in a diet intervention—A qualitative study of women in Northern Sweden. *BMC Women's Health* **2014**, *14*. [CrossRef] [PubMed]
67. Rosenstock, I.M. Why people use health services. *The Millbank Quartely.* **1966**, *44*, 1107–1108. [CrossRef]
68. Fishbein, M.; Ajzen, I. *Belief, Attitude, Intention, and Behavior: An Introduction to Theory and Research*; Addison Welsey: Boston, MA, USA, 1975.
69. Prochaska, J.; Diclemente, C. Trans-theoretical therapy—Toward a more integrative model of change. *Psychoter. Theory Res. Pract.* **1982**, *19*, 276–288. [CrossRef]
70. Michie, S.; van Stralen, M.; West, R. The behavior change wheel: A new method for characterizing and designing behavior change interventions. *Implement. Sci.* **2011**, *6*. [CrossRef]
71. Chung, S.-J.; Hoerr, S.; Levine, R.; Coleman, G. Processes underlying young women's decisions to eat fruits and vegetables. *J. Hum. Nutr. Dietet.* **2006**, *19*, 287–298. [CrossRef] [PubMed]

72. Jacka, F.N.; O'Neil, A.; Opie, R.; Itsiopoulos, C.; Cotton, S.; Mohebbi, M.; Castle, D.; Dash, S.; Mihalopoulos, C.; Chatterton, M.L.; et al. A randomized controlled trial of dietary improvement for adults with major depression (the SMILES trial). *BMC Med.* **2017**, *15*. [CrossRef] [PubMed]
73. Parletta, N.; Zarnowiecki, D.; Cho, J.; Wilson, A.; Bogomolova, S.; Villani, A.; Itsiopoulos, C.; Niyonsenga, T.; Blunden, S.; Meyer, B.; et al. A Mediterranean-style dietary intervention supplemented with fish oil improved diet quality and mental health in people with depression: A randomized controlled trial (HELFIMED). *Nutr. Neurosci.* **2017**. [CrossRef] [PubMed]
74. Mikkelsen, T.B.; Osterdal, M.L.; Knudsen, V.K.; Haugen, M.; Meltzer, H.M.; Bakketeig, L.; Olsen, S.F. Association between a Mediterranean-type diet and risk of preterm birth among Danish women: A prospective cohort study. *Acta Obset. Gynecol. Scand.* **2008**, *87*, 325–330. [CrossRef] [PubMed]
75. Chatzi, L.; Torrent, M.; Romieu, I.; Garcia-Esteban, R.; Ferrer, C.; Vioque, J.; Kogevinas, M.; Sunyer, J. Mediterranean diet in pregnancy is protective for wheeze and atopy in childhood. *Thorax* **2008**, *63*, 507–513. [CrossRef] [PubMed]
76. Kermack, A.J.; Calder, P.C.; Houghton, F.D.; Godfrey, K.M.; Macklon, N.S. A randomized controlled trial of a preconceptional dietary intervention in women undergoing IVF treatment (PREPARE trial). *BMC Women's Health* **2014**, *14*. [CrossRef] [PubMed]
77. Forster, J.; Higgins, E.T.; Idon, L.C. Approach and avoidance strength during goal attainment: Regulatory focus and the "Goal Looms Larger" effect. *J. Pers. Soc. Psychol.* **1998**, *75*, 1115–1131. [CrossRef] [PubMed]
78. Frederick, S.; Loewenstein, G.; O'Donoghue, T. Time discounting and time preference: A critical review. *J. Econ. Lit.* **2002**, *40*, 351–401. [CrossRef]
79. Peetz, J.; Wilson, A.E.; Strahan, E.J. So far away: The role of subjective temporal distance to future goals in motivation and behavior. *Soc. Cogn.* **2009**, *27*, 475–495. [CrossRef]
80. Munt, A.E.; Partridge, S.R.; Allman-Fairnelli, M. The barriers and enablers of healthy eating among young adults: A missing piece of the obesity puzzle: A scoping review. *Obes. Rev.* **2016**, *18*, 1–17. [CrossRef] [PubMed]
81. Craig, P.; Dieppe, P.; Macintyre, S.; Michie, S.; Nazareth, I.; Petticrew, M.; Medical Research Council Guidance. Developing and evaluating complex interventions: The new Medical Research Council guidance. *BMJ* **2008**, *337*, a1655. [CrossRef] [PubMed]
82. Baker, S.E.; Edwards, R. *How Many Qualitative Interviews Is Enough? Expert Voices and Early Career Reflections on Sampling and Cases in Qualitative Research*; National Center for Research Methods, 2012. Available online: http://eprints.ncrm.ac.uk/2273/ (accessed on 14 October 2018).

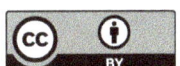

© 2018 by the authors. Licensee MDPI, Basel, Switzerland. This article is an open access article distributed under the terms and conditions of the Creative Commons Attribution (CC BY) license (http://creativecommons.org/licenses/by/4.0/).

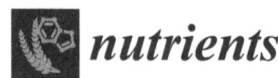

Article

Does the Mediterranean Diet Protect against Stress-Induced Inflammatory Activation in European Adolescents? The HELENA Study

Kenia M. B. Carvalho [1,*], Débora B. Ronca [1], Nathalie Michels [2], Inge Huybrechts [2,3], Magdalena Cuenca-Garcia [4], Ascensión Marcos [5], Dénes Molnár [6], Jean Dallongeville [7], Yannis Manios [8], Beatriz D. Schaan [9], Luis Moreno [10], Stefaan de Henauw [2] and Livia A. Carvalho [11]

1. Graduate Program in Human Nutrition, University of Brasília, Brasília 70910-900, Brazil; deboraronca@gmail.com
2. Department of Public Health, Faculty of Medicine and Health Sciences, Ghent University, 9000 Ghent, Belgium; Nathalie.Michels@UGent.be (N.M.); HuybrechtsI@iarc.fr (I.H.); stefaan.dehenauw@ugent.be (S.d.H.)
3. International Agency for Research on Cancer, 69372 Lyon, France
4. Department of Medical Physiology, School of Medicine, University of Granada, 18071 Granada, Spain; magdalena.cuenca@uca.es
5. ICTAN-CSIC Spanish National Research Council, 28040 Madrid, Spain; amarcos@ictan.csic.es
6. Department of Paediatrics, Medical School, University of Pécs, 7623 Pécs, Hungary; denes.molnar@aok.pte.hu
7. Institut Pasteur de Lille, 59800 Lille, France; jean.dallongeville@pasteur-lille.fr
8. Department of Nutrition and Dietetics, Harokopio University, 17671 Athens, Greece; helena@hua.gr
9. Graduate Program in Medical-Sciences, Endocrinology, Federal University of Rio Grande do Sul, Porto Alegre 90035-003, Brazil; bschaan@hcpa.edu.br
10. GENUD (Growth, Exercise, Nutrition and Development) Research Group, 50013 Zaragoza, Spain; lmoreno@unizar.es
11. Department of Clinical Pharmacology, William Harvey Research Institute, Barts and The London Hospital, Queen Mary University of London, London E1 4NS, UK; l.carvalho@qmul.ac.uk
* Correspondence: kenia@unb.br; Tel.: +55-613-1071-858

Received: 28 September 2018; Accepted: 10 November 2018; Published: 15 November 2018

Abstract: Stress increases inflammation but whether adherence to Mediterranean diet counteracts this association and how early can these effects be observed is not well known. We tested whether (1) cortisol is associated to inflammation, (2) cortisol is associated to the adolescent Mediterranean diet score (aMDS), (3) aMDS lessens inflammation, (4) aMDS associates with cortisol levels and inflammation. Two hundred and forty-two adolescents (137 females; 12.5–17.5 years old) provided salivary cortisol, blood and 2-day 24-h dietary recall from which aMDS was derived. Cortisol levels were associated with increased tumor necrosis factor (TNF-α B = 11.887, p = 0.001) when adjusted for age, gender, parental education and body mass index (BMI). Moreover, cortisol levels were inversely associated to adherence to the Mediterranean Diet (B = -1.023, p = 0.002). Adolescents with higher adherence to aMDS had lower levels of interleukins (IL) IL-1, IL-2, IL-6 and TNF-α, compared to those who did not adhere. The association between cortisol and TNF-α was no longer significant when aMDS was included in the model (B = 6.118, p = 0.139). In addition, comparing lower and higher aMDS groups, the association between cortisol and TNF-α was only observed in those with lower aMDS adherence. Our study suggests that adherence to the Mediterranean Diet may counteract the effect of stress on inflammatory biomarkers which may contribute to decreasing the risk of future mental health.

Keywords: diet quality; depressive symptoms; risk factors; epidemiology; immune system; prevention; hypothalamic–pituitary–adrenal-HPA axis

1. Introduction

During adolescence significant physical, emotional and physiological changes occur [1]. Stress may contribute towards unhealthy behaviors that poses mental health risk [2]. Approximately half of all psychiatric disorders start between late adolescence and early adulthood and predicts future psychopathology in adulthood [3–5]. There is now an extensive body of data showing that depression or stress are associated with a chronic low-grade inflammation [6,7]. Elevated levels of pro-inflammatory cytokines are observed in children and adolescents with major depressive disorder [8–10].

Diet is a modifiable behavior that impact levels of systemic inflammation [11–14]. The decreased systemic inflammation due to Mediterranean Diet can already be observed in adolescents [15]. Although not consistently observed [16], a systematic review shows an association between unhealthy diet with mental health disorders. In addition, an inflammatory dietary pattern based on lower levels of poly-saturated fatty acids (PUFA) n3 and higher levels of n6 is associated with risk of future depression [17]. Adherence to the Mediterranean diet attenuates the unfavorable effect of depression and anxiety on cardiovascular risk [18]. A healthy diet also protects the progression of inflammation and depression in the elderly [19]. In adolescents, better diet quality is also associated to depressed mood [20,21] but whether this is due to counteracting stress-induced inflammation is not yet known.

The aim of this study in adolescents was to test whether: 1—cortisol is associated with inflammation, 2—cortisol is associated with Mediterranean diet adherence, 3—Mediterranean diet adherence lessens inflammation, 4—Mediterranean diet adherence associates with cortisol biomarker and inflammation.

2. Materials and Methods

2.1. Study Design and Population

The HELENA-CSS (Healthy Lifestyle in Europe by Nutrition in Adolescence Cross-Sectional Study) is a multi-center study aiming to obtain reliable and comparable data on a broad variety of parameters related to nutrition and health in European adolescents [22]. The methodology used in this study has been published elsewhere [23]. Briefly, subjects aged 12.5–17.5 years were recruited from schools of 10 cities from nine countries across Europe (Greece, Germany, Belgium, France, Hungary, Italy, Sweden, Austria and Spain). Inclusion criteria included not participating simultaneously in any clinical trial, being free of any acute infection occurring within the week prior to the study and data being available concerning an individual's gender, height and weight. The enrollment of adolescents occurred at schools where students from the first two randomly chosen classes were invited to participate. In addition, the class attendance rate of at least 70% was considered for eligibility. The total eligible population consisted of 3528 adolescents. Blood and salivary sample was only collected in a random third of the population study. We have analyzed everyone who had complete data for the exposure, outcome and covariates used. Thus, we had complete data for 246 adolescents on diet, inflammatory markers and cortisol. We excluded subjects with C-reactive protein (CRP) >10 mg/L as a sign of acute infection ($n = 4$) so that the final sample consisted of 242 adolescents (Figure 1). In comparison to the total eligible HELENA-CSS population ($n = 3528$), this sample was less overweight and obese (14.0% vs. 23.9%, $p < 0.001$), had higher adherence to the Mediterranean diet (45.0% vs. 37.3%, $p = 0.019$), higher level of parental education (56.6% vs. 43.6% University degree, $p < 0.001$) but no differences in age ($p = 0.916$) or gender ($p = 0.164$).

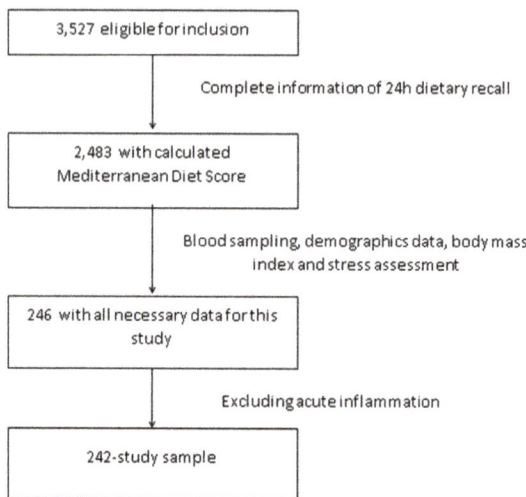

Figure 1. Flow chart of the selection procedure of the study sample among participants of Healthy Lifestyle in Europe by Nutrition in Adolescence Cross-Sectional Study (HELENA-CSS.)

2.2. Procedures

The Research Ethics Committees of each center involved approved the study protocol. Written informed consent was obtained from adolescents and their parents [24]. The fieldwork was carried out from October 2006 to December 2007 and consisted of clinical examination, blood and saliva sampling, questionnaires and dietary intake assessment [22]. All data was collected on the same day as the blood and saliva samples, measures needing repeat collection were conducted on the same week.

2.3. Measurements

2.3.1. Pubertal Stage, Nutritional Status and Socio-Demographics Characteristics

During the clinical examination, pubertal stage was assessed according to development of secondary sexual characteristics (breast/genitalia and pubic hair development) and using the five stages of development devised by Marshall and Tanner [25,26]. Body weight was determined to the nearest 100 g using a scale (SECA 861) with subjects in their underwear. Height was assessed to the nearest 0.1 cm with a stadiometer (SECA 225) while standing barefoot [27]. Body mass index (BMI) was calculated as weight (kg) divided by height (m) squared. The corresponding BMI z-score was calculated with reference to sex and age parameters and categorized in corresponding nutritional status [28]. BMI was coded (i) normal/underweight and (ii) overweight/obese [28]. The highest parental educational achievement was used and categorized in (i) lower education/higher secondary and (ii) University degree.

2.3.2. Salivary Cortisol Biomarkers

Baseline wake-up salivary free cortisol was measured in the adolescents as a biomarker for chronic stress according to previously published method [29]. Cortisol was measured in the accredited routine laboratory of Ghent University hospital on a Modular E 170 immunoanalyzer system (Roche Diagnostics, Mannheim, Germany) by the Roche Cobas Cortisol assay. The precise working mechanism and features of this analysis technique are described elsewhere [30]. This competitive electrochemiluminescence immunoassay had an inter-assay coefficient of variation of 3.9% and an intra-assay coefficient of variation of 1.9%, while for samples near the lower detection limit the coefficients of variation were respectively 12.7 and 10.2% (based on laboratory's internal quality assessment). Cortisol is the main hormonal end-product of the 'stress system.' Serum cortisol is the result of appraising all stress-inputs on the brain, coping and recovery from them and are influenced by several neuro-endocrine and physiological pathways. Unbound or free cortisol is also present in the saliva and is positively associated with acute and chronic stress. To reduce variance in cortisol biomarkers due to diurnal variations in salivary cortisol, baseline (without stimulation) salivary cortisol was measured immediately after awakening. In order to control individual variability in salivary cortisol, awakening samples from seven consecutive days were collected. Saliva was sampled during the same week as the inflammatory markers.

2.3.3. Inflammatory Markers

Blood samples were collected early morning after overnight fasting. For analysis of serum proteins, blood was collected in Vacutainer™ tubes (BD Biosciences, San Jose, CA, USA). Within the hour, serum was separated by centrifugation at 3500 rpm for 15 min; aliquots were made and sent to Bonn (Germany) in cooled containers on the same day and stored at −80 °C. At the end of the study, all samples were sent to Madrid (Spain) on dry ice and stored at −80 °C until analysis. The handling and transport system for fresh blood samples developed for the HELENA study assured stability of markers included in the analyses [29]. Serum levels of interleukin (IL)-1, IL-2, IL-4, IL-6 and tumor necrosis factor-α (TNF-α) were measured using the High Sensitivity Human Cytokine Milliplex™ MAP kit (MPXHCYTO-60K) (Millipore Corp., Billerica, MA, USA) and collected by flow cytometry (Luminex-100 v.2.3, Luminex Corporation, Austin, TX, USA). CRP levels were quantified by immunoturbidimetry (AU 2700, Olimpus, Rungis, France).

2.3.4. Adolescents Mediterranean Diet Score (aMDS)

Dietary intake was obtained with two non-consecutive 24-h dietary recalls via the HELENA-DIAT software (Dietary Assessment Tool; Ghent University, Ghent, Belgium) within a period of two weeks, comprising weekdays and weekend-days (except from Fridays and Saturdays), though not necessarily including a week and weekend-day for each individual [31]. Adolescents completed the program autonomously in the computer classroom during school time and dietary intake was referred to the day before the interview; therefore, no information on Fridays and Saturdays was available. Fieldworkers were present to give assistance if necessary.

The adherence to the Mediterranean dietary pattern was assessed by an adapted version of the traditional Mediterranean diet score (MDS) [32]. The MDS includes 9 components (vegetables, fruits and nuts, legumes, cereals, fish, monounsaturated fat/saturated fat ratio, dairy product, meat and poultry and wine); each component is assigned a score of 0 or 1 using the gender-specific medians as cut-off values (below and above, respectively). Dairy products and meat (including poultry), as detrimental components, are reverse scored, as well as the alcohol intake above the acceptable range. In this study, we modified the MDS to adapt it for adolescents (aMDS). The aMDS was calculated for each day and a mean of the daily scores was taken as the participant's global score. There were two dietary factors modified from the original MDS according to previously published work [33]. The alcohol component was removed because ethanol consumption is not recommended for children and adolescents. We also used age- and sex-specific median food intakes of the study's individuals as a cut-off value for each component. The possible range of scores was 0–8, with a higher score indicating higher adherence to Mediterranean diet. Based on these results, participants were categorized into two groups: low (<4 points) and high ($\geq$4 points) adherence.

2.3.5. Statistical Analyses

Descriptive characteristics are presented as mean (SD) and percentages for continuous and categorical variables, respectively. All immune variables were checked for normality of distribution by the Kolmogorov-Smirnov test; logarithmical transformation was used to achieve normality when needed. Analysis of variance (ANOVA) was performed in order to investigate association between cortisol biomarkers and aMDS. A multiple linear regression was applied to investigate the association between cortisol biomarkers and inflammatory cytokines. The model was adjusted for age, gender, parental education and BMI z-score. Then, aMDS was included in the model and finally, the analyses were performed separately by lower and higher aMDS groups. Results are presented as coefficients and p values. Analyses were carried out in SPSS 22 and statistical significance was set at $p \leq 0.05$.

3. Results

3.1. Characteristics of the Population

The social demographic characteristics of the study population divided by gender is presented in Table 1. There was significantly higher parental education level among boys (68.6% vs. 47.4% university degree; $p = 0.006$). There were no other differences between the sexes in relation to age, pubertal stage, BMI or adherence to aMDS (Table 1).

Table 1. Characteristics of the adolescent population studied.

Characteristics	Total	Boys	Girls	p *
	n = 242	n = 105	n = 137	
Age, years; mean (Standard Deviation, SD)	14.4 (1.1)	14.6 (1.1)	14.8(1.1)	0.222
Pubertal stage; %				0.091
Stage I	0.8	1.9	0.1	
Stage II	6.3	7.7	5.1	
Stage III	23.3	18.3	27.2	
Stage IV	35.4	31.7	38.2	
Stage V	34.2	40.4	29.4	
Parental education; %				0.006
Lower education-Higher secondary	43.4	31.4	52.6	
University degree	56.6	68.6	47.4	
BMI categories; %				0.485
Underweight/Normal weight	85.9	85.7	86.2	
Overweight/Obesity	14.1	14.3	13.8	
aMDS; mean (SD)	4.2 (1.5)	4.3 (1.5)	4.1 (1.5)	0.257

* p-values of independent samples t-tests for continuous variables and Pearson's chi-square tests for categorical variables. BMI, Body mass index; aMDS, adolescent Mediterranean diet score ranging 0–8, with a higher score indicating higher adherence to Mediterranean diet.

3.2. Inflammatory Markers, Cortisol and Adherence to the Mediterranean Diet

Increased levels of TNF-α were significantly associated with increased levels of cortisol when adjusted by age, gender, parental education and BMI ($B = 11.882$, $p = 0.001$). There was no association with other inflammatory markers. Cortisol biomarkers were inversely associated with adherence to the Mediterranean diet (overall ANOVA $F = 5.592$, $p = 0.004$, $B = -1.023$, $p = 0.002$).

Table 2 shows the unadjusted levels of inflammatory biomarkers according to adherence to Mediterranean diet. Lower IL-1, IL-2, IL-6 and TNF-α biomarkers were observed among adolescents with higher aMDS.

Table 2. Inflammatory markers in adolescents with low and high adherence to the Mediterranean diet.

Inflammatory Cytokines (mean, SD)	Low Mediterranean Diet Adherence n = 155	High Mediterranean Diet Adherence n = 87	p-Value *
IL-1 (pg/mL)	1.1 (2.3)	0.6 (1.0)	0.022
IL-2 (pg/mL)	7.4 (13.4)	4.8 (6.8)	0.049
IL-4 (pg/mL)	153.2 (300.5)	98.3 (214.0)	0.101
IL-6 (pg/mL)	24.2 (35.7)	15.8 (20.7)	0.020
TNF-α (pg/mL)	6.7 (3.8)	5.7 (2.4)	0.013
CRP (mg/L)	0.6 (0.9)	0.8 (1.2)	0.377

* p-values of independent samples t-tests. Mediterranean diet adherence groups: Lower than 4 meaning low adherence and equal to 4 or higher meaning high adherence to adolescent Mediterranean diet score (aMDS), IL, interleukin; TNF-α, tumor necrosis factor-α; CRP, C-reactive protein. Interleukins were logarithmical transformed to achieve normality.

3.3. Effect of Mediterranean Diet Adherence on Cortisol and Inflammatory Markers

The association between TNF-α and cortisol biomarkers was reduced to non-significant when we adjusted for adherence to aMDS ($F = 1.08$, $p = 0.362$, $B = 6.118$, $p = 0.139$). When we divided the groups in lower and higher adherence to aMDS the association between cortisol and TNF-α only observed in those who lower adherence to the aMDS ($B = 14.59$; $p = 0.028$) (Table 3).

Table 3. Association between cortisol biomarkers (nmol/L) and inflammatory cytokines, according to adherence to adolescent Mediterranean diet score (aMDS).

	Cortisol Biomarkers (nmol/L)			
	Low Mediterranean Diet Adherence n = 155		High Mediterranean Diet Adherence n = 87	
	B	p-Value	B	p-Value
IL-1 (pg/mL)	0.831	0.962	−2.9	0.737
IL-2 (pg/mL)	−0.323	0.931	3.189	0.240
IL-4 (pg/mL)	−0.308	0.760	0.064	0.921
IL-6 (pg/mL)	−0.714	0.718	1.001	0.419
IL-7 (pg/mL)	0.569	0.851	0.892	0.537
TNF-α (pg/mL)	14.59	0.028	7.853	0.131
CRP (mg/L)	75.06	0.383	−63.73	0.065

Mediterranean diet adherence: Lower than 4 meaning low adherence and equal a 4 or higher meaning high adherence to adolescent Mediterranean diet score (aMDS); B = standardized beta. Subjects with CRP > 10 mg/mL (acute inflammation) were excluded from the analysis. IL, interleukin; Interleukins were logarithmical transformed to achieve normality. Linear regression analysis adjusted for age, gender, parental education and body mass index categories.

4. Discussion

In the present study we have investigated the effect of adherence to the Mediterranean diet on the association between cortisol, a main end product of the stress system and inflammation in adolescents. We have found that cortisol was associated to TNF levels and that higher adherence to the Mediterranean diet counteracted this association. These results suggest that a healthy dietary patterns may exert a protective effect on the association between stress and inflammation.

The Mediterranean diet is a healthy dietary pattern and is defined by high intake of olive oil, fruits and vegetables, fish and seafood and a low intake of dairy and meat [34]. In general, adherence to the Mediterranean diet is associated with a reduced risk of several chronic diseases [34]. Despite its benefits, even in the Mediterranean region, adherence to the Mediterranean diet varies [35]. The effect of the Mediterranean diet on chronic diseases may be associated with the reduction of the inflammatory state, mainly measured by CRP and IL-6 markers in epidemiological adult cohorts [36] and adolescents [33]. Similar to such other studies, we also found adherence to the Mediterranean Diet associated to decreased levels of IL-6, IL-1, IL-2 and TNF-α. This study also agrees to previous HELENA analyses that evaluated Mediterranean diet food groups separately and found that IL-6 was negatively associated with cereal and roots and positively with dairy products consumption. There was also a positive association between IL-6 and both pulses and monounsaturated/saturated fat ratio [15]. Moreover, in a recent study conducted by Sureda et al. [12], the authors observed that among adolescent girls, higher adherence to Mediterranean diet was associated with lower levels of CRP. Although not the aim of our study, further studies are needed to clarify whether the same inflammatory marker are associated to Mediterranean diet in adults or adolescents.

Our study is also in accordance to a previous HELENA study which found that adolescents' perceived stress is a significant independent negative predictor of a healthy dietary pattern, as assessed by a diet quality index [37]. In older people, higher depressive symptoms is associated with increased IL-6 levels in those who did not adhere to Mediterranean diet, while in those who adhered had lower IL-6 levels [13]. TNF-α is a pro-inflammatory cytokine upstream to IL-6 and CRP is known to induce IL-6 levels. Although this protective role of Mediterranean diet may be due to combined properties of its components, some mechanistic hypotheses have been suggested from the key elements of the Mediterranean diet. Diets with higher n-6: n-3 PUFA ratios, for example, may enhance risk of both depression and inflammatory diseases, characterized by higher levels of IL-6 and TNF-α [38].

Some limitations of this study need to be considered. This study is cross-sectional and therefore we could not infer causality. We did not have smoking on our dataset and smoking may influence levels of inflammatory biomarkers. Nevertheless, to the best of our knowledge, this is the first study to evaluate stress biomarker, inflammation and adherence to the Mediterranean diet in adolescents and suggests that the Mediterranean diet may counteract stress-induced inflammation.

5. Conclusions

Higher adherence to the Mediterranean diet may counteract the effect of stress-induced inflammation and decrease risk of future mental health.

Author Contributions: Conceptualization, K.M.B.C., N.M. and L.A.C.; Data curation, K.M.B.C.; Formal analysis, K.M.B.C.; Methodology, I.H.; Project administration, L.M. and S.d.H.; Supervision, L.A.C.; Writing—original draft, K.M.B.C., D.B.R. and L.A.C.; Writing—review & editing, N.M., M.C.-G., A.M., J.D., Y.M., B.D.S., L.M. and S.d.H.

Funding: This work funded by CAPES—Brazilian Federal Agency for Support and Evaluation of Graduate Education within the Ministry of Education of Brazil to KMBC. This study was also funded by the Medical Research Council (UK) Immuno-Psychiatry Consortium grant awarded to University of Cambridge, University College London with industrial partnership funding from GlaxoSmithKline (GSK) and Janssen.

Conflicts of Interest: The authors declare no conflict of interest.

References

1. World Health Organization. Health for the World's Adolescents: A Second Chance in the Second Decade: Summary. Available online: https://www.WHO.int/adolescent/second-decade (accessed on 28 September 2018).
2. National Research Council; Institute of Medicine. Children's Health, The Nation's Wealth: Assessing and Improving Child Health. Available online: https://www.ncbi.nlm.nih.gov/books/NBK92206/ (accessed on 28 September 2018).
3. Jonsson, U.; Bohman, H.; von Knorring, L.; Olsson, G.; Paaren, A.; von Knorring, A.L. Mental health outcome of long-term and episodic adolescent depression: 15-year follow-up of a community sample. *J. Affect. Disord.* **2011**, *130*, 395–404. [CrossRef] [PubMed]
4. Nanni, V.; Uher, R.; Danese, A. Childhood maltreatment predicts unfavorable course of illness and treatment outcome in depression: A meta-analysis. *Am. J. Psychiatr.* **2012**, *169*, 141–151. [CrossRef] [PubMed]
5. Kessler, R.C.; Angermeyer, M.; Anthony, J.C.; De Graaf, R.O.N.; Demyttenaere, K.; Gasquet, I.; De Girolamo, G.; Gluzman, S.; Gureje, O.; Haro, J.M.; et al. Lifetime prevalence and age-of-onset distributions of mental disorders in the World Health Organization's World Mental Health Survey Initiative. *World Psychiatry* **2007**, *6*, 168. [PubMed]

6. Haapakoski, R.; Mathieu, J.; Ebmeier, K.P.; Alenius, H.; Kivimäki, M. Cumulative meta-analysis of interleukins 6 and 1β, tumour necrosis factor α and C-reactive protein in patients with major depressive disorder. *Brain Behav. Immun.* **2015**, *49*, 206–215. [CrossRef] [PubMed]
7. Zalli, A.; Jovanova, O.; Hoogendijk, W.J.G.; Tiemeier, H.; Carvalho, L.A. Low-grade inflammation predicts persistence of depressive symptoms. *Psychopharmacology* **2016**, *233*, 1669–1678. [CrossRef] [PubMed]
8. Carpenter, L.L.; Gawuga, C.E.; Tyrka, A.R.; Lee, J.K.; Anderson, G.M.; Price, L.H. Association between plasma IL-6 response to acute stress and early-life adversity in healthy adults. *Neuropsychopharmacology* **2010**, *35*, 2617. [CrossRef] [PubMed]
9. Gouin, J.P.; Glaser, R.; Malarkey, W.B.; Beversdorf, D.; Kiecolt-Glaser, J.K. Childhood abuse and inflammatory responses to daily stressors. *Ann. Behav. Med.* **2012**, *44*, 287–292. [CrossRef] [PubMed]
10. Mitchell, R.H.; Goldstein, B.I. Inflammation in children and adolescents with neuropsychiatric disorders: A systematic review. *J. Am. Acad. Child Adolesc. Psychiatry* **2014**, *53*, 274–296. [CrossRef] [PubMed]
11. Bosma-den Boer, M.M.; van Wetten, M.L.; Pruimboom, L. Chronic inflammatory diseases are stimulated by current lifestyle: How diet, stress levels and medication prevent our body from recovering. *Nutr. Metab.* **2012**, *9*, 32–44. [CrossRef] [PubMed]
12. Sureda, A.; Bibiloni, M.D.M.; Julibert, A.; Bouzas, C.; Argelich, E.; Llompart, I.; Pons, A.; Tur, J.A. Adherence to the Mediterranean Diet and Inflammatory Markers. *Nutrients* **2018**, *10*, 62. [CrossRef] [PubMed]
13. Milaneschi, Y.; Bandinelli, S.; Penninx, B.W.; Vogelzangs, N.; Corsi, A.M.; Lauretani, F.; Kisialiou, A.; Vazzana, R.; Terracciano, A.; Guralnik, J.M.; et al. Depressive symptoms and inflammation increase in a prospective study of older adults: A protective effect of a healthy (Mediterranean-style) diet. *Mol. Psychiatry* **2011**, *16*, 589–590. [CrossRef] [PubMed]
14. Kiecolt-Glaser, J.K.; Derry, H.M.; Fagundes, C.P. Inflammation: Depression fans the flames and feasts on the heat. *Am. J. Psychiatry* **2015**, *172*, 1075–1091. [CrossRef] [PubMed]
15. Arouca, A.; Michels, N.; Moreno, L.A.; González-Gil, E.M.; Marcos, A.; Gómez, S.; Díaz, L.E.; Widhalm, K.; Olnár, D.; Anios, Y.; et al. Associations between a Mediterranean diet pattern and inflammatory biomarkers in European adolescents. *Eur. J. Nutr.* **2018**, *57*, 1747–1760. [CrossRef] [PubMed]
16. Khalid, S.; Williams, C.M.; Reynolds, S.A. Is there an association between diet and depression in children and adolescents? A systematic review. *Br. J. Nutr.* **2016**, *116*, 2097–2108. [CrossRef] [PubMed]
17. Lucas, M.; Chocano-Bedoya, P.; Shulze, M.B.; Mirzaei, F.; O'Reilly, É.J.; Okereke, O.I.; Hu, F.B.; Willett, W.C.; Ascherio, A. Inflammatory dietary pattern and risk of depression among women. *Brain Behav. Immun.* **2014**, *36*, 46–53. [CrossRef] [PubMed]
18. Antonogeorgos, G.; Panagiotakos, D.B.; Pitsavos, C.; Papageorgiou, C.; Chrysohoou, C.; Papadimitriou, G.N.; Stefanadis, C. Understanding the role of depression and anxiety on cardiovascular disease risk, using structural equation modeling; the mediating effect of the Mediterranean diet and physical activity: The ATTICA study. *Ann. Epidemiol.* **2012**, *22*, 630–637. [CrossRef] [PubMed]
19. Luciano, M.; Mõttus, R.; Starr, J.M.; McNeill, G.; Jia, X.; Craig, L.C.; Deary, I.J. Depressive symptoms and diet: Their effects on prospective inflammation levels in the elderly. *Brain Behav. Immun.* **2012**, *26*, 717–720. [CrossRef] [PubMed]
20. Jacka, F.N.; Kremer, P.J.; Leslie, E.R.; Berk, M.; Patton, G.C.; Toumbourou, J.W.; Williams, J.W. Associations between diet quality and depressed mood in adolescents: Results from the Australian Healthy Neighbourhoods Study. *Aust. N. Z. J. Psychiatry* **2010**, *44*, 435–442. [CrossRef] [PubMed]
21. Kohlboeck, G.; Sausenthaler, S.; Standl, M.; Koletzko, S.; Bauer, C.P.; Von Berg, A.; Berdel, D.; Krämer, U.; Schaaf, B.; Lehmann, I.; et al. Food intake, diet quality and behavioral problems in children: Results from the GINI-plus/LISA-plus studies. *Ann. Nutr. Metab.* **2012**, *60*, 247–256. [CrossRef] [PubMed]
22. Moreno, L.A.; Gonzalez-Gross, M.; Kersting, M.; Molnar, D.; De Henauw, S.; Beghin, L.; Sjöström, M.; Hagströmer, M.; Manios, Y.; Gilbert, C.C.; et al. Assessing, understanding and modifying nutritional status, eating habits and physical activity in European adolescents: The HELENA (Healthy Lifestyle in Europe by Nutrition in Adolescence) Study. *Public Health Nutr.* **2008**, *11*, 288–299. [CrossRef] [PubMed]
23. Moreno, L.A.; De Henauw, S.; Gonzalez-Gross, M.; Kersting, M.; Molnar, D.; Gottrand, F.; Barrios, L.; Sjöström, M.; Manios, Y.; Gilbert, C.C.; et al. Design and implementation of the Healthy Lifestyle in Europe by Nutrition in Adolescence Cross-Sectional Study. *Int. J. Obes.* **2008**, *32*, S4–S11. [CrossRef] [PubMed]

24. Beghin, L.; Castera, M.; Manios, Y.; Gilbert, C.C.; Kersting, M.; De Henauw, S.; Kafatos, A.; Gottrand, F.; Molnar, D.; Sjöström, M.; et al. Quality assurance of ethical issues and regulatory aspects relating to good clinical practices in the HELENA Cross-Sectional Study. *Int. J. Obes.* **2008**, *32*, S12–S18. [CrossRef] [PubMed]
25. Marshall, W.A.; Tanner, J.M. Variations in Pattern of Pubertal Changes in Girls. *Arch. Dis. Child.* **1969**, *44*, 291–303. [CrossRef] [PubMed]
26. Marshall, W.A.; Tanner, J.M. Variations in Pattern of Pubertal Changes in Boys. *Arch. Dis. Child.* **1970**, *45*, 13–23. [CrossRef] [PubMed]
27. Nagy, E.; Vicente-Rodriguez, G.; Manios, Y.; Béghin, L.; Iliescu, C.; Censi, L.; Dietrich, S.; Ortega, F.B.; De Vriendt, T.; Plada, M.; et al. Harmonization process and reliability assessment of anthropometric measurements in a multicenter study in adolescents. *Int. J. Obes.* **2008**, *32*, S58–S65. [CrossRef] [PubMed]
28. Cole, T.J.; Freeman, J.V.; Preece, M.A. British 1990 growth reference centiles for weight, height, body mass index and head circumference fitted by maximum penalized likelihood. *Stat. Med.* **1998**, *17*, 407–429. [CrossRef]
29. González-Gross, M.; Breidenassel, C.; Gómez-Martínez, S.; Ferrari, M.; Beghin, L.; Spinneker, A.; Díaz, L.E.; Maiani, G.; Demailly, A.; Al-Tahan, J.; et al. Sampling and processing of fresh blood samples within a European multicenter nutritional study: Evaluation of biomarker stability during transport and storage. *Int. J. Obes.* **2008**, *32*, S66–S75. [CrossRef] [PubMed]
30. Van Aken, M.O.; Romijn, J.A.; Miltenburg, J.A.; Lentjes, E.G. Automated measurement of salivary cortisol. *Clin. Chem.* **2003**, *49*, 1408–1409. [CrossRef] [PubMed]
31. Vereecken, C.A.; Covents, M.; Sichert-Hellert, W.; Alvira, J.F.; Le Donne, C.; De Henauw, S.; De Vriendt, T.; Phillipp, M.K.; Béghin, L.; Manios, Y.; et al. Development and evaluation of a self-administered computerized 24-h dietary recall method for adolescents in Europe. *Int. J. Obes.* **2008**, *32*, S26–S34. [CrossRef] [PubMed]
32. Trichopoulou, A.; Costacou, T.; Bamia, C.; Trichopoulos, D. Adherence to a Mediterranean diet and survival in a Greek population. *N. Engl. J. Med.* **2003**, *348*, 2599–2608. [CrossRef] [PubMed]
33. Arouca, A.B.; Santaliestra-Pasías, A.M.; Moreno, L.A.; Marcos, A.; Widhalm, K.; Molnár, D.; Manios, Y.; Gottrand, F.; Kafatos, A.; Kersting, M.; et al. Diet as a moderator in the association of sedentary behaviors with inflammatory biomarkers among adolescents in the HELENA study. *Eur. J. Nutr.* **2018**, *2018*, 1–15. [CrossRef] [PubMed]
34. Grosso, G.; Mistretta, A.; Frigiola, A.; Gruttadauria, S.; Biondi, A.; Basile, F.; Vitaglione, P.; D'Orazio, N.; Galvano, F. Mediterranean diet and cardiovascular risk factors: A systematic review. *Crit. Rev. Food Sci. Nutr.* **2014**, *54*, 593–610. [CrossRef] [PubMed]
35. Naska, A.; Trichopoulou, A. Back to the future: The Mediterranean diet paradigm. *Nutr. Metab. Cardiovasc. Dis.* **2014**, *24*, 216–219. [CrossRef] [PubMed]
36. Smidowicz, A.; Regula, J. Effect of nutritional status and dietary patterns on human serum C-reactive protein and interleukin-6 concentrations. *Adv. Nutr.* **2015**, *6*, 738–747. [CrossRef] [PubMed]
37. De Vriendt, T.; Clays, E.; Huybrechts, I.; De Bourdeaudhuij, I.; Moreno, L.A.; Patterson, E.; Molnár, D.; Mesana, M.I.; Beghin, L.; Widhalm, K.; et al. European adolescents' level of perceived stress is inversely related to their diet quality: The Healthy Lifestyle in Europe by Nutrition in Adolescence study. *Br. J. Nutr.* **2012**, *108*, 371–380. [CrossRef] [PubMed]
38. Kiecolt-Glaser, J.K.; Belury, M.A.; Porter, K.; Beversdorf, D.; Lemeshow, S.; Glaser, R. Depressive symptoms, n-6: N-3 fatty acids, and inflammation in older adults. *Psychosom. Med.* **2007**, *69*, 217–224. [CrossRef] [PubMed]

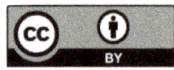

© 2018 by the authors. Licensee MDPI, Basel, Switzerland. This article is an open access article distributed under the terms and conditions of the Creative Commons Attribution (CC BY) license (http://creativecommons.org/licenses/by/4.0/).

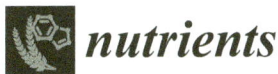

Article

Mediterranean Diet and Motivation in Sport: A Comparative Study Between University Students from Spain and Romania

Ramón Chacón-Cuberos [1], Georgian Badicu [2,*], Félix Zurita-Ortega [3] and Manuel Castro-Sánchez [3]

1. Department of Education. University of Almería, 04120 Almería, Spain; rchacon@ual.es
2. Department of Physical Education and Special Motility, Faculty of Physical Education and Mountain Sports, Transilvania University of Brasov, 500068 Brasov, Romania
3. Department of Didactics of Musical, Plastic and Corporal Expression, University of Granada, 18071 Granada, Spain; felixzo@ugr.es (F.Z.-O.); manuelcs@ugr.es (M.C.-S.)
* Correspondence: georgian.badicu@unitbv.ro; Tel.: +40-769-219-271

Received: 11 November 2018; Accepted: 20 December 2018; Published: 22 December 2018

Abstract: Background: The Mediterranean Diet (MD) is one of the healthiest dietary models worldwide, being an essential mean of preventing pathologies along with the practice of physical activity. Through a comparative study carried out across different countries, it has been demonstrated how this type of habits vary depending on the geographical context. The aim of this research was to evaluate the adherence to MD and its relationships with motivational climate in sport on a sample of university students from Spain and Romania; Methods: A cross-sectional study was conducted on a sample of university students [specialization: Physical Education (n = 605; 20.71 ± 2.42 years old)], using as main instruments the Mediterranean Diet Quality Index (KIDMED) for students and adolescents and the Perceived Motivational Climate in Sport Questionnaire-2 (PMCSQ-2); Results: It was shown that students from Spain had a high adherence to the MD (6.65 ± 2.63 vs. 5.06 ± 1.31). Spanish university students got higher scores in task-oriented motivational climate (4.03 ± 0.62 vs. 3.11 ± 0.55) while ego-oriented climate was higher in university students from Romania (3.24 ± 0.54 vs. 2.07 ± 0.75). Finally, it was observed that the task-oriented motivational climate was related to a lower adherence to MD in Spanish students (4.49 ± 0.37 vs. 3.98 ± 0.62). In contrast, in Romanian youth, a medium adherence to the MD was associated with higher scores for the ego-oriented motivational climate (3.27 ± 0.53 vs. 3.00 ± 0.54); Conclusions: As main conclusions, it was shown that the students from Spain had a high adherence to the MD. In addition, it has been demonstrated that ego-oriented climates are linked to a better adherence to MD, especially due to the importance of following a proper diet in sport contexts, as demonstrated by young Romanians.

Keywords: Mediterranean diet; motivational climate; sports; university students

1. Introduction

Being overweight (body mass index of 25 or higher) and its associated pathologies have become a problem in society nowadays, which is why the importance of following a healthy diet and lifestyle has gained much prominence [1–3]. The diet models that exist in the world are numerous and varied, each one with particular characteristics [3]. Dietary habits represent important elements for the quality of life and especially for young people [4]. Utilizing different dietary models, several authors state the importance of making a change in people's eating habits in European countries in order to reduce the risk of different types of diseases [5,6]. The Mediterranean Diet (MD) is one of the most studied model as it is associated with different benefits, such as a better health due to a high consumption of natural antioxidants and a low intake of fats. In addition, MD improves the cognitive function, decreases the risk of diabetes, bone diseases and overweight [6–8].

This dietary model is characterized by typical foods of the Mediterranean basin such as legumes, fruits, cereals and olive oil, with a moderate consumption of eggs, fish and dairy products [4,9,10]. It has been shown that people with a good adherence to MD have a high quality of life and life expectancy [11], as this diet has several benefits on public health [12], social relationships [13], sport performance [14] and emotional factors [15,16]. Furthermore, the influence of MD on young people living around the Mediterranean Sea has been studied in countries such as Cyprus, Italy, Greece, Turkey, Spain, Lebanon and Croatia [4,13,15–21]. Additionally, this dietary model has been analysed in various cultural and socio-economic contexts [10,22,23].

Several studies demonstrate the benefits of a high adherence to the MD [24–27]. This dietary model helps to improve body composition, favouring the decrease in the percentage of fat mass thanks to its low consumption in hypercaloric foods and foods rich in saturated fats [25]. In addition, MD helps to prevent diabetes, since this model is based on the consumption of foods with a low glycaemic index, such as fruits, vegetables and cereals [26]. Another benefit lies in the Non-alcoholic fatty liver disease, since Trovato et al. [27] demonstrated in an intervention study how a better adherence to MD improved the progress of this pathology due to a greater caloric restriction that generates temporary changes in the liver such as a better sensitivity to hepatic insulin or a lower content of triglycerides. Finally, O'Neil et al. [28] highlight some of the benefits of MD at cognitive level, such as an improvement of states of depression and anxiety or a better academic performance.

Regular and adequate Physical Activity (PA) in addition to following a healthy diet is essential for the improvement of health. Several studies show how performing a minimum of 90 minutes of moderate PA weekly helps to improve health, body composition or bone mineral density, as well as pulmonary and cardiovascular functions [29,30]. In addition, regular PA decreases anxiety and stress and improves self-concept, well-being and self-esteem [31,32]. For these reasons, promoting this type of habits is essential among university students, since many habits developed in early adulthood are reinforced later in life [21]. In this sense, it is essential to study the motivational aspects that allow to create adherence to the practice of PA, which will be linked to other healthy habits such as adopting a healthy diet.

The Achievement Goals Theory has been one of the most used explanatory models in order to explain the motivational processes involved in sports practice [33,34]. This theory establishes that people set objectives in sports, which will be related to the person's perception of their own abilities. Therefore, the goals pursued by an individual can be linked to motivational climates oriented toward the task or the ego [33,35]. In the first case, the task-oriented climate will be linked to team work, to higher levels of effort to learn and the assignment of an important role in the task [36]. The ego-oriented climate is related to people whose goals depend on the social recognition that they will achieve through competition within the sport context [36,37]. Considering the premises exposed by Ryan et al. [38] in the Self-Determination Theory, the task-oriented climate will be associated with intrinsic motivations, while the ego climate will be related to extrinsic motivations [39]. In this regard, it has been shown that certain types of motivations can be linked to healthy or non-healthy behaviours [40–42].

Studies such as those carried out by Chacón et al. [43] or Erturan-Ilker et al. [44] analyse the relationship between motivation in sport and different healthy habits, such as the consumption of harmful substances, the practice of PA or adherence to MD. Although the adherence to MD has been studied in association with physical and healthy lifestyles, a few studies connect it with motivation in sport, as well as with cultural-geography factors. Thus, it is interesting to study these variables in order to promote MD in non-Mediterranean populations [19,45,46]. In view of the above, the present study will provide novel data about the importance of the MD in relation to sociodemographic and motivational parameters in a sample of university students of Physical Education from two countries: Spain and Romania.

The present study establishes two aims: (a) to assess the level of adherence to MD in a sample of university students from Spain and Romania; (b) to analyse the relationship between adherence to MD and motivational climate in sport depending on the country (Spain or Romania); (c) to contrast a structural equation model about the relationship between MD and motivational climate using multi-group analysis.

2. Materials and Methods

2.1. Subjects and Design

This non-experimental, cross-sectional and descriptive research was conducted on a sample of 651 university students from Spain and Romania, enrolled in the Physical Education degrees, aged between 18 and 24 years old (20.71 ± 2.42 years). The respondents participated voluntarily after receiving a detailed explanation of the objectives and nature of the study. Written informed consent was provided. We excluded from the analysis 46 participants that did not complete the inclusion criteria correctly (i.e., incomplete questionnaires, did not hand informed consent forms), thus the final sample was comprised of 605 subjects (368 males and 237 females): Romania ($n = 178$) and Spain ($n = 427$). The students from Romania were enrolled in the Transylvania University of Brasov, while the Spanish students were enrolled in the University of Granada. Finally, an assumed sampling error of 0.05 was taken into account, considering a random sampling by natural groups [47].

2.2. Instruments

Test of Adherence to Mediterranean Diet (KIDMED) [48]. This scale comprises 16 items with an affirmative or negative response; for example: "You eat fruit every day", which are related to patterns associated with the MD. Twelve of these items have positive connotations (+1) while the other four have negative values (−1). The final score ranges from −4 to +12. This instrument has a reliability of $\alpha = 0.86$.

Perceived Motivational Climate in Sport Questionnaire (PMCSQ-2, [49,50]). This instrument is composed by 33 items which are scored by a five-point Likert-scale, ranging from 1 to 5 (Strongly Disagree-Strongly agree). The scale comprised two factors, higher-order dimensions, each containing three indicators. For task-oriented climate the indicators were: effort/improvement, cooperative learning and important role. For ego-oriented climate the indicators were: unequal recognition, member rivalry and punishment for mistakes. The internal consistency for this questionnaire was $\alpha = 0.85$ for task-climate and $\alpha = 0.82$ for ego-climate.

2.3. Procedure

First, we proceeded to request the approval of the study by the Ethics Committee of the University of Granada, which was granted with code "641/CEIH/2018". Subsequently, the collaboration of educational centres was requested through an informative letter elaborated by the Area of Corporal Expression of the University of Granada. In addition, the informed consent of the respondents was requested through a document in which the nature of the study was detailed.

The data was collected during regular classes in the different university campus. Different research assistants were present in the data collection in order to ensure that questionnaires were properly completed, to provide guidance on the completion of scales and to answer questions. Furthermore, participants receive any incentives.

2.4. Data Analysis

Statistical analysis was conducted using the software IBM SPSS®22.0 (IBM Corp., Armonk, NY, USA). Frequencies and medians were used for basic descriptors, whereas the association between the variables detailed were analysed using T-test and ANOVA-test. In addition, the Kolmogorov–Smirnov's test was used in order to check the normality of data, as well as the Lillieforts' correction. Levene's test was employed in order to check homoscedasticity. Finally, Cronbach's Alpha coefficient was used to analyse the internal reliability of the instruments used, establishing the Reliability Index at 95%. In addition, AMOS version 23.0 (IBM Corp., Armonk, NY, USA) is used for the structural equation analysis.

The Structural Equation Model (SEM) is composed by seven observed variables and two latent variables (Figure 1). Task-involved climate (TC) and ego-involved climate (EC) represent the exogenous variables, which is inferred by three indicators. Effort/Improvement (EI), Cooperative learning (CL) and Important Role (RI) are the indicators for task-oriented climate while Unequal Recognition (UR), Member Rivalry (MR) and Punishment for Mistakes (PM) are the indicators for ego-oriented climate. On the contrary, the Mediterranean diet (MD) was the observed endogenous variable. The bi-directional arrow (covariance) relates exogenous variables, while the unidirectional arrows are lines of influence between the latent and observable indicators and are interpreted as multivariate regression coefficients. In addition, error prediction terms are associated with endogenous variables. The method of maximum likelihood (ML) was used to estimate relationships between variables. We chose this method because it is consistent, unbiased and invariant to types of scale given variables with a normal distribution.

Model fit was tested using several indices. Chi-squared analysis followed when non-significant p-values indicated good model fit. Normalized Fit Index (NFI), Comparative Fit Index (CFI) and Increase Fit Index (IFI) values higher than 0.90 indicate acceptable model fit while values higher than 0.95 indicate excellent model fit. Root Mean Square Error of Approximation (RMSEA) values below 0.08 indicate acceptable model fit while values below 0.05 indicate excellent model fit.

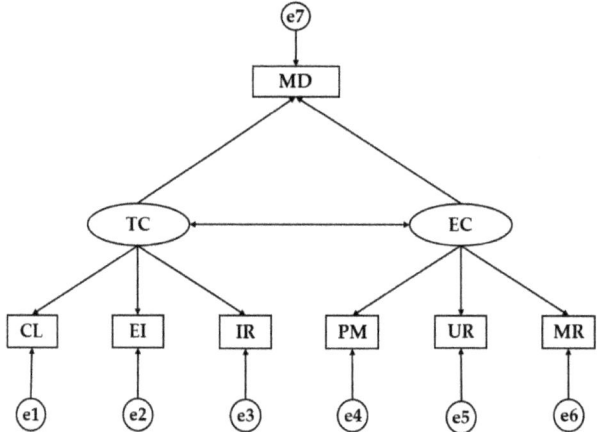

Figure 1. Theoretical model. TC, Task Climate; EC, Ego Climate; CL, Cooperative Learning; EI, Effort/Improvement; IR, Important Role; PM, Punishment for Mistakes; UR, Unequal Recognition; MR, Member Rivalry; MD, Mediterranean Diet.

3. Results

Table 1 shows the average scores obtained in each item of the test on adherence to the MD, according to the country of origin of the university students enrolled in Physical Education degrees. In this way, statistically significant differences ($p < 0.05$) were found in fruit and daily fruit juice consumption (0.27 ± 0.44 vs. 0.77 ± 0.41) and in the intake of a daily second fruit (0.78 ± 0.41 vs. 0.42 ± 0.49), obtaining a higher score for Spanish students in the first case and in Romanians in the second. Moreover, Spanish students obtained higher scores for fish consumption (0.42 ± 0.49 vs. 0.67 ± 0.46), pulses more than once a week (0.63 ± 048 vs. 0.71 ± 0.45), cereal consumption (0.71 ± 0.45 vs. 0.86 ± 0.34) and dairy consumption (0.26 ± 0.44 vs. 0.81 ± 0.39), showing statistically significant differences in all the relationships. In addition, students from Romania obtained higher mean values than Spaniards in vegetable consumption (0.88 ± 0.33 vs. 0.33 ± 0.47), pasta and rice consumption (0.76 ± 0.42 vs. 0.42 ± 0.49) and nut use (0.93 ± 0.25 vs. 0.50 ± 0.50). Nevertheless, Romanian students got the highest scores on negative items, showing a higher absolute mean value for fast food (−0.56 ± 0.49 vs. −0.34 ± 0.47), jumping breakfast (−0.46 ± 0.49) vs. −0.31 ± 0.46), processed food intake (−0.89 ± 0.31 vs. −0.12 ± 0.32) and sweets intakes (−0.79 ± 0.40 vs. −0.17 ± 0.37). Finally, Spanish students obtained a higher average value in the total score for adherence to the MD (5.06 ± 1.31 vs. 6.65 ± 2.63).

Table 1. Dietary patterns depending on country.

Items of Adherence to MD	Country	A	SD	Levene's Test F	Levene's Test Sig.	T-Test Sig.
I1. To eat a fruit or fruit juice every day	Romania	0.27	0.44	4.65	0.031	***
	Spain	0.77	0.41			
I2. To have a second fruit every day	Romania	0.78	0.41	119.95	0.000	***
	Spain	0.42	0.49			
I3. To eat fresh or cooked vegetables regularly once a day	Romania	0.55	0.49	6.91	0.009	0.109
	Spain	0.62	0.48			
I4. To consume fresh or cooked vegetables more than once a day	Romania	0.88	0.33	181.53	0.000	***
	Spain	0.33	0.47			
I5. Regular fish consumption (at least 2–3/week)	Romania	0.42	0.49	14.27	0.000	***
	Spain	0.67	0.46			
I6. To go > 1/ week to a fast food restaurant (hamburger)	Romania	−0.56	0.49	14.83	0.000	***
	Spain	−0.34	0.47			
I7. Pulses > 1/week	Romania	0.63	0.48	13.77	0.000	*
	Spain	0.71	0.45			
I8. To eat pasta or rice almost every day (5 or more per week)	Romania	0.76	0.42	106.34	0.000	***
	Spain	0.42	0.49			
I9. To have cereals or grains (bread, etc.) for breakfast	Romania	0.71	0.45	66.35	0.000	***
	Spain	0.86	0.34			
I10. To consume nuts regularly (at least 2–3/week)	Romania	0.93	0.25	1266.61	0.000	***
	Spain	0.50	0.50			
I11. To use olive oil at home	Romania	0.99	0.07	0.86	0.353	0.643
	Spain	0.99	0.09			
I12. No breakfast	Romania	−0.46	0.49	24.63	0.000	**
	Spain	−0.31	0.46			
I13. To have a dairy product for breakfast (yoghurt, milk, etc.)	Romania	0.26	0.44	15.15	0.000	***
	Spain	0.81	0.39			
I14. To eat commercially baked goods or pastries for breakfast	Romania	−0.89	0.31	0.42	0.513	***
	Spain	−0.12	0.32			
I15. To consume two yoghurts and/or some cheese (40 g) daily	Romania	0.56	0.49	2.42	0.120	0.070
	Spain	0.48	0.50			
I16. To have sweets and candy several times every day	Romania	−0.79	0.40	5.64	0.018	***
	Spain	−0.17	0.37			
Global score in adherence to MD	Rumanía	5.06	1.31	101.88	0.000	***
	España	6.65	2.63			

* Statistically significant differences at level $p < 0.05$; ** Statistically significant differences at level $p < 0.01$; *** Statistically significant differences at level $p < 0.001$. A, Average; SD, Standard Deviation. MD, Mediterranean Diet.

Scores obtained for motivational climate according to the country are shown in Table 2, showing statistically significant differences at level $p < 0.001$ for all relationships. University students from Spain got higher values for Task-oriented Climate (3.11 ± 0.55 vs. 4.03 ± 0.62) and its categories: Cooperative Learning (2.93 ± 0.75 vs. 4.06 ± 0.72), Effort/Improvement (3.34 ± 0.53 vs. 3.97 ± 0.63) and Important Role (2.87 ± 0.86 vs. 4.10 ± 0.73). Furthermore, students from Romania showed the highest scores in Ego-oriented Climate (3.24 ± 0.24 vs. 2.07 ± 0.75) and its categories: Punishment for Mistakes (3.24 ± 0.61 vs. 1.93 ± 0.79), Unequal Recognition (3.17 ± 0.70 vs. 1.98 ± 0.89) and Member Rivalry (3.39 ± 0.80 vs. 2.56 ± 0.95).

Table 2. Motivational climate in sport depending on country.

Dimensions of Motivational Climate	Country	A	SD	Levene's Test F	Sig.	T-Test Sig.
TC	Romania	3.11	0.55	2.720	0.100	***
	Spain	4.03	0.62			
CL	Romania	2.93	0.75	4.363	0.037	***
	Spain	4.06	0.72			
EI	Romania	3.34	0.53	4.477	0.035	***
	Spain	3.97	0.63			
IR	Romania	2.87	0.86	8.223	0.004	***
	Spain	4.10	0.73			
EC	Romania	3.24	0.54	18.175	0.000	***
	Spain	2.07	0.75			
PM	Romania	3.24	0.61	14.471	0.000	***
	Spain	1.93	0.79			
UR	Romania	3.17	0.70	6.259	0.013	***
	Spain	1.98	0.89			
MR	Romania	3.39	0.80	14.872	0.000	***
	Spain	2.56	0.95			

*** Statistically significant differences at level $p < 0.001$. TC, Task-oriented Climate; CL, Cooperative Learning; EI, Effort/Improvement; IR, Important Role; EC, Ego-oriented Climate; PM, Punishment for Mistakes; UR, Unequal Recognition; MR, Member Rivalry. A, Average; SD, Standard Deviation.

Table 3 shows the relationships between adherence to MD and motivational climate in the university students of both countries. Romanian students revealed statistical differences at level $p < 0.05$ for Ego-oriented Climate (3.27 ± 0.53 vs. 3.00 ± 0.54) and punishment for Mistakes (3.28 ± 0.61 vs. 2.96 ± 0.50) showing higher scores for medium adherence to MD than for higher adherence. In addition, statically significant differences at level $p < 0.01$ were found for Member Rivalry with a high average for medium adherence (3.45 ± 0.76 vs. 2.93 ± 0.96. Moreover, Spanish students showed significant differences at level $p < 0.05$ with higher values for low adherence to MD than medium adherence in Task-oriented Climate (4.49 ± 0.37 vs. 3.98 ± 0.62), Cooperative Learning (4.60 ± 0.37 vs. 4.01 ± 0.72) and Effort/Improvement (4.37 ± 0.53 vs. 3.90 ± 0.65).

Table 3. Adherence to MD according to motivational climate and country.

Level of Adherence to MD According to Motivational Climate		Romania A	Romania DT	Romania P	Spain A	Spain DT	Spain P
TC	Low adherence	-	-		4.49	0.37	
	Medium adherence	3.12	0.54	0.263	3.98	0.62	*
	High adherence	2.98	0.56		4.06	0.62	
CL	Low adherence	-	-		4.60	0.37	
	Medium adherence	2.94	0.73	0.677	4.01	0.72	*
	High adherence	2.87	0.90		4.10	0.71	
EI	Low adherence	-	-		4.37	0.53	
	Medium adherence	3.35	0.52	0.313	3.90	0.65	*
	High adherence	3.23	0.61		4.02	0.60	
IR	Low adherence	-	-		4.60	0.37	
	Medium adherence	2.90	0.88	0.253	4.10	0.71	0.305
	High adherence	2.68	0.67		4.08	0.76	
EC	Low adherence	-	-		1.87	0.81	
	Medium adherence	3.27	0.53	*	2.04	0.71	0.491
	High adherence	3.00	0.54		2.11	0.78	
PM	Low adherence	-	-		1.66	0.39	
	Medium adherence	3.28	0.61	*	1.89	0.75	0.391
	High adherence	2.96	0.50		1.98	0.82	
UR	Low adherence	-	-		1.85	1.16	
	Medium adherence	3.19	0.71	0.400	1.97	0.86	0.885
	High adherence	3.05	0.70		2.00	0.92	
MR	Low adherence	-	-		2.33	1.17	
	Medium adherence	3.45	0.76	**	2.49	0.90	0.225
	High adherence	2.93	0.96		2.64	0.99	

* Statistically significant differences at level $p < 0.05$; ** Statistically significant differences at level $p < 0.01$. TC, Task-oriented Climate; CL, Cooperative Learning; EI, Effort/Improvement; IR, Important Role; EC, Ego-oriented Climate; PM, Punishment for Mistakes; UR, Unequal Recognition; MR, Member Rivalry. MD, Mediterranean Diet. A, Average; SD, Standard Deviation.

Finally, a structural equation model is developed in order to compare the relationships between all the analysed factors according to the country (Figures 2 and 3). Almost all fit indices of model suggested good fit. A significant chi-square value was obtained ($\chi^2 = 126.85$; df = 5.28; $p < 0.001$). Nevertheless, as this index has no upper limit and may also be sensitive to sample size, we also considered other standardized indices which are less sensitive to sample size. The NFI was 0.93, indicating an acceptable fit to the model. The CFI yielded a value of 0.94 and the IFI got a value of 0.94. Finally, RMSEA value was 0.74, indicating acceptable fit.

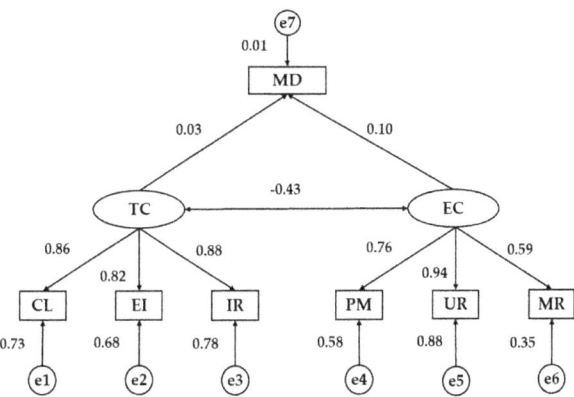

Figure 2. Structural Equation Model for Spanish students. TC, Task Climate; EC, Ego Climate; CL, Cooperative Learning; EI, Effort/Improvement; IR, Important Role; PM, Punishment for Mistakes; UR, Unequal Recognition; MR, Member Rivalry; MD, Mediterranean Diet.

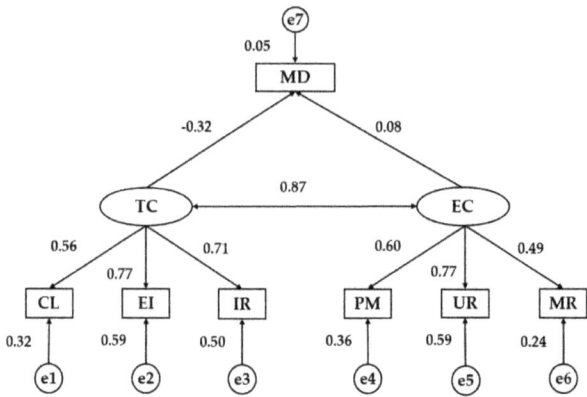

Figure 3. Structural Equation Model for Romanian students. TC, Task Climate; EC, Ego Climate; CL, Cooperative Learning; EI, Effort/Improvement; IR, Important Role; PM, Punishment for Mistakes; UR, Unequal Recognition; MR, Member Rivalry; MD, Mediterranean Diet.

Table 4 shows the standardized weights of university students from Spain and Romania. A significant negative relationship was found between the two dimensions of motivational climate for university students from both countries, being negative in Spaniards ($p < 0.001$, $b = -0.429$) and positive in Romanians ($p < 0.001$, $b = 0.872$). In relation to the indicators and their association with the exogenous variables, the variable that showed the highest regression weight for the task-oriented climate in Spanish students was the important role ($p < 0.001$, $b = 0.884$), while in the students from Romania it was the effort / improvement ($p < 0.001$, $b = 0.765$). In the case of the ego-oriented climate, the indicator with the highest regression weight was unequal recognition for Spaniards and Romanians ($p < 0.001$, $b = 0.940$; $p < 0.001$; $b = 0.765$).

Finally, the relationship between adherence to MD and motivational climate in sport is analysed (Table 4). A significant and positive relationship was obtained between the ego-oriented climate and the level of adherence to MD ($p < 0.05$, $b = 0.103$) in young Spaniards, whereas this association was not significant for young Romanians. On the contrary, there was a statistically significant association between the task-oriented climate and the level of adherence to the MD, which was negative ($p < 0.001$, $b = 0.315$). Nevertheless, this relationship was not statistically significant for Spanish university students.

Table 4. Structural equation model: multi-group analysis according to country.

Relationship between Variables			R.W.			S.R.W.
			Estimations	S.E.	C.R.	Estimations
Weights and standardized regression weights of students from Spain						
CL	←	TC	1.000	-	-	0.856 ***
EI	←	TC	0.848	0.042	19.996	0.823 ***
IR	←	TC	1.057	0.049	21.424	0.884 ***
PM	←	EC	1.000	-	-	0.759 ***
UR	←	EC	1.403	0.096	14.656	0.940 ***
MR	←	EC	0.936	0.078	12.016	0.589 ***
MD	←	TC	0.115	0.247	0.465	0.027
MD	←	EC	0.451	0.252	2.786	0.103 *
EC	↔	TC	-0.159	0.024	-6.723	-0.429 ***
Weights and standardized regression weights of students from Romania						
CL	←	TC	1.000	-	-	0.562 ***
EI	←	TC	0.959	0.133	7.219	0.765 ***
IR	←	TC	1.434	0.208	6.905	0.708 ***
PM	←	EC	1.000	-	-	0.601 ***
UR	←	EC	1.479	0.188	7.883	0.765 ***
MR	←	EC	1.085	0.191	5.669	0.494 ***
MD	←	TC	-0.977	1.337	-3.731	-0.315 ***
MD	←	EC	0.294	1.531	0.192	0.082
EC	↔	TC	0.167	0.032	5.286	0.872 ***

R.W., Regression Weights; S.R.W., Standardized Regression Weights; S.E., Estimation of Error; C.R., Critical Ratio. TC, Task Climate; CL, Cooperative Learning; EI, Effort/Improvement; IR, Important Role; EC, Ego Climate; PM, Punishment for Mistakes; UR, Unequal Recognition; MR, Member Rivalry; MD, Mediterranean Diet. * $p < 0.05$; *** $p < 0.001$. ←, Relationships between latent and observable indicators; ↔, Relationships between exogenous variables.

4. Discussion

Adherence to the MD has been studied in many countries [4,13,15–21]. Nevertheless, there are few studies comparing dietary habits and other aspects, such as motivational factors related to the practice of sport. The global score obtained for adherence to the MD was higher for Spanish students. This is due to Romania being a non-coastal country, located further north than Spain. This geographical location, which comes with a different climate and cultural customs, does not enable the cultivation of many of the typical foods of the Mediterranean basin (that constitute the MD) in Romania [6,9,12]. Nevertheless, there is a good amount of food exports in the countries of the European Union, which make these differences less important to the level of adherence to MD, as Baylis et al. [51] show.

It was found that the consumption of vegetables, fruits and juice is higher in Spanish students than in the Romanian students. This is due to the geographical and cultural characteristics of the Spanish region, as these products are frequently cultivated given the better climatological conditions, an easy access and a low price [12,52]. Furthermore, there is a large production of oranges in Spain. The importance of the intake of this fruit is established in society and juice is one of the most frequent methods of consumption. The benefits of consuming these foods are known since they are rich in vitamins and antioxidants, which encourage their consumption by the Spanish population [52,53].

In addition, it was shown that Romanian students ate fruit or vegetables more than once a day with higher frequency than Spanish students. It has been observed that Spanish students follow a better diet and the consumption of these foods is globalized in general. Nevertheless, they did not achieve much higher scores in the consumption of fruit or vegetables. However, the higher consumption of vegetables and fruit among Romanian students may be justified by the participants who follow a healthy lifestyle. Moreover, the scores can be explained by the anthropometric characteristics of people from Eastern

Europe and by the climatic conditions that require a higher food intake. Studies carried out around the world have highlighted the differences that exist between different countries [9,12,54–56].

The geographical situation of Spain and its climate favour the consumption of food such as fish, milk or cereals more consumed among its students, whereas the diet model of Romanian students is more oriented towards the consumption of pasta or rice. On the other hand, it is worrisome that the consumption of sweets, processed foods or fast food is higher in Romanian students. This is because they have not adopted the Mediterranean diet within their dietary models and this promotes little or no consumption of these foods [13,52].

The motivational climate in sports practice has been studied in different contexts, mainly the field of Physical Education, competitive sports and healthy habits [36,57,58]. In the present study, higher scores have been observed in the task-oriented motivational climate of Spanish students, whereas Romanian students obtained higher scores in the ego-oriented motivational climate in all its dimensions. This could be explained by the type of sports that are practiced most frequently in these countries. Team sports such as football or basketball are more common in Spain, promoting factors that are more linked to the task climate, such as cooperation or teamwork [50,59]. On the contrary, there is a greater tendency for the practice of individual sports such as wrestling, sports gymnastics or weightlifting in Romania, making them stand out in a greater competitive context with the disappearance of the hedonistic factor [40,60,61]. Therefore, although both sports may link all kinds of motivations, those that involve greater social interaction and collaborative work will be related to more self-determined motivations. This idea, along with the cultural influences of each country, will justify these findings [33,34,60].

In the relationship between the motivational climate and MD, those students who are oriented towards the task are those who have a lower adherence to MD. This can be explained by students that are intrinsically predisposed to the pleasure of physical activity and, thus, do not follow a diet of quality in order to improve their sport performance [41,62]. Nevertheless, the students who got higher scores for ego-oriented climate were those with a medium or high adherence to MD, may propitiated by the importance that has the feeding and the nutrition for the sports performance [6,63]. In addition, the scores in ego-oriented climate showed an increase in relation to medium adherence to MD in Romanian students, which is produced because they do not have low adherence in any case and the importance given to get good results in sport context [41]. On the contrary, the statistical differences are shown in task-oriented climate in Spanish university students. In this students an increase of the average scores of the task climate was linked to a low adherence to the MD. This can be justified by the intrinsic motivations of this group, who do not prioritize nutrition as much as they should, as they do not aim at a better performance like their competitors [64–68].

First, the limitations found in this study are determined by the cross-sectional design of this study, where data is collected at a specific time, not allowing to establish causal explanation of this variables. Another limitation is associated with the sample size, since data cannot be generalized to the general population of these countries. Only students between 18 and 24 years of age, enrolled in Physical Education and who have knowledge of nutrition have been analysed. It would also have been interesting to apply the PREDIMED questionnaire but this test that analyses the adherence to the MD in people older than 21 years was not appropriate for our participants (who were mostly less than that age). The variables selected represent another limitation since it would have been of interest to include the socio-economic level and the place of residence of the students in order to know their influence on the level of adherence to the MD. Lastly, with KIDMED being a self-report questionnaire, some comprehension errors could be found, although this is not impeding its application [41–48].

5. Conclusions

The present study show evidence for a higher adherence to MD among Spanish students, as indicated by a higher intake of fruit, vegetables, cereals and fish. On the contrary, Romanian students ate more pasta, rice and processed products such as sweets or fried foods. In relation to the motivational climate, it was observed that students from Spain obtained higher scores in task climate and students from Romania achieved higher scores in ego climate, due to the type of sports practiced. The relationship between these two variables suggested that the task-oriented motivational climate was related to a diet of poorer quality in young Spaniards, observing the opposite in students from Romania. Finally, the structural equation model revealed how the task-oriented climate exerted a negative influence on the adherence to DM in Romanian students, while the ego-oriented climate exerted a positive influence on the quality of the diet of Spanish students.

It has been shown that the existence of extrinsic motivations can be linked to better nutrition, both for health purposes and the achievement of better sports performance. Although the motivations of intrinsic type are linked to healthier habits associated with sport practice, these were not related to nutrition. While further research is necessary to substantiate the findings from this study, there are adequate indications to pursue development of intervention programs aimed at improving the quality of diet, especially among students in Romania. On the other hand, such programs are also of vital importance for Spanish students, in order to obtain a better quality of the diet in those intrinsically motivated.

Author Contributions: R.C.-C., G.B., F.Z.-O. and M.C.-S. conceived the hypothesis of this study. F.Z.-O., R.C.-C. and G.B. participated in data collection. R.C.-C., M.C.-S. and F.Z.-O. analysed the data. All authors contributed to data interpretation of the statistical analysis. F.Z.-O., M.C.-S. and G.B. wrote the paper with significant input from R.C.-C. All authors read and approved the final manuscript.

Funding: This research received no external funding.

Conflicts of Interest: The authors declare no conflict of interest.

References

1. Redondo, M.P.; De Mateos, B.; Carreno, L.; Marugan, J.M.; Fernández, M.; Camina, M.A. Dietary intake and adherence to the Mediterranean diet in a group of university students depending. *Nutr. Hosp.* **2016**, *33*, 1172–1178. [CrossRef]
2. Belogianni, K.; Ooms, A.; Ahmed, H.; Nikoletou, D.; Grant, R.; Makris, D.; Moir, H.J. Rationale and design of an Online educational program using game-based learning to improve nutrition and physical activity outcomes among university students in the United Kingdom. *J. Am. Coll. Nutr.* **2018**, 1–8. [CrossRef] [PubMed]
3. Torstveit, M.K.; Johansen, B.T.; Haugland, S.H.; Stea, T.H. Participation in organized sports is associated with decreased likelihood of unhealthy lifestyle habits in adolescents. *Scand. J. Med. Sci. Sports* **2018**, *28*, 2384–2396. [CrossRef] [PubMed]
4. Zurita, F.; San Roman, S.; Chacon, R.; Castro, M.; Muros, J.J. Adherence to the Mediterranean Diet is associated with physical activity, self-concept and sociodemographic factors in university student. *Nutrients* **2018**, *10*, 966. [CrossRef] [PubMed]
5. Erwin, C.M.; McEvoy, C.T.; Moore, S.E.; Prior, L.; Lawton, J.; Kee, F.; Cupples, M.E.; Young, I.S.; Appleton, K.; McKinley, M.C.; et al. A qualitative analysis exploring preferred methods of peer support to encourage adherence to a Mediterranean diet in a Northern European population at high risk of cardiovascular disease. *BMC Public Health* **2017**, *18*, 213. [CrossRef] [PubMed]
6. Lotrean, L.M.; Stan, O.; Lencu, C.; Laza, V. Dietary patterns, physical activity, body mass index, weight-related behaviours and their interrelationship among Romanian university students-trends from 2003 to 2016. *Nutr. Hosp.* **2018**, *35*, 375–383. [CrossRef] [PubMed]
7. Esposito, K.; Maiorino, M.I.; Bellastella, G.; Panagiotakos, D.B.; Giugliano, D. Mediterranean diet for type 2 diabetes: Cardiometabolic benefits. *Endocrine* **2017**, *56*, 27–32. [CrossRef] [PubMed]
8. Godos, J.; Rapisarda, G.; Marventano, S.; Galvano, F.; Mistretta, A.; Grosso, G. Association between polyphenol intake and adherence to the Mediterranean diet in Sicily, southern Italy. *NFS J.* **2017**, *8*, 1–7. [CrossRef]
9. Yahia, N.; Achkar, A.; Abdallah, A.; Rizk, S. Eating habits and obesity among Lebanese university students. *Nutr. J.* **2008**, *7*, 32. [CrossRef]

10. Ortiz-Moncada, R.; Norte, A.I.; Zaragoza, A.; Fernández, J.; Davo, M.C. Mediterranean diet patterns follow Spanish university students. *Nutr. Hosp.* **2012**, *27*, 1952–1959. [CrossRef]
11. García, S.; Herrera, N.; Rodríguez, C.; Nissensohn, M.; Román, B.; Serra-Majem, L. KIDMED test; prevalence of low adherence to the Mediterranean diet in children and young; a systematic review. *Nutr. Hosp.* **2015**, *32*, 2390–2399. [CrossRef]
12. Baldini, M.; Pasqui, F.; Bordoni, A.; Maranesi, M. Is the Mediterranean lifestyle still a reality? Evaluation of food consumption and energy expenditure in Italian and Spanish university students. *Public Health Nutr.* **2008**, *12*, 148–155. [CrossRef] [PubMed]
13. Noale, M.; Nardi, M.; Limongi, F.; Siviero, P.; Caregaro, L.; Crepaldi, G.; Maggi, S. Mediterranean Diet Foundation Study Group. Adolescents in southern regions of Italy adhere to the Mediterranean diet more than those in the northern regions. *Nutr. Res.* **2014**, *34*, 771–779. [CrossRef] [PubMed]
14. Muros, J.J.; Cofre-Bolados, C.; Arriscado, D.; Zurita-Ortega, F.; Knox, E. Mediterranean diet adherence is associated with lifestyle, physical fitness, and mental wellness among 10-y-olds in Chile. *Nutrition* **2017**, *35*, 87–92. [CrossRef] [PubMed]
15. Sánchez-Villegas, A.; Ruiz-Canela, M.; Gea, A.; Lahortiga, F.; Martínez-González, M.A. The association between the Mediterranean lifestyle and depression. *Clin. Psychol. Sci.* **2016**, *4*, 1085–1093. [CrossRef]
16. Mosconi, L.; Walters, M.; Sterling, J.; Quinn, C.; McHugh, P.; Andrews, R.; Matthews, D.C.; Ganzer, C.; Osorio, R.S.; Isaacson, R.S.; et al. Lifestyle and vascular risk effects on MRI-based biomarkers of Alzheimer´s disease: A cross-sectional study of middle-aged adults from the broader New York City area. *BMJ Open* **2018**, *8*, e019362. [CrossRef] [PubMed]
17. Santomauro, F.; Lorini, C.; Tanini, T.; Indiani, L.; Lastrucci, V.; Comodo, N.; Bonaccorsi, G. Adherence to Mediterranean diet in a simple of Tuscan adolescents. *Nutrition* **2014**, *30*, 1379–1383. [CrossRef]
18. Baydemir, C.; Ozgur, E.G.; Balci, S. Evaluation of adherence to Mediterranean diet in medical students at Kocaeli University, Turkey. *J. Int. Med. Res.* **2018**, *46*, 1585–1594. [CrossRef]
19. Kyriacou, A.; Evans, J.M.; Economides, N.; Kyriacou, A. Adherence to the Mediterranean diet by the Greek and Cypriot population: A systematic review. *Eur. J. Public Health* **2015**, *25*, 1012–1018. [CrossRef]
20. Roccaldo, R.; Censi, L.; D'Addezio, L.; Toti, E.; Martone, D.; D'Addesa, D.; Cernigliaro, A. ZOOM8 Study group. Adherence to the Mediterranean diet in Italian school children (the ZOOM8 study). *Int. J. Food Sci. Nutr.* **2014**, *65*, 621–628. [CrossRef]
21. Chacón-Cuberos, R.; Castro-Sánchez, M.; Muros-Molina, J.J.; Espejo-Garcés, T.; Zurita-Ortega, F.; Linares-Manrique, M. Adherence to Mediterranean diet in university students and its relationship with digital leisure habits. *Nutr. Hosp.* **2016**, *33*, 405–410. [CrossRef]
22. Padial-Ruz, R.; Viciana-Garófano, V.; Palomares, J. Adherence to the Mediterranean diet, physical activity and its relationship with the BMI, in university students of the grade of Primary, mention in Physical Education of Granada. *Educ. Sport Health Phys. Act.* **2018**, *2*, 30–49.
23. Stefan, L.; Cule, M.; Milinovic, I.; Juranko, D.; Sporis, G. The relationship between lifestyle factors and body compositionin young adults. *Int. J. Environ. Res. Public Health* **2017**, *14*, 893. [CrossRef]
24. Tognon, G.; Hebestreit, A.; Lanfer, A.; Moreno, L.A.; Pala, V.; Siani, A.; Tornaritis, M.; De Henauw, S.; Veidebaum, T.; Molnár, D.; et al. Mediterranean diet, overweight and body composition in children from eight European countries: Cross-sectional and prospective results from the IDEFICS study. *Nutr. Metab. Cardiovasc. Dis.* **2014**, *24*, 205–213. [CrossRef] [PubMed]
25. Abenavoli, L.; Greco, M.; Milic, N.; Accattato, F.; Foti, D.; Gulletta, E.; Luzza, F. Effect of Mediterranean diet and antioxidant formulation in non-alcoholic fatty liver disease: A randomized study. *Nutrients* **2017**, *9*, 870. [CrossRef] [PubMed]
26. Salas-Salvadó, J.; Bulló, M.; Babio, N.; Martínez-González, M.Á.; Ibarrola-Jurado, N.; Basora, J.; Estruch, R.; Covas, M.I.; Corella, D.; Arós, F.; et al. Erratum. Reduction in the Incidence of Type 2 Diabetes with the Mediterranean Diet: Results of the PREDIMED-Reus nutrition intervention randomized trial. *Diabetes Care* **2018**, *34*, 14–19. [CrossRef] [PubMed]
27. Trovato, F.M.; Catalano, D.; Martines, G.F.; Pace, P.; Trovato, G.M. Mediterranean diet and non-alcoholic fatty liver disease: The need of extended and comprehensive interventions. *Clin. Nutr.* **2015**, *34*, 86–88. [CrossRef]
28. O'neil, A.; Quirk, S.E.; Housden, S.; Brennan, S.L.; Williams, L.J.; Pasco, J.A.; Berk, M.; Jacka, F.N. Relationship between diet and mental health in children and adolescents: A systematic review. *Am. J. Public Health* **2014**, *104*, e31–e42. [CrossRef]

29. Warburton, D.E.; Nicol, C.W.; Bredin, S.S. Health benefits of physical activity: The evidence. *Can. Med. Assoc. J.* **2006**, *174*, 801–809. [CrossRef]
30. Lewis, B.A.; Napolitano, M.A.; Buman, M.P.; Williams, D.M.; Nigg, C.R. Future directions in physical activity intervention research: Expanding our focus to sedentary behaviors, technology, and dissemination. *J. Behav. Med.* **2017**, *40*, 112–126. [CrossRef]
31. McMahon, E.M.; Corcoran, P.; O'Regan, G.; Keeley, H.; Cannon, M.; Carli, V.; Wasserman, C.; Hadlaczky, G.; Sarchiapone, M.; Apter, A.; et al. Physical activity in European adolescents and associations with anxiety, depression and well-being. *Eur. Child Adol. Psychiatr.* **2017**, *26*, 111–122. [CrossRef] [PubMed]
32. Krøll, L.S.; Hammarlund, C.S.; Westergaard, M.L.; Nielsen, T.; Sloth, L.B.; Jensen, R.H.; Gard, G. Level of physical activity, well-being, stress and self-rated health in persons with migraine and co-existing tension-type headache and neck pain. *J. Headache Pain* **2017**, *18*, 46. [CrossRef] [PubMed]
33. Roberts, G.C.; Treasure, D.C.; Balague, G. Achievement goals in sport: The development and validation of the Perception of Success Questionnaire. *J Sports Sci.* **1998**, *16*, 337–347. [CrossRef] [PubMed]
34. Ring, C.; Kavussanu, M. The impact of achievement goals on cheating in sport. *Psychol. Sport Exerc.* **2018**, *35*, 98–103. [CrossRef]
35. Lochbaum, M.; Kallinen, V.; Konttinen, N. Task and Ego Goal Orientations across the Youth Sports Experience. *Stud. Sport.* **2017**, *11*, 99–105. [CrossRef]
36. McLaren, C.D.; Newland, A.; Eys, M.; Newton, M. Peer-initiated motivational climate and group cohesion in youth sport. *J. Appl. Sport Psychol.* **2017**, *29*, 88–100. [CrossRef]
37. Chacón-Cuberos, R.; Muros-Molina, J.J.; Cachón, J.; Zagalaz, M.L.; Castro-Sánchez, M.; Zurita-Ortega, F. Physical activity, Mediterranean diet, maximal oxygen uptake and motivational climate towards sports in schoolchildren from the province of Granada: A structural equation model. *Nutr. Hosp.* **2018**, *35*, 774–781. [CrossRef]
38. Ryan, R.M.; Deci, E.L. *Self-Determination Theory: Basic Psychological Needs in Motivation, Development, and Wellness*; Guilford Publications: New York, NY, USA, 2017.
39. Hancox, J.E.; Quested, E.; Ntoumanis, N.; Thøgersen-Ntoumani, C. Putting self-determination theory into practice: Application of adaptive motivational principles in the exercise domain. *Qual. Res. Sport Exerc. Health* **2018**, *10*, 75–91. [CrossRef]
40. Hulleman, C.S.; Schrager, S.M.; Bodmann, S.M.; Harackiewicz, J.M. A meta-analytic review of achievement goal measures: Different labels for the same constructs or different constructs with similar labels? *Psychol. Bull.* **2010**, *136*, 422–449. [CrossRef]
41. Chacon, R.; Zurita, F.; Puertas, P.; Knox, E.; Cofre, C.; Viciana, V.; Muros, J.J. Relationship between healthy habits and perceived motivational climate in sport among university students: A structural equation model. *Sustainability* **2018**, *10*, 938. [CrossRef]
42. Moore, S.E.; McEvoy, C.T.; Prior, L.; Lawton, J.; Patterson, C.C.; Kee, F.; Cupples, M.; Young, I.S.; Appleton, K.; McKinley, M.C.; et al. Barriers to adopting a Mediterranean diet in Nothern European adults at high risk of developing cardiovascular disease. *J. Hum. Nutr. Diet* **2017**, *31*, 451–462. [CrossRef] [PubMed]
43. Chacón-Cuberos, R.; Zurita-Ortega, F.; Martínez-Martínez, A.; Olmedo-Moreno, E.; Castro-Sánchez, M. Adherence to the Mediterranean Diet Is Related to Healthy Habits, Learning Processes, and Academic Achievement in Adolescents: A Cross-Sectional Study. *Nutrients* **2018**, *10*, 1566. [CrossRef] [PubMed]
44. Erturan-Ilker, G.; Yu, C.; Alemdaroğlu, U.; Köklü, Y. Basic psychological needs and self-determined motivation in PE to predict health-related fitness level. *J. Sport Health Res.* **2018**, *10*, 91–100.
45. Dare, C.; Viebig, R.F.; Batista, N.S. Body composition and components of Mediterranean diet in Brazilian and European University Students. *RBONE* **2017**, *11*, 557–566.
46. Bottcher, M.R.; Marincic, P.Z.; Nahay, K.L.; Baerlocher, B.E.; Willis, A.W.; Park, J. Nutrition knowledge and Mediterranean diet adherence in the southeast United States: Validation of a field-based survey instrument. *Appetite* **2017**, *111*, 166–176. [CrossRef] [PubMed]
47. Merino-Marban, R.; Mayorga-Vega, D.; Fernandez-Rodríguez, E.; Estrada, F.; Viciana, J. Effect of a physical education-based stretching programme on sit-andreach score and its posterior reduction in elementary schoolchildren. *Eur. Phys. Educ. Rev.* **2015**, *21*, 83–92. [CrossRef]
48. Serra-Majem, L.; Ribas, L.; Ngo, J.; Ortega, R.M.; Garcia, A.; Pérez-Rodrigo, C.; Aranceta, J. Food, youth and the Mediterranean diet in Spain. Development of KIDMED, Mediterranean diet quality index in children and adolescents. *Public Health Nutr.* **2004**, *7*, 931–935. [CrossRef]

49. Newton, M.; Duda, J.; Yin, Z. Examination of the psychometric properties of the Perceived Motivational in Sport Questionnaire-2 in a sample of female athletes. *J. Sports Sci.* **2000**, *18*, 275–290. [CrossRef]
50. González-Cutre, C.D.; Sicilia, A.; Moreno, J.A. The social-cognitive model of achievement motivation in physical education. *Psicothema* **2008**, *20*, 642–651.
51. Baylis, K.; Nogueira, L.; Pace, K. Food import refusals: Evidence from the European Union. *Am. J. Agric. Econ.* **2010**, *93*, 566–572. [CrossRef]
52. Celis-Morales, C.; Livingstone, K.M.; Affleck, A.; Navas-Carretero, S.; San Cristobal, R.; Martínez, J.A.; Marsaux, C.F.; Saris, W.H.M.; O'Donovan, C.B.; Forster, H.; et al. Correlates of overall and central obesity in adults from seven European countries: Findings from the Food4Me Study. *Eur. J. Clin. Nutr.* **2018**, *72*, 207–219. [CrossRef] [PubMed]
53. Berry, E.M.; Arnoni, Y.; Aviram, M. The Middle Eastern and biblical origins of the Mediterranean diet. *Public Health Nutr.* **2011**, *14*, 2288–2295. [CrossRef] [PubMed]
54. Mantziki, K.; Renders, C.M.; Seidell, J.C. Water Consumption in European Children: Associations with Intake of Fruit Juices, Soft Drinks and Related Parenting Practices. *Int. J. Environ. Res. Public Health* **2017**, *14*, 583. [CrossRef] [PubMed]
55. Basu, S.; McKee, M.; Galea, G.; Stuckler, D. Relationship of soft drink consumption to global overweight, obesity, and diabetes: A cross-national analysis of 75 countries. *Am. J. Public Health* **2013**, *103*, 2071–2077. [CrossRef] [PubMed]
56. Bauman, A.; Bull, F.; Chey, T.; Craig, C.L.; Ainsworth, B.E.; Sallis, J.F.; Bowles, H.R.; Hagstromer, M.; Sjostrom, M.; Pratt, M.; et al. The international prevalence study on physical activity: Results from 20 countries. *Int. J. Behav. Nutr. Phys. Act.* **2009**, *6*, 1–11. [CrossRef] [PubMed]
57. Al-Yaaribi, A.; Kavussanu, M. Consequences of prosocial and antisocial behaviors in adolescent male soccer players: The moderating role of motivational climate. *Psychol. Sport Exerc.* **2018**, *37*, 91–99. [CrossRef]
58. Jaakkola, T.; Yli-Piipari, S.; Barkoukis, V.; Liukkonen, J. Relationships among perceived motivational climate, motivational regulations, enjoyment, and PA participation among Finnish physical education students. *Int. J. Sport Exerc. Psychol.* **2017**, *15*, 273–290. [CrossRef]
59. Harwood, C.G.; Keegan, R.J.; Smith, J.M.; Raine, A.S. A systematic review of the intrapersonal correlates of motivational climate perceptions in sport and physical activity. *Psychol. Sport Exerc.* **2015**, *18*, 9–25. [CrossRef]
60. Curran, T.; Hill, A.P.; Hall, H.K.; Jowett, G.E. Relationships between the coach-created motivational climate and athlete engagement in youth sport. *J. Sport Exerc. Psychol.* **2015**, *37*, 193–198. [CrossRef]
61. Gagea, A.; Marinescu, G.; Cordun, M.; Gagea, G.; Szabo, G.; Paunescu, M. Recreational sport culture in Romania and some European countries. *Rev. Cercet. Interv. Soc.* **2010**, *31*, 54–63.
62. Craig, C.L.; Marshall, A.L.; Sjostrom, M.; Bauman, A.E.; Booth, M.L.; Ainsworth, B.E.; Pratt, M.; Ekelund, U.; Yngve, A.; Sallis, J.F.; et al. International physical activity questionnaire: 12-country reliability and validity. *Med. Sci. Sports Exerc.* **2003**, *35*, 1381–1395. [CrossRef] [PubMed]
63. González-Valero, G.; Zurita-Ortega, F.; Puertas-Molero, P.; Chacón-Cuberos, R.; Garcés, T.E.; Sánchez, M.C. Education for health: Implementation of the program "Sportfruits" in schools of Granada. *SPORT TK* **2017**, *6*, 137–146. [CrossRef]
64. Heemsoth, T.; Retelsdorf, J. Student-student relations from the teacher versus student perspective: A multi-level confirmatory factor analysis. *Meas. Phys. Educ. Exerc. Sci.* **2018**, *22*, 48–60. [CrossRef]
65. Sánchez-Garcia, C.; López-Sánchez, G.F.; González-Carcelén, C.M.; Ibáñez-Ortega, E.J.; Díaz-Suárez, A. Physical fitness and body image of sports science students. *Educ. Sport, Health, Phys. Act.* **2018**, *2*, 92–104.
66. Ivashchenko, O.V.; Khudolii, O.M.; Yermakova, T.S.; Veremeenko, V.Y. Power abilities: The structure of development in girls of 12–14 years old. *Pedagog. Psychol. Med.-Biol. Probl. Phys. Train. Sports* **2018**, *4*, 195–202. [CrossRef]
67. Badau, A.; Badau, D.; Talaghir, L.G.; Rus, V. The impact of the needs and roles of nutrition counselling in sport. *Hum. Sport. Med.* **2018**, *18*, 88–96. [CrossRef]
68. Badicu, G. Physical Activity and Sleep Quality in Students of the Faculty of Physical Education and Sport of Braşov, Romania. *Sustainability* **2018**, *10*, 2410. [CrossRef]

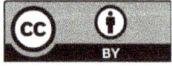

© 2018 by the authors. Licensee MDPI, Basel, Switzerland. This article is an open access article distributed under the terms and conditions of the Creative Commons Attribution (CC BY) license (http://creativecommons.org/licenses/by/4.0/).

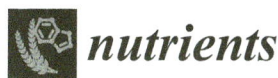

Review

Metabolomics and Microbiomes as Potential Tools to Evaluate the Effects of the Mediterranean Diet

Qi Jin [1], Alicen Black [1], Stefanos N. Kales [2], Dhiraj Vattem [1,3], Miguel Ruiz-Canela [4,5,6] and Mercedes Sotos-Prieto [1,2,7,*]

1. Division of Food Sciences and Nutrition, School of Applied Health Sciences and Wellness, Ohio University, Athens, OH 45701, USA; qj196613@gmail.com (Q.J.); ab914017@ohio.edu (A.B.); vattem@ohio.edu (D.V.)
2. Department of Environmental Health, Harvard T.H Chan School of Public Health, 677 Huntington Avenue, Boston, MA 02115, USA; skales@hsph.harvard.edu
3. Edison Biotechnology Institute, Ohio University, Athens, OH 45701, USA
4. Department of Preventive Medicine and Public Health, University of Navarra, 31008 Pamplona, Spain; mcanela@unav.es
5. IDISNA, Navarra Health Research Institute, 31008 Pamplona, Spain
6. CIBER Fisiopatología de la Obesidad y Nutrición (CIBER Obn), Instituto de Salud Carlos III, 28029 Madrid, Spain
7. Diabetes Institute, Ohio University, Athens, OH 45701, USA
* Correspondence: sotospri@ohio.edu; Tel.: +1-740-593-9943

Received: 14 December 2018; Accepted: 17 January 2019; Published: 21 January 2019

Abstract: The approach to studying diet–health relationships has progressively shifted from individual dietary components to overall dietary patterns that affect the interaction and balance of low-molecular-weight metabolites (metabolome) and host-enteric microbial ecology (microbiome). Even though the Mediterranean diet (MedDiet) has been recognized as a powerful strategy to improve health, the accurate assessment of exposure to the MedDiet has been a major challenge in epidemiological and clinical studies. Interestingly, while the effects of individual dietary components on the metabolome have been described, studies investigating metabolomic profiles in response to overall dietary patterns (including the MedDiet), although limited, have been gaining attention. Similarly, the beneficial effects of the MedDiet on cardiometabolic outcomes may be mediated through gut microbial changes. Accumulating evidence linking food ingestion and enteric microbiome alterations merits the evaluation of the microbiome-mediated effects of the MedDiet on metabolic pathways implicated in disease. In this narrative review, we aimed to summarize the current evidence from observational and clinical trials involving the MedDiet by (1) assessing changes in the metabolome and microbiome for the measurement of diet pattern adherence and (2) assessing health outcomes related to the MedDiet through alterations to human metabolomics and/or the microbiome.

Keywords: Mediterranean diet; metabolomics; microbiome

1. Introduction

The Mediterranean diet (MedDiet) is a dietary pattern that emphasizes the intake of vegetables, fruits, nuts, whole grains, fish, and unsaturated fats and vegetable oils (mainly olive oil) and aims to limit the intake of butter, sweets, and red and processed meat [1,2]. Multiple studies have found evidence of lower risk and incidence of and mortality from chronic metabolic diseases with adherence to the MedDiet [3–6]. The United States (US) Department of Agriculture and Health and Human Services recognized the MedDiet as a healthy dietary pattern in the 2015–2020 Dietary Guidelines for Americans [7,8], and this dietary pattern has been successfully adapted into workplace interventions [9]. Notwithstanding the MedDiet's growing acceptance for health improvement, the accurate assessments of exposure and adherence to the MedDiet in epidemiological studies and clinical interventions, respectively, continue to be major hurdles in advancing our understanding of the MedDiet's efficacy. Additionally, the underlining molecular and metabolic mechanisms that influence health outcomes in response to the MedDiet have not been elucidated.

The inherent subjectivity in the self-administered instruments used for dietary adherence/compliance assessment, such as food frequency questionnaires, multiple-day food records, and 24-h dietary recall, creates susceptibility to the introduction of bias and errors into data collection, ultimately impacting study outcomes [10–12]. There is an increasing consensus that employing objective measurement approaches (e.g., biomarkers and metabolic signatures) and robust research design (controlling for regression to the mean) concurrently with self-administered instruments may significantly improve data quality and validate study outcomes. However, logistical challenges, the economic burden, and the absence of reliable and sensitive biomarkers for dietary patterns, as opposed to an individual nutrient/ingredient, have limited the inclusion of objective analytical approaches in study methodologies. In this regard, leveraging rapid advances in high-throughput, big data omics technologies may overcome such pitfalls in nutritional epidemiology and intervention studies. Specifically, metabolomics (the study of low-molecular-weight metabolites in biological samples) and the research of microbiomes (the study of host-enteric microbial ecology) may facilitate the discovery and validation of specific biomarker signatures of dietary behavior and probe the complex interactions between food, lifestyle, and disease [13,14]. Generally, the most commonly used techniques in metabolomics analysis are mass spectrometry (MS), usually coupled with gas or liquid chromatography, and nuclear magnetic resonance (NMR) spectroscopy [15]. Each of these techniques has its own advantages and disadvantages. Both can be used to identify the structure of metabolites and measure the absolute and relative concentrations of metabolites. However, NMR has higher reproducibility and is more reliable for determining concentrations, while MS is more sensitive [15,16]. As for the analysis of the microbiome, techniques have evolved from culture-dependent methodologies to novel, next generation sequencing tools. The latter has allowed for the taxonomic and phylogenetic evaluation of the bacterial community based on 16S RNA gene amplicon analysis [17].

There is a growing body of knowledge on the metabolic signatures of individual food groups, such as fruit (proline betaine as a biomarker of citrus fruits) [18–22], vegetables (S-methyl-L-cysteine sulphoxide and its derivatives for cruciferous vegetables) [23–26], and whole grains (urinary excretions of alkylresorcinols and benzoxazinoid) [23,27–29] (Supplemental Table S1). However, notwithstanding the scientific interest in the matter, the literature on the metabolomics of overall diet patterns (including the MedDiet) is limited [30].

The importance of the gut microbiome in food digestion, nutrient metabolism, micronutrient production, enteric immunity, and gut function have been known for a long time [31,32]. Seminal papers published in the past two decades have expanded the understanding of the gut microbiome to overall human health and exposed the multilevel dimensional complexity of the diet–environment–microbiome–host interactions that impact human health [33–35]. The rapid expansion in this research area, in this regard, has disrupted the functional locality of the microbiome and highlighted its systemic effects beyond the gut, which are mediated by a combination of direct (physical) interactions of the microbes with the host and indirect processes via the production of metabolites, de novo or from diet. Moreover, the plasticity of the microbial ecology in response to diet and the growing evidence of the association between an altered ecological profile of the microbiome (dysbiosis) and disease have positioned the targeted and directed modulation of the gut microbiome as an exciting therapeutic target for a wide variety of pathologies, including acute infections (*Clostridium difficle*) [36], chronic illnesses (metabolic disease) [37], and mental health [38].

Sustained scientific exploration of the direct manipulation of gut ecology has identified strain-level specificity of microorganisms (e.g., lactic acid bacteria) for different health indications, as well as diet-derived natural or synthetic compounds that can stimulate colonization (fructooligosaccharides) and delivery mechanisms (encapsulation) to ensure survival and viability during gastrointestinal transit. The relative simplicity of this approach, favorable consumer perception, and historical correlation of fermented diets with health has allowed for the successful commercial exploitation of these principles by the food and beverage industry on a global scale. The rapid proliferation of consumer products (probiotic/prebiotics) and the dramatic growth of the size of this market continue to raise new instances of regulatory scrutiny and topics of policy debate [39].

The body of knowledge on the 'indirect' interactions between diet, the microbiome, and health via metabolite production is, on the other hand, relatively nascent [40]. The chemical complexity of diet, gut microbial diversity, and host-related genetic and lifestyle factors have been hurdles that have impeded investigations that attempt to reliably study even just the interaction of an individual dietary ingredient with health. Moreover, these challenges are amplified when attempting to delineate the effects of dietary patterns (e.g., the MedDiet) as opposed to one specific dietary ingredient (e.g., polyunsaturated fatty acid (PUFA)) on health outcomes. These problems are compounded when a potential metabolite of interest is produced both in the host and by the microbiome. For example, levels of trimethylamine oxide-N-oxide (TMAO) and its precursors choline and carnitine have been correlated with cardiovascular outcomes. However, establishing the relative contributions of the host, diet, and microbial dysbiosis have proven to be challenging in nutrition studies.

The application of big data and high-throughput omics approaches have successfully transformed physical, medical, forensic, and environmental sciences [41–43]. The combination of metabolomics and the study of the microbiome using powerful big data statistics can be leveraged to improve our understanding of the relationship between the MedDiet and health. In this narrative review, we summarize current scientific evidence from epidemiological studies focused on (1) the assessment of changes in the metabolome and microbiome for the measurement of adherence to the MedDiet pattern and (2) the understanding of the effect of the MedDiet on health outcomes through alterations in human metabolomics and/or the microbiome.

2. Metabolomics and the Mediterranean Diet—The Present Status

Strong evidence supports the use of the MedDiet as a preventive strategy to lower the risk of cardiovascular diseases (CVD) [44–46]. However, the characterization of the dietary pattern has been hindered due to the complex interactions between the human genome and diet [30,45]. Recent research in nutritional metabolomics has focused on discovering new biomarkers of nutritional exposure, nutritional status, and nutritional impacts on disease [47]. There is general consensus that establishing reliable biomarkers is imperative to facilitate the development of "precision nutrition", in which omics techniques can be applied to a personalized diet for the prevention and management of disease. Although relevant scientific literature is emerging on this topic, with several studies pursuing the identification of metabolic signatures for overall dietary patterns, few have focused specifically on the MedDiet [30]. Moreover, a collective endeavor in this regard can also be extended to discover biomarkers of health outcomes following a MedDiet intervention or dietary approaches [48]. Along these lines, this section will summarize the current status of the research on using metabolomics to assess the MedDiet pattern and to understand the associations between the MedDiet and health.

2.1. Metabolomics Approach as an Assessment of Adherence to the Mediterranean Diet

A recent review of the use of nutritional metabolomics to assess dietary intake found 16 studies on dietary patterns and metabolomics, of which only three specifically assessed the MedDiet pattern [30]. Here, we include three additional articles regarding metabolomics and dietary patterns in general [49,50] and four specifically about the MedDiet [51–53]. Metabolomics profiles have been characterized in multiple dietary patterns, including the New Nordic diet, low-fat diet, low glycemic index diet, very-low-carbohydrate diet, a diet concordant with World Health Organization (WHO) healthy eating guidelines, prudent diet, etc. A recent study assessing overall dietary patterns was a randomized, controlled, crossover study that used a targeted metabolomics method to assess concentrations of 333 plasma metabolites of three hypocaloric dietary patterns—low-fat, low glycemic index, and very-low-carbohydrate diets—to evaluate compliance with each for a 4-week period [49]. Using four types of constructed, Bayesian network classifiers, the plasma metabolites that were different from at least one other diet were diacylglycerols (DAG), triacylglycerols (TAG), and branched-chain amino acids (BCAA) [49]. For example, the low glycemic index diet had an intermediate concentration of most metabolites (105 out of 152), which differentiated it from the other two diets [49]. These metabolites included hippurate 5-aminolevulinic acid, pipecolic acid, cytosine, triacylglycerides, and hydroxyproline [49]. Another study identified two distinct dietary patterns using dietary and urinary metabolomics data obtained from the National Adult Nutrition Survey [50]. They used two-step cluster analysis in both urine and dietary data and identified in the latter a "healthy" and an "unhealthy" cluster [50]. Consistent with the previous studies, the authors found higher levels of hippurate and also betaine, anserine, N-phenylacetylglutamine, 3-hydroxybutyrate, citrate, tryptophan, and 2-aminoadipate in the healthy cluster [50]. Higher creatinine, glycylproline, N-aceytalglutamate, and theophylline were found in the unhealthy cluster, and the two dietary patterns were further supported by subsequent validation in the NutriTech food intake study [50]. Recently, the serum metabolic profile of the Dietary Approaches to Stop Hypertension (DASH) pattern identified the top 10 most influential known metabolites, which differed significantly between participants randomly assigned to the DASH diet compared with both the control diet and the fruit and vegetables diet [54].

With regards to the MedDiet pattern, while still emerging, the evidence about metabolomics and the MedDiet–health association remains limited [48]. Compared with general dietary patterns, the number of published studies exploring the metabolomics signatures of the MedDiet is relatively small. In addition to those studies addressed by Guasch et al. [30], we describe here the evidence of four additional studies. Table 1 provides a more detailed summary of the evidence from studies using metabolomics to assess potential biomarkers for the MedDiet. González-Guardia and colleagues investigated biomarkers in a crossover study with four isocaloric diets: the MedDiet supplemented with Coenzyme Q_{10} (Med + CoQ), the MedDiet, the Western diet high in saturated fat, and a low-fat, high-carbohydrate diet rich in n-3 polyunsaturated fat [55]. Greater urinary hippurate levels after the adherence to the Med + CoQ diet and greater phenylacetylglycine levels after adherence to the Western diet high in saturated fat were found in female participants [55]. This higher level of hippurate was reported to positively correlate with CoQ and plasma β-carotene levels and negatively correlate with gene expression of transcription factor Nrf2, thioredoxin, superoxide dismutase 1, and the gp91phox subunit of NADPH (nicotinamide adenine dinucleotide phosphate) oxidase gene expression [55].

Another cross-sectional study, using a targeted metabolomics approach explored the association between the effect of the interaction between polymorphisms and the MedDiet on the levels of 14 specific serum metabolites that could be related to dietary adherence [56]. These metabolites played key roles in gene-encoding enzymes modulated by nine previously genotyped polymorphisms [57–59]. The results showed that a 1 unit increase in adherence to the MedDiet pattern was associated with a 5% increase in 5-Methylfolate (5-MTHF) [56]. Finally, another cross-sectional study found that urine microbial metabolites (phenylacetylglutamine, p-cresol, and 4-hydroxyphenylacetate) defined high adherence to the MedDiet [60].

Table 1. Metabolomics as an assessment of the Mediterranean diet (MedDiet) dietary pattern.

	Study Design	Participants	Dietary Pattern/Intervention	Follow-Up	Biological Sample/Metabolomics Approach/Technique	Biomarkers Identified	Main Conclusion
Playdon et al., 2017 [51]	5 nested case-control studies (within the Alpha-Tocopherol, Beta-Carotene Cancer Prevention Study)	Male Finnish smokers n = 1336, aged 50–69 years	HEI [1] 2010, aMED [2], HDI [3], and BSD [4]	3 years	Serum Untargeted MS	HEI 2010, HDI and BSD: associated with 17, 11, and 10 identified metabolites, respectively. aMED: associated with 21 identifiable metabolites: 4 aminoacids (indolebutyrate, tryptophan betaine, N-methylproline, 3-Hydroxy-2-ethylpropionate); 1 carbohydrate (threitol); 2 co-factors (threonate, γ-CEHC [5]); 3 xenobiotics (stachydrine, Phytanate, ergothionein) 11 lipids (1-myristoleoylglycerophosphocholine (14:1), Scyllo-inositol, Mead acid (20:3n-9), g-CEHC, cis-4-Decenoyl carnitine, 3-Carboxy-4-methyl-5-propyl-2-furanpropanoate, linoleate (18:2n-6), linolenate (α or γ; 18:3n-3 or 18:3n-6), chiro-inositol, 1-linoleoylglycerol, DHA, methyl palmitate	The HEI-2010, aMED, HDI, and BSD were correlated with metabolites correlated with foods that are used to evaluate adherence to each score.
Vázquez-Fresno et al., 2015 [53]	Parallel-group, single-blind, multicenter, randomized, controlled feeding trial. A follow-up in the PREDIMED [6] study.	Clinically identified non-diabetic participants at high CVD [7] risk n = 98 aged 55–80 years	MedDiet [8] + EVOO [9] (n = 41) (MedDiet + nuts (n = 27) LFD [10] (n = 30)	3 years	Urine (baseline, 1 year, and 3 year of the intervention) Untargeted NMR	MedDiet: carbohydrates (3-HB [11], citrate, and cisaconitate), creatine, creatinine, amino acids (proline, N-acetylglutamine, glycine, branched-chain amino acids, and derived metabolites), lipids (oleic and suberic acids), and microbial cometabolites (PAGN [12] and p-cresol) LFD: hippurate, TMAO [13], anserine, histidine and derivates (3-MH [14], 1-MH, carnosine, anserine), and xanthosine.	The MedDiet groups had distinct metabolic profiles compared to the baseline and control group related to carbohydrate and lipid metabolism, amino acids, and microbial cometabolites (PAGN and p-cresol).
Bondia-Pons et al., 2015 [52]	Randomized controlled dietary intervention	Individuals with high BMI and at least two features of metabolic syndrome. N = 72	RESMENA [15] diet (n = 47) (based on MedDiet). 7 meals/day. (40% CHO [16], 30%protein, 30% lipid). Control diet (n = 45) (American Heart Association guidelines). 5 meals/day (55% CHO 55%, 15% protein, 30% lipid)	6-month (2-month nutritional learning followed by a 4-month self-control period)	Plasma Non-targeted MS-Liquid	Lipids, mainly phospholipids and lysophospholipids. lactic acid, L-isoleucine, alloisoleucine, hydroxyvaleric acid, hypaphorine, paraxanthine, hippuric acid, furancarboxylic acid, LysoPC [17] (14:0), LysoPC (20:5), LysoPE [18] (16:1), LysoPC (22:6), LysoPE (20:4), LysoPC (18:2), LysoPC (16:0), Linoleamide, LysoPC (20:3), LysoPE (18:1), LysoPC (18:1), LysoPC (20:4), Eicosapentaenoic acid, LysoPC (15:0), Lithocholic acid, Oleamide, 1-Monopalmitin, LysoPC (18:0), GPL [19] containing (18:2), Palmitic acid, PC [20], and PE [21]	The major discriminative markers between the two groups were the plasmalogen PC (p 22, 18:1/20:3) after 2 months and palmitic acid after 6 months.

127

Table 1. Cont.

	Study Design	Participants	Dietary Pattern/Intervention	Follow-Up	Biological Sample/Metabolomics Approach/Technique	Biomarkers Identified	Main Conclusion
González-Guardia et al., 2015 [55]	Randomized, crossover	Men ($n = 5$) and women ($n = 5$) aged 65 years or older. $n = 10$	MedDiet+ 200mg/d CoQ [23], MedDiet without CoQ, Western diet rich in SFA [24], Low-fat, high-carbohydrate diet enriched in n-3 PUFA [25]	4 weeks	Urine and plasma Targeted NMR	CoQ and β-carotene plasma levels and isoprostanes urinary levels were determined. Higher levels of hippurate and lower levels of phenylacetylglycine were found when comparing the MedDiet + CoQ and the SFA.	The MedDiet supplemented with CoQ is associated with increased levels of excreted hippurate and decreased levels of phenylacetylglycine compared with a SFA-rich diet.
Kakkoura et al., 2017 [56]	Cross-sectional study.	Greek-Cypriot control women who have previously participated in the population-based case-control study of BC, MASTOS [61]. $n = 564$	MedDiet (highest and lowest adherence to MedDiet)	N/A	Serum Targeted. UPLC-MS/MS	5-MTHF [26], riboflavin, FMN [27], PA, methionine, methionine sulfoxide, SAM [28], SAH [29], total HCY [30], cystathionine, total cysteine, γ-glu-cys, total GSH [31] and α-hydroxybutyrate.	Higher adherence to the MedDiet was associated with an increase in antioxidant-related metabolites, 5-MTHF.

[1] HEI: Healthy Eating Index. [2] aMED: Mediterranean diet score. [3] HDI: the WHO Healthy Diet Indicator. [4] BSD: the Baltic Sea Diet. [5] CEHC: carboxyethyl hydroxychroman. [6] PREDIMED: Prevención con Dieta Mediterránea. [7] CVD: cardiovascular disease. [8] MedDiet: Mediterranean diet. [9] EVOO: extra virgin olive oil. [10] LFD: a control, low-fat diet. [11] HB: hydroxybutyrate. [12] PAGN: phenylacetylglutamine. [13] TMAO: Trimethylamine N-oxide. [14] MH: Methylhistidine [15] RESMENA: Metabolic Syndrome Reduction in Navarra. [16] CHO: Carbohydrates. [17] LysoPC: lysophosphatidylcholine. [18] LysoPE: lysophosphatidylethanolamine. [19] GPL: glycerophospholipid. [20] PC: phosphatidylcholine. [21] PE: phosphatidylethanolamine. [22] P: plasmalogen. [23] CoQ: coenzyme Q. [24] SFA: Saturated fatty acids. [25] PUFA: polyunsaturated fatty acids. [26] 5-MTHF: L-Methylfolate. [27] FMN: flavin mononucleotide. [28] SAM: S-adenosylmethionine. [29] SAH: S-adenosylhomocysteine. [30] HCY: Homocysteine. [31] GSH: glutathione. MS: Mass spectrometry; DHA: Docosahexaenoic Acid; NMR: nuclear magnetic resonance; BMI: Body mass index. 5-MTHF: 5-Methylfolate.

2.2. Metabolomics, the Mediterranean Diet, and the Association with Health

Several studies have investigated the role of metabolites on the etiological and patho-physiological processes implicated in cardiovascular disease and related morbidities. For example, in a meta-analysis, the results from prospective studies support robust positive associations of BCAAs (leucine, isoleucine, and valine) and aromatic amino acids (tyrosine and phenylalanine) and inverse associations of glycine and glutamine with incident type 2 diabetes (T2D) [62]. Similarly, the results from a systematic review showed that the metabolites associated with CVD risk were acylcarnitines and dicarboxylacylcarnitines, TMAO, and several amino acids, such as phenylalanine, glutamate, and several lipid classes [63]. Although it is known that the MedDiet is associated with lower risk of CVD, attempts to correlate MedDiet-adherence-derived metabolites with CVD-associated biomarkers and clinical outcomes have proved inconclusive. For example in the randomized, controlled OmniHeart study, blood pressure was found to be significantly associated with six urinary metabolites reflecting dietary intake [64], and among those following the New Nordic Diet, higher levels of vaccenic acid and 3-hydroxybutanoic acid were related to higher weight loss, while higher concentrations of salicylic, lactic, and N-aspartic acids and 1,5-anhydro-d-sorbitol were related to lower weight loss [65]. Evidence from studies specifically addressing the MedDiet come from the PREDIMED (Prevención con Dieta Mediterránea) study (a randomized, controlled trial with a 4.8-year follow-up) that has focused on baseline and 1-year changes in metabolites after following the MedDiet supplemented with extra virgin olive oil (EVOO) or nuts in comparison with a low-fat diet and its association with CVD and T2D. In this section, we summarized the evidence of metabolomics relating to the MedDiet pattern and its association with CVD and T2D (Table 2).

All the studies evaluating the metabolites in the PREDIMED study followed a nested case–cohort study design, by which between 10–20% of the original study participants were randomly selected along with all the incident cases of CVD (n = 229–233) or diabetes (n = 251). The studies focusing on CVD, were assessing most of the metabolites already identified to be associated with CVD, including the following: BCAAs, choline pathway, different classes of lipids, ceramides, tryptophan, acylcarnitines, and glutamine. Higher concentrations of short and medium acylcarnitines [66], choline pathway metabolites (TMAO, betaine, choline, phosphocholine, and α-glycerophosphocholine) [67], kynurenine risk score [68], ceramides [69], glutamine [70], and some lipids (monoacylglicreol (MAG), DAG, short-chain triacylglycerol (TAG)) [71] were associated with increased CVD risk at the baseline. On the contrary, higher tryptophan, cholesterol esters (CE), glutamine/glutamate ratio, and polyunsaturated phosphatidylcholines were associated with lower risk of CVD (Figure 1). When the one-year changes in the metabolites were assessed, their associations with CVD were less clear. Only changes in acylcarnitynes [66] and phosphatidylethanolamine [71] were associated with the composite of CVD risk. Similarly, the role of the MedDiet in mediating the association seemed to be more significant when baseline metabolites were assessed. The MedDiet counteracted the deleterious effect of the high tryptophan risk score [68] and modulated the risk at the baseline for acylcarnitines [66], choline [67], ceramides [69], and glutamine [70], demonstrating the cardioprotective effects of the MedDiet by shedding some light on the biological mechanisms.

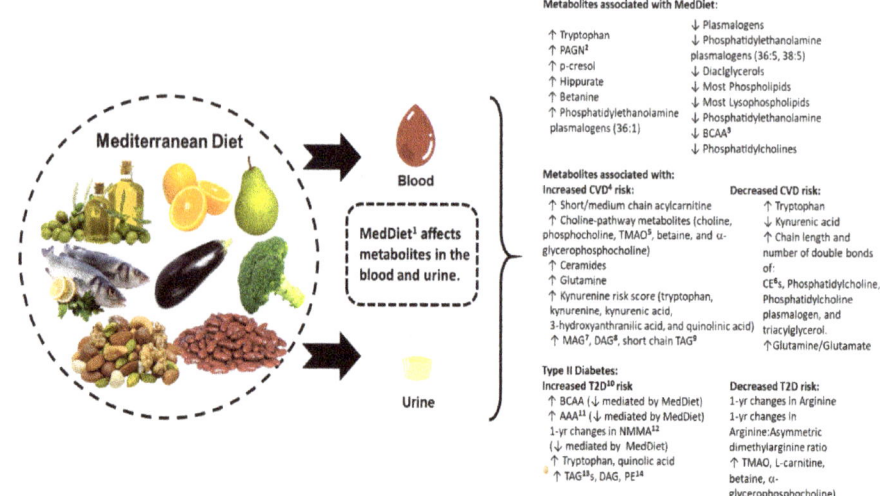

Figure 1. Depiction of the metabolites associated with adherence to the MedDiet in the absence and presence of disease. All the increases in the metabolite profiles are identified with an up arrow, and all the decreases are identified with a down arrow. In general, the results from the PREDIMED study suggest that the MedDiet may counteract the deleterious effect of metabolites related to CVD and diabetes and that it is able to reduce the levels of some of them (e.g., tryptophan and BCAA) after one-year of intervention in comparison with the control group. [1] MedDiet: Mediterranean diet. [2] PAGN: phenylacetylglutamine. [3] BCAA: branched-chain amino acids. [4] CVD: cardiovascular disease. [5] TMAO: Trimethylamine N-oxide. [6] CE: cholesterol ester. [7] MAG: monoacylglycerols. [8] DAG: diacylglycerols. [9] TAG: Triacylglycerol. [10] T2D: type 2 diabetes. [11] AAA: aromatic amino acid. [12] NMMA: N-methylmalonamic acid. [13] TAG: triacylglycerols; [14] PE: phosphatidylethanolamines. ↓: decreased with the consumption of MedDiet. ↑: increased with consumption of MedDiet.

As with CVD, some metabolites have been associated with T2D (nested case–cohort PREDIMED study with around 250–251 cases of T2D) (Table 2). Higher concentrations of BCAAs, aromatic amino acid (phenylalanine and tyrosine) [72], changes in ornitin and citrulline [73], triacylglycerols (TAG), DAG, phosphatidylethanolamines (PE) [74], tryptophan, and one-year changes in quinolic [75] were associated with higher risk of T2D. In contrast, TMAO, L-carnitine, betaine, α-glycerophosphocholine [76], and arginine: asymmetric dimethylarginine (ADMA) [73] were associated with lower risk of T2D. Only BCAAs, aromatic amino acid, and tryptophan interacted with the MedDiet + EVOO intervention to modulate the risk of T2D [72] (Figure 1).

In summary, the above studies demonstrated extensive variability in the metabolomic signatures of the MedDiet pattern, disease biomarkers, and clinical health outcomes (Figure 1). These may result from disparities in the biological samples (urine versus plasma/serum), the frequency of metabolite analysis, the analytical methods/techniques, inter-laboratory variability, and differences in the study design, the participant health status, and the MedDiet composition (e.g., Mediterranean countries have a higher consumption of olive oil than non-Mediterranean countries). Furthermore, different self-reported dietary assessment tools and inherent recall errors and biases exacerbate metabolomic profile inconsistencies across different MedDiet studies. Future approaches should attempt to standardize the above stated methodological discrepancies and also validate the findings in wider populations, especially for the MedDiet, for which little information is available outside of the PREDIMED study.

Table 2. Metabolomics, the Mediterranean diet pattern, and its association with CVD and T2D.

Author	Study Design	Study Population	Dietary Pattern/Intervention	Follow-Up	Biological Sample/Metabolomics Approach	Metabolites Examined	Main Conclusion
Guasch-Ferré et al., 2016 [66]	Case-cohort study within the PREDIMED [1] study	Participants aged 55–80 years at high risk of CVD [2]. n = 980 (229 cases CVD cases).	MedDiet [3] groups: (MedDiet + EEVO [4] and MedDiet + mixed nuts. Control group: low-fat diet.	4.8 years	Plasma. (baseline and after 1 year) Targeted	28 acylcarnitines: short-chain acylcarnitines (C2–C7), medium-chain acylcarnitines (C8–C14), and long-chain acylcarnitines (C16–C26).	An increased level of acylcarnitines metabolic profiles is independently associated with total CVD risk and risk of stroke. MedDiet interventions may attenuate the association between acylcarnitines and CVD risk.
Guasch-Ferré et al., 2017 [67]	Case-cohort study within the PREDIMED study	Participants aged 55–80 years at high risk of CVD. n = 980 (229 CVD cases)	MedDiet groups: (MedDiet + EEVO and MedDiet + mixed nuts. Control group: low-fat diet.	4.8 years	Plasma (baseline and after 1 year) Targeted	Metabolites of the choline pathway: TMAO [5], betaine, choline, phosphocholine, and a-glycerophosphocholine. A choline metabolite score was created.	The baseline choline metabolite score was associated with increased risk of CVD. The one-year changes in plasma metabolites were not significantly associated with CVD. The participants in the highest metabolite score quartile and assigned to low-fat diets had higher risk of CVD than those in the lowest metabolite quartile and in the MedDiet group. No significant interaction was found between the continuous choline score, the betaine/choline ratio, and the intervention group and CVD
Yu et al., 2017 [68]	Case-cohort study within the PREDIMED study, controlled trial	Participants aged 55–80 at high risk of CVD. n = 985 (231 CVD cases)	MedDiet groups: (MedDiet + EEVO and MedDiet + mixed nuts. Control group: low-fat diet.	4.7 year	Plasma (baseline and after 1 year) Targeted	Tryptophan, kynurenine, kynurenic acid, 3-hydroxyanthranilic acid, and quinolinic acid concentrations. A KRS [6] was created.	The positive association between the KRS and CVD risk is stronger in the control group, indicating that the MedDiet may attenuate the effect of a high KRS score.
Toledo et al., 2017 [77]	Case-cohort study within the PREDIMED study	Participants aged 55–80 years at high risk of CVD. n = 983 (230 CVD cases)	MedDiet groups: (MedDiet + EEVO and MedDiet + mixed nuts. Control group: low-fat diet.	4.8 years	Plasma (baseline and after 1 year) Untargeted lipidome	202 lipid species	The baseline concentrations of cholesterol esters (CEs) were inversely associated with CVD. The MedDiet interventions resulted in changes in the lipidome at 1 year; however, they were not found to be associated with subsequent CVD risk. Lipid metabolites with a longer acyl chain and a higher number of double bonds at the baseline were significantly and inversely associated with the risk of CVD.
Wang et al., 2017 [69]	Case-cohort study within the PREDIMED study	Participants aged 55–80 years at high risk of CVD. n = 980 (230 CVD cases)	MedDiet groups: (MedDiet + EEVO and MedDiet + mixed nuts. Control group: low-fat diet.	≤7.4 years	Plasma (baseline and after 1 year) Targeted	4 different ceramides: ceramide (d [7] 18:1/16:0), ceramide (d18:1/22:0), ceramide (d18:1/24:0), and ceramide (d18:1/24:1). A ceramide score was calculated.	The ceramide score was positively associated with the risk of CVD. The MedDiet may alleviate the potential negative effects of increased plasma ceramide levels on CVD.

Table 2. Cont.

Author	Study Design	Study Population	Dietary Pattern/Intervention	Follow-Up	Biological Sample/ Metabolomics Approach	Metabolites Examined	Main Conclusion
Zheng et al., 2017 [70]	Case-cohort study within the PREDIMED study	Participants aged 55–80 years at high risk of CVD. $n = 980$ (788 subcohort, 192 incident external cases)	MedDiet groups (intervention diets): (MedDiet + EEVO and MedDiet + mixed nuts. Control group: low-fat diet.	4.8 years	Plasma (baseline and after 1 year) Targeted	Glu[14] Gln[15], Glu/Gln ratio	A positive association between Glu levels and CVD risk (43% increased risk) and a negative association between Gln/Glu and risk of CVD (25% decreased risk) were found. The interventions effectively lowered CVD risk for the participants with high baseline Glu, while no effects were found among the participants with low baseline Glu. No significant effect of the intervention on one-year changes in the metabolites. No effect of the changes themselves on the CVD risk was apparent.
Razquin et al., 2018 [71]	Unstratified case-cohort design within the PREDIMED study.	$n = 983$ participants (233 CVD cases).	MedDiet groups: (MedDiet + EEVO and MedDiet + mixed nuts. Control group: low-fat diet.	4.8 years	Plasma (baseline and after 1 year)	Lipid group A: PC [10] (PCs, LysoPC[11]s and PC-plasmalogens with ≥5 double bonds); CE [12] with N3 double bonds; and TAG [13] with ≥52 carbon atoms containing ≥6 double bonds. Lipid group B: MAG [14], DAG [15], short-chain, TAGs containing ≤4 double bonds; PEs [16] except those with saturated fatty acids; hydroxyPC. PC, CE, long-chain TAG, MAG and DAG, short-chain TAG, PE, and Hpc [17] scores were calculated.	The metabolites from lipid group A were inversely associated with CVD; the metabolites from lipid group B were directly associated with CVD. The baseline phosphatidylethanolamines (PEs) and their one-year changes tended to be associated with higher CVD risk. No significant effect of the MedDiet intervention was found on the metabolite scores.
Ruiz-Canela et al., 2016 [78]	Case-cohort study within the PREDIMED study	$n = 970$ (226 CVD cases)	MedDiet groups: (MedDiet + EEVO and MedDiet + mixed nuts. Control group: low-fat diet.	4.8 years	Plasma (baseline and after 1 year)	BCAAs	Higher concentrations of baseline BCAAs were associated with increased risk of CVD. No significant effect of the intervention on one-year changes in BCAAs or any association between one-year changes in BCAAs and CVD were observed.
Yu et al., 2017 [73]	Case-cohort study within the PREDIMED study	$n = 984$ (231 CVD cases)	MedDiet groups: (MedDiet +EEVO and MedDiet + mixed nuts. Control group: low-fat diet.	4.7 years	Plasma (baseline and after 1 year)	arginine, ornithine, citrulline, ADMA [18], symmetric dimethylarginine (SDMA [19]), and NG-monomethylarginine (NMMA [20])	A higher baseline arginine/asymmetric dimethylarginine ratio was associated with lower CVD incidence. No significant modification by the MedDiet after one-year intervention was observed.
Guasch-Ferre et al., 2018 [79]	Case-cohort study in the PREDIMED study	$n = 892$ participants (251 T2D cases)	MedDiet groups: (MedDiet + EEVO and MedDiet + mixed nuts. Control group: low-fat diet	3.8 years	Plasma (baseline and after 1 year)	Short-chain acylcarnitines (C2–C7), medium-chain acylcarnitines (C8–C14), and long-chain acylcarnitines (C16–C26).	The acylcarnitines profile, specifically short- and long- chain acylcarnitines, was significantly associated with a higher risk of T2D.

Table 2. Cont.

Author	Study Design	Study Population	Dietary Pattern/Intervention	Follow-Up	Biological Sample/ Metabolomics Approach	Metabolites Examined	Main Conclusion
Yu et al., 2018 [73]	Case-cohort study in the PREDIMED study	n = 892 participants (251 T2D cases)	MedDiet groups: (MedDiet + EEVO and MedDiet + mixed nuts. Control group: low-fat diet	1 year	Plasma	Arginine, citrulline, ornithine, ADMA, SDMA, and NMMA	The one-year changes in arginine and the arginine/ADMA ratio were negatively associated with the risk of T2D [21]. Positive changes in ornithine and citrulline and negative changes in SDMA and GABR were inversely associated with concurrent changes in HOMA-IR [22]. The MedDiet significantly modified the association between one-year changes in NMMA and T2D risk.
Ruiz-Canela et al., 2018 [72]	Case-cohort study in the PREDIMED study	n = 945 participants (251 T2D cases)	MedDiet groups: (MedDiet + EEVO and MedDiet + mixed nuts. Control group: low-fat diet	3.8 years	Plasma (baseline and after 1 year)	The baseline BCAA [23] (leucine, isoleucine and valine) and AAA [24] (phenylalanine and tyrosine) scores were associated with a higher risk of T2D. Increases in the BCAA score after one year were associated with higher T2D risk only in the control group.	The MedDiet rich in EVOO significantly reduced the levels of BCAA and attenuated the positive association between plasma BCAA levels and T2D incidence.
Papandreou et al. 2018 [76]	Case-cohort study in the PREDIMED study	n = 945 participants (251 T2D cases)	MedDiet groups: (MedDiet + EEVO and MedDiet + mixed nuts. Control group: low-fat diet	3.8 years	Plasma (baseline and after 1 year)	TMAO, L-carnitine, betaine, LPC and LPE species, phosphocholine, α-glycerophosphocholine, and choline. Higher baseline concentrations of TMAO, L-carnitine, betaine, α-glycerophosphocholine, and several LPC [25] and LPE [26] species were associated with a lower risk of T2D development.	There was no significant difference in the association of most of the one-year changes in the metabolites with T2D risk in the MedDiet intervention and control groups. The intervention diets did not appear to significantly change the study metabolite levels during the intervention.
Razquin et al. (2018) [74]	Case-cohort study in the PREDIMED study	n = 942 participants (250 T2D cases)	MedDiet groups: (MedDiet + EEVO and MedDiet + mixed nuts. Control group: low-fat diet	3.8 years	Plasma (baseline and after 1 year)	The baseline TAGs, DAGs, and PEs were positively associated with T2D risk. TAGs with odd-chain fatty acids showed inverse associations with T2D after adjusting for total TAGs.	The one-year changes in the baseline metabolites associated with T2D were not significant. The changes in LP [27], PC-PL [28], SM [29], and CE scores showed no apparent mediating effects.
Yu et al., 2018 [75]	Case-cohort study in the PREDIMED study	n = 892 participants (251 T2D cases)	MedDiet groups: (MedDiet + EEVO and MedDiet + mixed nuts. Control group: low-fat diet	3.8 years	Plasma (baseline and after 1 year) Targeted	Tryptophan, kynurenine, kynurenic acid, 3-hydroxyanthranilic acid, and quinolinic acid concentrations. A KRS score was created.	The baseline tryptophan and one-year increases in quinolinic acid were positively associated with incident T2D. No effect of the MedDiet was observed.

[1] PREDIMED: Prevención con Dieta Mediterránea. [2] CVD: cardiovascular disease. [3] MedDiet: Mediterranean diet. [4] EVOO: extra virgin olive oil. [5] TMAO: trimethylamine N-oxide. [6] KRS: kynurenine risk score. [7] d: shorthand notation of sphingolipids refer to 1,3 dihydroxy. [8] Glu: glutamate. [9] Gln: glutamine. [10] PC: phosphatidylcholines. [11] LysoPC: lysophosphatidylcholine. [12] CE: cholesterol esters. [13] TAG: long-chain triacylglycerols. [14] MAG: monoacylglycerols. [15] DAG: diacylglycerols. [16] PE: phosphatidylethanolamine. [17] hPC: hydroxyPC. [18] ADMA: asymmetric dimethylarginine. [19] SDMA: symmetric dimethylarginine. [20] NMMA: N-monomethyl-l-arginine. [21] T2D: type 2 diabetes. [22] HOMA-IR: homeostatic model assessment of insulin resistance. [23] BCAA: branched-chain amino acids. [24] AAA: aromatic amino acids. [25] LPC: lyso-phosphatidylcholine. [26] LPE: lyso-phosphatidylethanolamine. [27] LP: lysophospholipids. [28] PC-PL: phosphatidylcholine-plasmalogens. [29] SM: sphingomyelins.

3. Microbiome and the Mediterranean Diet—The Present Status

The human gut is a highly diverse ecosystem consisting of 10–100 trillion microbial cells that are mostly bacteria, but it also includes viruses, archaea, fungi, and others [46,80]. Quantitatively, the total number of microbial genes in the gut or 'gut microbiome' outnumbers the host (human) genome by 100 to 1 [81], and they may significantly impact the host's physiology and ultimately health. Recent advances in 16S rRNA-based sequencing technologies have facilitated species-level identification of several of these non-culturable bacteria, with the majority belonging to the phyla Firmicutes, Bacteroidetes, Actinobacteria, and Proteobacteria [46,82,83]. Evidence suggests that there are complex and dynamic associations between the host's health, diet, lifestyle, and environment and the composition of the host's gut microbiome throughout the host's lifespan [84]. Elucidating causal relationships between intrinsic/extrinsic host factors on the gut microbiome and the impact of the gut microbiome on metabolic functions, immunity, and health outcomes is currently an area of active investigation globally [85–90].

It has been estimated that about 57% of the microbiome's entire variation is due to dietary habits, emphasizing the importance of diet in gut microbial ecology [91]. However, studies exploring the relationship between the gut microbiome and diet have primarily focused on single nutrients or foods and microbial response [92]. The literature describing the influence of dietary patterns, a more comprehensive determinant of health, on the microbiome is very limited. For example, with respect to the MedDiet, several studies have assessed the impact of olive oil [93], red wine [94], whole grains [95], or other individual components on microbiota, but few have analyzed the MedDiet pattern in its entirety [92]. Research on the MedDiet's effects on the composition of the microbiome and the contribution of the composition of the microbiome to MedDiet-related health outcomes will be reviewed in the next two sections.

3.1. Mediterranean Diet Effects on General Microbiome Composition

Although microbiome changes in response to habitual dietary intake are not very well understood, general associations between some dietary components/patterns and microbiota have been noted in the literature. For example, elevated levels of *Bacteroides sp.* in the gut have been observed with a Western-style dietary pattern that is rich in animal protein and saturated fat, while gut *Prevotella sp.* have been shown to increase with the consumption of carbohydrates, especially from vegetables and grains, or a more Mediterranean-style diet [46,96,97]. As described above, the physiological effects of the microbiome are mediated by a combination of direct (physical) interactions of the microbe with the host and indirect processes via the production of fermentation metabolites, *de novo* or from diet. The profile of gut bacterial metabolites from fermentation is a function of both the bacterial ecology and the substrate (i.e., fermentation of dietary fiber and other complex carbohydrates, which are prominent in the MedDiet, or other plant-based foods results in short-chain fatty acids (SCFA) as opposed to TMAO, which is usually seen in populations consuming diets rich in red meats). Table 3 lists studies that evaluated the consumption of the MedDiet and its effects on the microbial composition in healthy individuals. A recent, comparative, cross-sectional study explored the differences between two groups of teenagers from different geographical locations (Egypt versus United States) with respect to their microbial ecology, enterotype clustering function, and metabolite production in response to their dietary intake. The authors found that in the group of Egyptian teenagers, who were primarily exposed to a Mediterranean-style diet, all the gut microbial communities belonged to the *Prevotella* enterotype. In contrast, almost all of the American teenagers in the study had gut microbial communities belonging to the *Bacteroides* enterotype [96]. In an earlier 10-day controlled-feeding study that examined gut microbial enterotypes as a result of high-fat/low-fiber or low-fat/high-fiber diets, Wu et al. found similar results but additionally observed that the enterotype of the host microbiome remained unaltered as the relative distributions (abundance) of bacterial phyla and genera levels changed within 24 h of initiating a new diet pattern [97]. However, the magnitude of the changes was modest and was not sufficient to switch the individuals between the enterotype clusters associated with protein/fat and carbohydrates, suggesting an association between a long-term Mediterranean-style diet and enterotype partitioning [97].

In a randomized controlled trial, Djuric and colleagues explored the relationship between carotenoid concentrations and mucosal colonic bacteria in healthy individuals at an increased risk of colon cancer. Colonic biopsy samples ($n = 88$ at baseline, $n = 82$ after dietary intervention) were obtained from the Healthy Eating study, in which the participants were assigned to one of two dietary interventions, a MedDiet or a Healthy Eating diet for 6 months, with the primary difference being the total fat content of the diet [98,99]. The researchers found that after the interventions, the colonic mucosal bacteria was not significantly altered. However, 11 operational taxonomic units were significantly associated with increased serum carotenoid concentrations, including lower Firmicutes taxa and higher Proteobacteria abundance. Additionally, an increased abundance of *Prevotella sp.* was observed in the highest carotenoid tertile [100]. These findings are consistent with other "short-term" dietary intervention studies on the microbiome and suggest that long-term dietary patterns may have a greater impact on changes in microbial ecology. The results from other cross-sectional studies also evidence the higher abundance of *Prevotella sp.* with greater adherence to the MedDiet [92,101]. De Filippis et al. found that *Prevotella sp.* was specifically associated with fiber-degrading Firmicutes and increased levels of fecal SCFA, which has been associated with health benefits [40]. Consistent with the previous section, higher urinary TMAO was associated with lower adherence to the MedDiet. Another cross-sectional study assessing the association between the MedDiet and microbial-derived phenolic compounds in stool samples ($n = 74$) found that subjects with greater MedDiet scores had statistically higher levels of *Clostridium* cluster XIVa and *Faecalibacterium prausnitzii*, which is a butyrate producer with proposed anti-inflammatory properties. This suggests the MedDiet may produce more beneficial bacteria in the gut, which produces healthy metabolites. They also found that *Akkermansia sp.*, Bacteroides-*Prevotella-Porphirimonas sp.*, and *Bifidobacterium sp.* trended higher in the 42 subjects scoring ≥4 on the MedDiet score (range 0–8); however, there was a smaller presence of the *Lactobacillus sp.* group in the greater MedDiet adherence group [102].

In an earlier cross-sectional study, Gutierrez-Diaz and colleagues explored the effects of the MedDiet in 31 healthy subjects. The study found that several individual components of the MedDiet were associated with an abundance of specific gut taxa. For example, cereals were linked to *Bifidobacterium sp.* and *Faecalibacterium sp.*, olive oil with Tenericutes and *Dorea sp.*, red wine with *Faecalibacterium sp.*, vegetables with Rikenellaceae, *Dorea sp.*, *Alistipes sp.*, and *Ruminococcus sp.*, and legumes with *Coprococcus sp*. The study also observed direct associations between the MedDiet classifications and the abundance of the phylum Bacteroidetes and family Prevotellaceae. Additionally, the genus *Prevotella sp.* was found to be inversely related to the phylum Firmicutes and the genus *Ruminococcus sp.* [92]. This lower ratio of Firmicutes–Bacteroides with higher adherence to the MedDiet was also shown in a recent study with 27 healthy individuals [103]. In agreement with the previous research, higher concentrations of fecal propionate and butyrate were detected, corroborating the potential mediated health effects of the MedDiet by SCFA production.

In summary, the MedDiet affects the composition of the gut microbiota (such as higher *Prevotella sp.*, *Clostridium* cluster XIVa, *F. Pprausnitzii*, Bacteroides, and *Bifidobaterium sp.* or lower Firmicutes and Bacteroides) and can affect the functionality, diversity, and activity of some bacteria, whose metabolites can have health benefits (such as SFCA). Further studies evaluating temporal changes to the colonization, stability, and enterotype changes of the gut microbiota in clinical studies are still warranted to establish a gut microbiota composition as a marker of MedDiet adherence.

Table 3. Effects of a Mediterranean diet on microbiome composition.

Author	Study Design	Study Population	Dietary Pattern/Intervention	Follow-up	Sample	Microbiota Observed	Results/Conclusion
Gutierrez-Diaz et al., 2016 [92]	Cross-sectional	Adults with a non-declared pathology; $n = 31$ (23 females, 8 males, mean age of 42.1 years)	MedDiet [1] score (0-8 points; > 4 = High adherence)	N/A	Stool	Bifidobacterium, Faecalibacterium, Tenericutes, Dorea, Rikenellaceae, Alistipes, Ruminococcus (Lechnospiraceae family), Coprococcus, Bacteroidetes, Prevotel-laceae, Prevotella, and Firmicutes	The MedDiet score was associated with a higher abundance of Bacteroidetes, Prevotel-laceae, and Prevotella and a lower concentration of Firmicutes and Lachnospiraceae.
Gutierrez-Diaz et al., 2017 [102]	Cross-sectional	Healthy men ($n = 20$) and women ($n = 54$) older than 50 years of age	MedDiet	N/A	Stool	Akkermansia, Bacteroides-Prevotella-Porphiromonas, Bifidobacterium, Clostridium cluster XIVa, Lactobacillus group, and F. prausnitzii	Higher levels of Clostridium cluster XIVA and F. prausnitzii were found in subjects with MDS [2] scores ≥4 and were positively correlated with fecal concentrations of benzoic and 3-hydroxyphenylacetic acids and the intake of polyphenols and fibers.
De Filippis et al., 2016 [101]	Cross-sectional study	Healthy Volunteers $n = 153$	MedDiet Vegan Vegetarian Omnivore	N/A	Stool, urine	Lachnospira, Prevotella, Roseburia, and Ruminococcus	Plant-based diets appear to increase fecal SCFAs, while Prevotella specifically was associated with fiber-degrading Firmicutes. Higher urinary trimethylamine oxide levels were found to be higher in those with lower MedDiet adherence. Beneficial microbiome-related metabolic profiles were associated with the increased consumption of plant-based foods, consistent with a MedDiet.
Garcia-Mantrana et al., 2018 [103]	Cross-sectional study	Healthy individuals $n = 27$, mean age 39.5 years	MedDiet	N/A	Stool samples	Enterobacteriaceae family, Bifidobacterium group, Bacteroides-Prevotella-Porphyromonas group, Bacteroides fragilis group, Blautia coccoides group, Methanobrevibacter smithii, and Faecalibacterium prausnitzii	A higher ratio of Firmicutes–Bacteroidetes was related to lower adherence to the MedDiet, and greater presence of Bacteroidetes was associated with lower animal protein intake. Better adherence to the MedDiet was associated with significantly higher levels of total SCFA [3].
Shankar et al., 2017 [96]	Comparative cross-sectional stud	Healthy Egyptian male teenagers $n = 28$, mean age 13.9 years Healthy American male teenagers $n = 14$, mean age 12.9 years	MedDiet Western diet	N/A	Stool	Egyptian: Gammaproteobacteria, Methanobacteria, Prevotella, Megasphaera, Eubacterium, Mitsuokella, Catenibacterium U.S.: Clostridia, Verrucomicrobia, Bacteroides, Ruminococcus, Coprococcus, Blautia, Bilophila, Akkermansia, and Faecalibacterium,	Egyptian gut microbial communities belonged to Prevotella in all the subjects with increased polysaccharide-degrading microbes and end products of polysaccharide fermentation. United States (US) gut microbial communities mostly belonged to Bacteroides with increased proteolytic microbes and end products of protein and fat metabolism.

Table 3. Cont.

Author	Study Design	Study Population	Dietary Pattern/Intervention	Follow-up	Sample	Microbiota Observed	Results/Conclusion
Djuric et al., 2018 [100]	Randomized control trial	n = 88 baseline samples n = 82 post-intervention (men and women) Mean age 53 years	MedDiet (30% kcals form fat, PUFA/SAT/MUFA [4] ratios of 1:2.5, foods high in n-3 fatty acids 2x/week, 3 servings/day whole grains, 7–9.5 cup s/day F [5]+V [6]) including at least one cup dark green or orange F or V). Healthy Eating diet (5.5 cup servings/day F + V, 3 s/day whole grains, <10% kcals from sat. fat.	6 months	Blood, colon biopsy	Firmicutes, Proteobacteria, Lachnospiraceae, Blautia, Roseburia, Prevotella, and Bacteroides,	A total of 11 operational taxonomic units were significantly associated with increased serum carotenoid levels. The Bacteria in the colonic mucosa was resistant to change after both diet interventions The intestinal microbiota did not show significant changes after 6 months of diet intervention; however, an abundance of specific OTUs [7] was significantly associated with serum carotenoid concentrations at the baseline, suggesting that long-term dietary exposures may have more of an influence on bacteria in the colonic mucosa.

[1] MedDiet: Mediterranean diet. [2] MDS: Mediterranean Diet Score. [3] SCFA: Short Chain Fatty Acids. [4] PUFA/SAT/MUFA: polyunsaturated fatty acids/saturated fatty acids/mono-unsataurated fatty acids. [5] F: Fruits. [6] V: Vegetables. [7] OTUs: Operational Taxonomic Unit.

3.2. Microbiome, the Mediterranean Diet, and the Association with Health

While extensive research exists in the literature regarding the health benefits of following a MedDiet pattern, there is limited knowledge regarding the MedDiet's impact on microbiome-mediated disease outcomes. In this section, the literature on microbiome changes as they relate to MedDiet consumption in individuals with known diseases and the contribution of microbiome changes to disease risk will be reviewed and summarized in Table 4.

Emerging evidence is showing that the adherence to a MedDiet is associated with more gut microbial diversity. In the CORonary Diet Intervention with Olive Oil and Cardiovascular PREVention (CORDIOPREV) study, 138 participants with metabolic syndrome (MetS) and 101 without MetS were randomized into two groups. For 2 years, both groups underwent either a MedDiet or a low-fat diet intervention. At basal time, a higher abundance of *Bacteroides*, *Eubacterium* and *Lactobacillus* generas were found while *Bacteroides fragilis* group, *Parabacteroides. distasonis*, *Bacteroides thetaiotaomicron*, *Faecalibacterium prausnitzii*, *Fusobacterium. nucleatum*, *Bifidobacterium. longum*, *Bifidobacterium adolescentis*, *Ruminococcus flavefaciens* subgroupm and *Eubacterium rectale* were decreased in the participants with MetS when compared to those without. After the two-year intervention, MedDiet adherence increased the abundance of *P. distasonis*, *B. thetaiotaomicron*, *F. prausnitzii*, *B. adolescentis*, and *B. longum* in the MetS patients, suggesting that a long-term MedDiet partially restored the dysbiosis in the gut microbiota in the MetS patients, although the MetS persisted.

In another study conducted by the same research team, the effects of both a MedDiet and a low-fat diet were examined but this time on the restoration of the microbiome in three different groups of participants. A total of 106 subjects were evaluated: 33 were obese with MetS, 32 were obese without MetS, and 41 were not obese and did not have MetS. The researchers found that the MedDiet and low-fat diet consumption restored the microbiota in the MetS–obese participants to the gut microbiome found in metabolically healthy people. However, no significant changes in gut microbial composition occurred if MetS was absent (non-MetS–non-obese or non-MetS–Obese). Specifically, the study showed that the Firmicutes/Bacteroidetes ratio (which has been linked to obesity) was related to the presence or absence of metabolic traits and not with obesity itself. The Met–Obese group, previously described with a reduction of genera with saccharolytic activity, showed increases in *Bacteroides*, *Prevotella* (both forming bacteroidetes phylum), *Faecalibacterium*, *Roseburia*, *Ruminococcus* generas, and *P. distasonis* and *F. prausnitzii*, a decreasing Firmicutes/ Bacteroidetes ratio, and no effect on the abundance of Streptococcus or Clostridium. This is important because the restoration of saccharolytic activity genera are associated with an increase in fermentation capacity to SCFA, for which health benefits have previously been described. Consistent with those results, an increased abundance of *Roseburia sp.* and *Oscillospira sp.* and insulin sensitivity were found in 20 obese subject after following a one-year MedDiet intervention [104]. This butyrate-producing genus (*Roseburia*) has been found to have anti-inflammatory effects and has a lower abundance in T2D [105,106]. Interestingly, *F. prausnitzii*, which in the previous literature had been significantly increased with MedDiet consumption [102,107], increased significantly only in the low-fat diet group. This study also showed that some changes in fecal and plasma metabolites could also be linked to changes in gut microbiota [102]. Overall, the results of this study suggested that a MedDiet could be used to prevent and manage T2D, although more research is necessary to associate these therapeutic effects with microbiome-related factors [104].

Other studies exploring the MedDiet's influence on inflammation associated with Crohn's disease (CD) found that 6 weeks of MedDiet intervention had no significant effect on the microbial ecology relative to the control group. However, a trend towards "normal" composition (Bacteroidetes and *Clostridium* clusters IV and XIVa increased, and the abundance of Proteobacteria decreased as did Bacillaceae) was found in this study. Notwithstanding the lower number of subjects ($n = 8$), shorter duration, and absence of a significant alteration in the microbial ecology in this particular study, it should be noted that study participants were already under dietary management of CD, which may have altered their microbiota before the study [83]. Finally, Mitsou et al. explored the relationship between MedDiet adherence with gut microbiota composition and gastrointestinal (GI) symptomology.

A profiling analysis showed that participants with high adherence to the MedDiet had significantly less *Escherichia coli*, a higher ratio of *Bifidobacteria to E. Coli*, and increased levels of *Candida albicans* and SCFA [108]. Interestingly, the MedDiet was also correlated with the alleviation of undesirable GI symptoms and fecal moisture.

The present literature reveals that consuming a global MedDiet leads to alterations in the microbiome; however, the extent to which these changes occur likely depends on numerous factors. The study duration, disease risk, progression and severity, and dietary adherence potentially impact the observed microbial changes. Furthermore, smoking, alcohol consumption, physical activity, and other lifestyle behaviors may also be important determinants in influencing gut microbial composition. It is well known and widely accepted that consumers of healthy dietary patterns often engage in a variety of positive health practices, thus restricting the credibility of intervention studies as an appropriate evaluation method of the MedDiet's microbial influence on health [92]. Further research is necessary to better identify the general outcome of MedDiet consumption on the microbiome and to identify contributing factors to microbial changes. Figure 2 provides a summary of the evidence of the previous two sections.

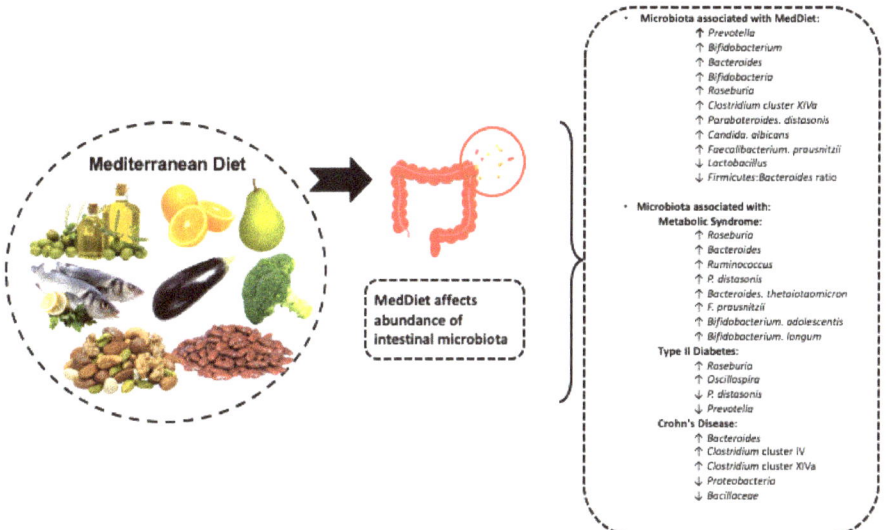

Figure 2. Depiction of the microbiota associated with MedDiet consumption in the absence and presence of disease. All the increases in the microbial changes are identified with an up arrow, and all the decreases are identified with a down arrow. General alterations in the microbiota were only indicated if two or more studies identified that same bacterial change. Research on microbial responses to MedDiet intervention in different disease states is limited, but what has been observed is listed under each respective disease. ↓: decreased with the consumption of MedDiet. ↑: increased with consumption of MedDiet.

Table 4. Mediterranean diet effects on the microbiomes of diseased subjects.

	Design	Participant Characteristics	Dietary Pattern/Treatment	Length	Sample	Microbiota Observed	Results/Conclusion
Haro et al., 2016 [109]	Randomized control trial	n = 138 with metabolic syndrome (MetS) and n = 101 without MetS; male and female patients within the CORDIOPREV study with CHD [1], who had their last coronary event over 6 months before enrolling, in addition to conventional treatment for CHD.	MedDiet group:35% fat (22% MUFA, 6% PUFA, 7% SAT). Low-fat high-complex carb (LFHCC) diet group: 28% fat (12% MUFA, 8% PUFA, 8% SAT).	2 years	Stool, blood	Bacteroides, Eubacterium, Lactobacillus, Bacteroides fragilis group, Parabacteroides distasonis, Bacteroides thetaiotaomicron, Faecalibacterium prausnitzii, Fusobacter- ium nucleatum, Bifidobacterium longum, Bifidobacterium adolescentis, Ruminococcus flavefaciens subgroup, and Eubacterium rectale	The long-term consumption of the Mediterranean diet partially restores the population of P. distasonis, B. thetaiotaomicron, F. prausnitzii, B. adolescentis and B. longum in MetS patients although MetS persists.
Haro et al., 2016 [104]	Randomized control trial	n= 20, 40 total samples collected (20 at the baseline, 20 post-intervention) from obese men with CHD within the CORDIOPREV study	MedDiet group: 35% fat (22% MUFA, 6% PUFA, 7% SAT). Low-fat high-complex carb (LFHCC) diet group: 28% fat (12% MUFA, 8% PUFA, 8% SAT).	1 year	Blood, stool	Bacteroides, Prevotella, unknown Lachnospiraceae, Faecalibacterium, unknown Clostridiales, unknown Ruminococcaceae, Oscillospira, Parabacteroides, and unknown Bacteroidales	Both diet changes increased insulin sensitivity and appeared to exert protective effects on the development of T2DM [2] based off of specific changes in gut microbiota. Changes in feces include mostly amino acids, peptides, and shingolipid metabolism, which may be linked to changes occurring in the gut microbiota.
Haro et al., 2017 [107]	Randomized control trial	n = 33 obese patients with severe MetS-OB [3], n = 32 obese patients without non-MetS-OB, and 41 non-obese subjects (non-MetS-non-OB).	MedDiet group: 35% fat (22% MUFA, 6% PUFA, <10% SAT). Low-fat diet group: <30% total fat (<10% SAT, 12–14% MUFA, 6–8% PUFA).	2 years	Stool	Actinobacteria, Bacteroidetes, Firmicutes, Bacteroides, Prevotella, Ruminococcus, Faecalibacterium, Roseburia, Streptococcus, Clostridium, P. distasonis, and F. prausnitzii	Both diets were associated with partially restored gut microbiome dysbiosis, converting MetS-OB microbiota patterns to microbiota patterns similar to those found in (metabolically) healthy people, after 2 years of nutrition intervention in participants with coronary heart disease. The degree of participants' metabolic dysfunction may alter the effectiveness of nutrition therapy.
Marlow et al., 2014 [83]	Non-randomized trial	n = 8 Crohn's patients with no history of bowel surgery who were not taking prednisone or similar anti-inflammatory medication and had no changes in medication over the last 3 months.	MedDiet	6 weeks	Stool, blood	Firmicutes, Bacteroidetes, Actinobacteria, Proteo- bacteria, Fusobacteria, and Verrucomicrobia	The Mediterranean-inspired diet appeared to benefit the health of people with Crohn's disease. The participants showed a trend for reduced markers of inflammation and normalization of the microbiota; however, the changes were not significant.

Table 4. Cont.

	Design	Participant Characteristics	Dietary Pattern/Treatment	Length	Sample	Microbiota Observed	Results/Conclusion
Mitsu et al., 2017 [108]	Cross-sectional	$n = 120$ Men and women, age 18–65 years	MedDiet Tertiles of adherence based on MedDiet score: Low tertile score = 19–30 ($n = 31$) Medium tertile score = 31–33 ($n = 29$) High tertile score = 34–41 ($n = 40$)	N/A	Stool	*E. coli*, bifidobacteria, and *Candida albicans*	The findings support a link between MedDiet adherence and the gut microbiota profile. Those with high adherence had lower *E. coli* counts, a higher bifidobacterial/*E. coli* ratio, and increased levels and prevalence of *Candida albicans* when compared to those with low adherence
Garcia-Mantrana et al., 2018 [103]	Cross-sectional study	Healthy individuals $n = 27$, mean age 39.5 years	MedDiet		Stool samples	Enterobacteriaceae family, *Bifidobacterium* group, *Bacteroides-Prevotella-Porphyromonas* group, *Bacteroides fragilis* group, *Blautia coccoides* group, *Methanobrevibacter smithii*, and *Faecalibacterium prausnitzii*	*Butyricimonas*, *Desulfovibrio*, and *Oscillospira* genera were associated with a BMI of <25 and the genus *Catenibacterium* was associated with a higher adherence to the MedDiet.

[1] CHD: coronary heart disease. [2] T2DM: type II diabetes. [3] OB: Obese subjects.

4. Conclusions, Implications, and Future Directions

In recent years, high-throughput metabolomic and microbiome analysis techniques have emerged as promising, objective tools to aid and complement the traditional epidemiology methods used to assess diet. Due to the complexity of the diet–disease relationship, assessing both the metabolome and microbiome of an individual may help provide information regarding dietary patterns in light of the information provided in Food Frequency Questionarries (FFQs), food diaries, and interviews. In addition, metabolomics can help to document compliance in dietary intervention studies, although it should be recognized that unlike in drug studies, blinding and/or randomization of the participants may be difficult in nutrition research. Currently, metabolomic literature has identified numerous metabolites related to the consumption of individual dietary components and has begun to identify metabolomic patterns in response to global dietary patterns. Identifying specific physiologically relevant small metabolites derived after the ingestion of unique diets may provide insight into health status and merits further investigation. In order for metabolites to assist in dietary assessment, they must be stable and sensitive to dietary consumption and also reflect long-term usual intake. Subtle and intermittent fluctuations in metabolite concentrations, as well as a short half-life, may not only pose analytical challenges, but also may only be indicative of recent dietary intake and not a global dietary pattern.

The current MedDiet–microbiome literature, though promising, does not provide conclusive evidence on the relative contributions of the gut microbiome on the beneficial health outcomes associated with the MedDiet [110]. Emerging evidence from the literature points to the prominent role of the microbiome in human health, although the causality and governing mechanisms remain unclear. Moreover, differences in microbial profiles appear to be dependent upon several factors including age, habitual dietary consumption, overall health, disease risk, and underlying pathology [110–112]. Therefore, at this time, the analysis of microbial composition, though promising, cannot be recommended as a stand-alone tool for either dietary assessment or related health outcomes. It can, however, complement and strengthen the existing tools, and it holds significant potential as a promising tool in the future. Further research that comprehensively examines the relationships between dietary patterns, microbial changes, and disease outcomes should also focus on using standardized methods and reporting processes that are transferrable across different research groups [110]. Furthermore, systemic approaches that integrate both metabolomics and the microbiome will help researchers to understand their complex interrelationships and interactions with health. The evidence shows that some metabolites (e.g., SCFA production) are mediated by the gut microbiome [40,112]. For example, the CORDIOPREV study found that changes in the metabolites in feces were accompanied by changes in the gut microbiota [101], and a recent investigation within the Malmö Offspring Study found an association between four gut microbiota genera and body mass index-predicted plasma metabolites, including glutamine and BCAAs [113]. Thus, evidence is emerging in this regard, and recent and future studies will further elucidate these relationships/associations (such as the potential effect of the microbial amino acid metabolism on obesity [114]).

It is undeniable that emerging, big data, multi-omics approaches will improve our understanding of the distinctive metabolomics/microbial characteristics that contribute to our overall health and disease risk at an individual and population level. Each method is accompanied by its own strengths and limitations, but when used together, subjective dietary assessments, metabolomic assessments, and microbiome assessments may be able to provide a much more complete picture of the diet–health relationship. This knowledge can have a significant impact on the shaping of policy and the advancement of targeted precision/personalized nutrition-based therapeutic approaches for the prevention and management of chronic diseases [110,115].

Supplementary Materials: The following are available online at http://www.mdpi.com/2072-6643/11/1/207/s1, Table S1: Main findings and evidence from metabolites associated with food.

Author Contributions: Conceptualization, M.S.-P.; Methodology, Q.J., A.B., and M.S.-P.; Review Process, Q.J., A.B., and M.S.-P.; Original Draft Preparation, Q.J., A.B., M.S.-P., and D.V.; Review and Editing of Final Manuscript, M.S.-P., D.V., M.R.-C., and S.N.K.; and Supervision, M.S.-P., D.V., M.R.-C., and S.N.K.

Funding: This research received no external funding.

Conflicts of Interest: The authors declare no conflict of interest.

References

1. Mitrou, P.N.; Kipnis, V.; Thiébaut, A.C.M.; Reedy, J.; Subar, A.F.; Wirfält, E.; Flood, A.; Mouw, T.; Hollenbeck, A.R.; Leitzmann, M.F.; et al. Mediterranean dietary pattern and prediction of all-cause mortality in a US population: Results from the NIH-AARP Diet and Health Study. *Arch. Intern. Med.* **2007**, *167*, 2461–2468. [CrossRef]
2. Benjamin, E.J.; Blaha, M.J.; Chiuve, S.E.; Cushman, M.; Das, S.R.; Deo, R.; De, S.F.; Floyd, J.; Fornage, M.; Gillespie, C.; et al. Heart Disease and Stroke Statistics-2017 Update: A Report From the American Heart Association. *Circ. Circ.* **2017**, *135*, e146. [CrossRef] [PubMed]
3. Grosso, G.; Marventano, S.; Yang, J.; Micek, A.; Pajak, A.; Scalfi, L.; Galvano, F.; Kales, S.N. A comprehensive meta-analysis on evidence of Mediterranean diet and cardiovascular disease: Are individual components equal? *Crit. Rev. Food Sci. Nutr.* **2017**, *57*, 3218–3232. [CrossRef] [PubMed]
4. Schwingshackl, L.; Missbach, B.; König, J.; Hoffmann, G. Adherence to a Mediterranean diet and risk of diabetes: A systematic review and meta-analysis. *Public Health Nutr.* **2015**, *18*, 1292–1299. [CrossRef] [PubMed]
5. Schwingshackl, L.; Schwedhelm, C.; Galbete, C.; Hoffmann, G. Adherence to Mediterranean Diet and Risk of Cancer: An Updated Systematic Review and Meta-Analysis. *Nutrients* **2017**, *9*, 1063. [CrossRef] [PubMed]
6. Sofi, F.; Abbate, R.; Gensini, G.F.; Casini, A. Accruing evidence on benefits of adherence to the Mediterranean diet on health: An updated systematic review and meta-analysis. *Am. J. Clin. Nutr.* **2010**, *92*, 1189–1196. [CrossRef]
7. USDA. *Scientific Report of the 2015 Dietary Guidelines Advisory Committee*; USDA: Washington, DC, USA, 2015.
8. Shen, J.; Wilmot, K.A.; Ghasemzadeh, N.; Molloy, D.L.; Burkman, G.; Mekonnen, G.; Gongora, M.C.; Quyyumi, A.A.; Sperling, L.S. Mediterranean Dietary Patterns and Cardiovascular Health. *Annu. Rev. Nutr.* **2015**, *35*, 425–449. [CrossRef]
9. Korre, M.; Sotos-Prieto, M.; Kales, S.N. Survival Mediterranean Style: Lifestyle Changes to Improve the Health of the US Fire Service. *Front. Public Health* **2017**, *5*, 331. [CrossRef]
10. Praticò, G.; Gao, Q.; Scalbert, A.; Vergères, G.; Kolehmainen, M.; Manach, C.; Brennan, L.; Pedapati, S.H.; Afman, L.A.; Wishart, D.S.; et al. Guidelines for Biomarker of Food Intake Reviews (BFIRev): How to conduct an extensive literature search for biomarker of food intake discovery. *Genes Nutr.* **2018**, *13*, 3. [CrossRef]
11. Thompson, F.E.; Subar, A.F.; Loria, C.M.; Reedy, J.L.; Baranowski, T. Need for technological innovation in dietary assessment. *J. Am. Diet. Assoc.* **2010**, *110*, 48–51. [CrossRef]
12. Frobisher, C.; Maxwell, S.M. The estimation of food portion sizes: A comparison between using descriptions of portion sizes and a photographic food atlas by children and adults. *J. Hum. Nutr. Diet. Off. J. Br. Diet. Assoc.* **2003**, *16*, 181–188. [CrossRef]
13. Jenab, M.; Slimani, N.; Bictash, M.; Ferrari, P.; Bingham, S.A. Biomarkers in nutritional epidemiology: Applications, needs and new horizons. *Hum. Genet.* **2009**, *125*, 507–525. [CrossRef]
14. O'Sullivan, A.; Gibney, M.J.; Brennan, L. Dietary intake patterns are reflected in metabolomic profiles: Potential role in dietary assessment studies. *Am. J. Clin. Nutr.* **2011**, *93*, 314–321. [CrossRef] [PubMed]
15. Nicholson, J.K.; Lindon, J.C. Systems biology: Metabonomics. *Nature* **2008**, *455*, 1054–1056. [CrossRef] [PubMed]
16. Wishart, D.S. Metabolomics: Applications to food science and nutrition research. *Trends Food Sci. Technol.* **2008**, *19*, 482–493. [CrossRef]
17. Panek, M.; Paljetak, H.Č.; Barešić, A.; Perić, M.; Matijašić, M.; Lojkić, I.; Bender, D.V.; Krznarić, Ž.; Verbanac, D. Methodology challenges in studying human gut microbiota—Effects of collection, storage, DNA extraction and next generation sequencing technologies. *Sci. Rep.* **2018**, *8*, 5143. [CrossRef] [PubMed]
18. Atkinson, W.; Downer, P.; Lever, M.; Chambers, S.T.; George, P.M. Effects of orange juice and proline betaine on glycine betaine and homocysteine in healthy male subjects. *Eur. J. Nutr.* **2007**, *46*, 446–452. [CrossRef]

19. Pujos-Guillot, E.; Hubert, J.; Martin, J.-F.; Lyan, B.; Quintana, M.; Claude, S.; Chabanas, B.; Rothwell, J.A.; Bennetau-Pelissero, C.; Scalbert, A.; et al. Mass spectrometry-based metabolomics for the discovery of biomarkers of fruit and vegetable intake: Citrus fruit as a case study. *J. Proteome Res.* **2013**, *12*, 1645–1659. [CrossRef]
20. Heinzmann, S.S.; Brown, I.J.; Chan, Q.; Bictash, M.; Dumas, M.-E.; Kochhar, S.; Stamler, J.; Holmes, E.; Elliott, P.; Nicholson, J.K. Metabolic profiling strategy for discovery of nutritional biomarkers: Proline betaine as a marker of citrus consumption. *Am. J. Clin. Nutr.* **2010**, *92*, 436–443. [CrossRef]
21. May, D.H.; Navarro, S.L.; Ruczinski, I.; Hogan, J.; Ogata, Y.; Schwarz, Y.; Levy, L.; Holzman, T.; McIntosh, M.W.; Lampe, J.W. Metabolomic Profiling of Urine: Response to a Randomized, Controlled Feeding Study of Select Fruits and Vegetables, and Application to an Observational Study. *Br. J. Nutr.* **2013**, *110*, 1760–1770. [CrossRef]
22. Lloyd, A.J.; Beckmann, M.; Favé, G.; Mathers, J.C.; Draper, J. Proline betaine and its biotransformation products in fasting urine samples are potential biomarkers of habitual citrus fruit consumption. *Br. J. Nutr.* **2011**, *106*, 812–824. [CrossRef] [PubMed]
23. Brennan, L.; Gibbons, H.; O'Gorman, A. An Overview of the Role of Metabolomics in the Identification of Dietary Biomarkers. *Curr. Nutr. Rep.* **2015**, *4*, 304–312. [CrossRef]
24. Edmands, W.M.B.; Beckonert, O.P.; Stella, C.; Campbell, A.; Lake, B.G.; Lindon, J.C.; Holmes, E.; Gooderham, N.J. Identification of human urinary biomarkers of cruciferous vegetable consumption by metabonomic profiling. *J. Proteome Res.* **2011**, *10*, 4513–4521. [CrossRef] [PubMed]
25. Andersen, M.-B.S.; Reinbach, H.C.; Rinnan, Å.; Barri, T.; Mithril, C.; Dragsted, L.O. Discovery of exposure markers in urine for Brassica-containing meals served with different protein sources by UPLC-qTOF-MS untargeted metabolomics. *Metabolomics* **2013**, *9*, 984–997. [CrossRef]
26. Guertin, K.A.; Moore, S.C.; Sampson, J.N.; Huang, W.-Y.; Xiao, Q.; Stolzenberg-Solomon, R.Z.; Sinha, R.; Cross, A.J. Metabolomics in nutritional epidemiology: Identifying metabolites associated with diet and quantifying their potential to uncover diet-disease relations in populations. *Am. J. Clin. Nutr.* **2014**, *100*, 208–217. [CrossRef] [PubMed]
27. Aubertin-Leheudre, M.; Koskela, A.; Samaletdin, A.; Adlercreutz, H. Plasma alkylresorcinol metabolites as potential biomarkers of whole-grain wheat and rye cereal fibre intakes in women. *Br. J. Nutr.* **2010**, *103*, 339–343. [CrossRef] [PubMed]
28. Landberg, R.; Townsend, M.K.; Neelakantan, N.; Sun, Q.; Sampson, L.; Spiegelman, D.; van Dam, R.M. Alkylresorcinol metabolite concentrations in spot urine samples correlated with whole grain and cereal fiber intake but showed low to modest reproducibility over one to three years in U.S. women. *J. Nutr.* **2012**, *142*, 872–877. [CrossRef] [PubMed]
29. Guyman, L.A.; Adlercreutz, H.; Koskela, A.; Li, L.; Beresford, S.A.A.; Lampe, J.W. Urinary 3-(3,5-dihydroxyphenyl)-1-propanoic acid, an alkylresorcinol metabolite, is a potential biomarker of whole-grain intake in a U.S. population. *J. Nutr.* **2008**, *138*, 1957–1962. [CrossRef]
30. Guasch-Ferré, M.; Bhupathiraju, S.N.; Hu, F.B. Use of Metabolomics in Improving Assessment of Dietary Intake. *Clin. Chem.* **2018**, *64*, 82–98. [CrossRef]
31. Slemc, L.; Kunej, T. Transcription factor HIF1A: Downstream targets, associated pathways, polymorphic hypoxia response element (HRE) sites, and initiative for standardization of reporting in scientific literature. *Tumour Biol. J. Int. Soc. Oncodev. Biol. Med.* **2016**, *37*, 14851–14861. [CrossRef]
32. Roberfroid, M.; Gibson, G.R.; Hoyles, L.; McCartney, A.L.; Rastall, R.; Rowland, I.; Wolvers, D.; Watzl, B.; Szajewska, H.; Stahl, B.; et al. Prebiotic effects: Metabolic and health benefits. *Br. J. Nutr.* **2010**, *104* (Suppl. S2), S1–S63. [CrossRef] [PubMed]
33. Guarner, F.; Malagelada, J.-R. Gut flora in health and disease. *Lancet Lond. Engl.* **2003**, *361*, 512–519. [CrossRef]
34. Human Nutrition, the Gut Microbiome and the Immune System | Nature. Available online: https://www-nature-com.ezp-prod1.hul.harvard.edu/articles/nature10213 (accessed on 28 November 2018).
35. Marchesi, J.R.; Adams, D.H.; Fava, F.; Hermes, G.D.A.; Hirschfield, G.M.; Hold, G.; Quraishi, M.N.; Kinross, J.; Smidt, H.; Tuohy, K.M.; et al. The gut microbiota and host health: A new clinical frontier. *Gut* **2016**, *65*, 330–339. [CrossRef] [PubMed]
36. Leffler, D.A.; Lamont, J.T. Clostridium difficile Infection. *N. Engl. J. Med.* **2015**, *373*, 287–288. [CrossRef] [PubMed]

37. Round, J.L.; Mazmanian, S.K. The gut microbiota shapes intestinal immune responses during health and disease. *Nat. Rev. Immunol.* **2009**, *9*, 313–323. [CrossRef] [PubMed]
38. Schmidt, C. Thinking from the Gut. *Nature* **2015**, *518*, S12. [CrossRef] [PubMed]
39. Markowiak, P.; Śliżewska, K. Effects of Probiotics, Prebiotics, and Synbiotics on Human Health. *Nutrients* **2017**, *9*, 1021. [CrossRef] [PubMed]
40. Tindall, A.M.; Petersen, K.S.; Kris-Etherton, P.M. Dietary Patterns Affect the Gut Microbiome-The Link to Risk of Cardiometabolic Diseases. *J. Nutr.* **2018**, *148*, 1402–1407. [CrossRef]
41. Castillo-Peinado, L.S.; Luque de Castro, M.D. Present and foreseeable future of metabolomics in forensic analysis. *Anal. Chim. Acta* **2016**, *925*, 1–15. [CrossRef]
42. Xia, J.; Broadhurst, D.I.; Wilson, M.; Wishart, D.S. Translational biomarker discovery in clinical metabolomics: An introductory tutorial. *Metabolomics* **2013**, *9*, 280–299. [CrossRef]
43. Bundy, J.G.; Davey, M.P.; Viant, M.R. Environmental metabolomics: A critical review and future perspectives. *Metabolomics* **2008**, *5*, 3. [CrossRef]
44. Dam, R.M.V.; Li, T.; Spiegelman, D.; Franco, O.H.; Hu, F.B. Combined impact of lifestyle factors on mortality: Prospective cohort study in US women. *BMJ* **2008**, *337*, a1440. [CrossRef] [PubMed]
45. Fitó, M.; Konstantinidou, V. Nutritional Genomics and the Mediterranean Diet's Effects on Human Cardiovascular Health. *Nutrients* **2016**, *8*, 218. [CrossRef] [PubMed]
46. Del Chierico, F.; Vernocchi, P.; Dallapiccola, B.; Putignani, L. Mediterranean Diet and Health: Food Effects on Gut Microbiota and Disease Control. *Int. J. Mol. Sci.* **2014**, *15*, 11678–11699. [CrossRef] [PubMed]
47. Rezzi, S.; Ramadan, Z.; Fay, L.B.; Kochhar, S. Nutritional metabonomics: Applications and perspectives. *J. Proteome Res.* **2007**, *6*, 513–525. [CrossRef] [PubMed]
48. Martínez-González, M.Á.; Ruiz-Canela, M.; Hruby, A.; Liang, L.; Trichopoulou, A.; Hu, F.B. Intervention Trials with the Mediterranean Diet in Cardiovascular Prevention: Understanding Potential Mechanisms through Metabolomic Profiling. *J. Nutr.* **2016**, *146*, 913S–919S. [CrossRef]
49. Esko, T.; Hirschhorn, J.N.; Feldman, H.A.; Hsu, Y.-H.H.; Deik, A.A.; Clish, C.B.; Ebbeling, C.B.; Ludwig, D.S. Metabolomic profiles as reliable biomarkers of dietary composition. *Am. J. Clin. Nutr.* **2017**, *105*, 547–554. [CrossRef] [PubMed]
50. Gibbons, H.; Carr, E.; McNulty, B.A.; Nugent, A.P.; Walton, J.; Flynn, A.; Gibney, M.J.; Brennan, L. Metabolomic-based identification of clusters that reflect dietary patterns. *Mol. Nutr. Food Res.* **2017**, *61*, 1601050. [CrossRef] [PubMed]
51. Playdon, M.C.; Moore, S.C.; Derkach, A.; Reedy, J.; Subar, A.F.; Sampson, J.N.; Albanes, D.; Gu, F.; Kontto, J.; Lassale, C.; et al. Identifying biomarkers of dietary patterns by using metabolomics. *Am. J. Clin. Nutr.* **2017**, *105*, 450–465. [CrossRef] [PubMed]
52. Bondia-Pons, I.; Martinez, J.A.; de la Iglesia, R.; Lopez-Legarrea, P.; Poutanen, K.; Hanhineva, K.; de los Ángeles Zulet, M. Effects of short- and long-term Mediterranean-based dietary treatment on plasma LC-QTOF/MS metabolic profiling of subjects with metabolic syndrome features: The Metabolic Syndrome Reduction in Navarra (RESMENA) randomized controlled trial. *Mol. Nutr. Food Res.* **2015**, *59*, 711–728. [CrossRef] [PubMed]
53. Vázquez-Fresno, R.; Llorach, R.; Urpi-Sarda, M.; Lupianez-Barbero, A.; Estruch, R.; Corella, D.; Fitó, M.; Arós, F.; Ruiz-Canela, M.; Salas-Salvadó, J.; et al. Metabolomic Pattern Analysis after Mediterranean Diet Intervention in a Nondiabetic Population: A 1- and 3-Year Follow-up in the PREDIMED Study. *J. Proteome Res.* **2015**, *14*, 531–540. [CrossRef]
54. Rebholz, C.M.; Lichtenstein, A.H.; Zheng, Z.; Appel, L.J.; Coresh, J. Serum untargeted metabolomic profile of the Dietary Approaches to Stop Hypertension (DASH) dietary pattern. *Am. J. Clin. Nutr.* **2018**, *108*, 243–255. [CrossRef] [PubMed]
55. González-Guardia, L.; Yubero-Serrano, E.M.; Delgado-Lista, J.; Perez-Martinez, P.; Garcia-Rios, A.; Marin, C.; Camargo, A.; Delgado-Casado, N.; Roche, H.M.; Perez-Jimenez, F.; et al. Effects of the Mediterranean Diet Supplemented with Coenzyme Q10 on Metabolomic Profiles in Elderly Men and Women. *J. Gerontol. Ser. A* **2015**, *70*, 78–84. [CrossRef] [PubMed]
56. Kakkoura, M.G.; Sokratous, K.; Demetriou, C.A.; Loizidou, M.A.; Loucaides, G.; Kakouri, E.; Hadjisavvas, A.; Kyriacou, K. Mediterranean diet-gene interactions: A targeted metabolomics study in Greek-Cypriot women. *Mol. Nutr. Food Res.* **2017**, *61*, 1600558. [CrossRef]

57. Kakkoura, M.G.; Demetriou, C.A.; Loizidou, M.A.; Loucaides, G.; Neophytou, I.; Marcou, Y.; Hadjisavvas, A.; Kyriacou, K. Single-nucleotide polymorphisms in one-carbon metabolism genes, Mediterranean diet and breast cancer risk: A case-control study in the Greek-Cypriot female population. *Genes Nutr.* **2015**, *10*, 453. [CrossRef] [PubMed]
58. Kakkoura, M.G.; Demetriou, C.A.; Loizidou, M.A.; Loucaides, G.; Neophytou, I.; Malas, S.; Kyriacou, K.; Hadjisavvas, A. MnSOD and CAT polymorphisms modulate the effect of the Mediterranean diet on breast cancer risk among Greek-Cypriot women. *Eur. J. Nutr.* **2016**, *55*, 1535–1544. [CrossRef] [PubMed]
59. Kakkoura, M.G.; Loizidou, M.A.; Demetriou, C.A.; Loucaides, G.; Daniel, M.; Kyriacou, K.; Hadjisavvas, A. The synergistic effect between the Mediterranean diet and GSTP1 or NAT2 SNPs decreases breast cancer risk in Greek-Cypriot women. *Eur. J. Nutr.* **2017**, *56*, 545–555. [CrossRef]
60. Almanza-Aguilera, E.; Urpi-Sarda, M.; Llorach, R.; Vázquez-Fresno, R.; Garcia-Aloy, M.; Carmona, F.; Sanchez, A.; Madrid-Gambin, F.; Estruch, R.; Corella, D.; et al. Microbial metabolites are associated with a high adherence to a Mediterranean dietary pattern using a 1H-NMR-based untargeted metabolomics approach. *J. Nutr. Biochem.* **2017**, *48*, 36–43. [CrossRef]
61. Hadjisavvas, A.; Loizidou, M.A.; Middleton, N.; Michael, T.; Papachristoforou, R.; Kakouri, E.; Daniel, M.; Papadopoulos, P.; Malas, S.; Marcou, Y.; et al. An investigation of breast cancer risk factors in Cyprus: A case control study. *BMC Cancer* **2010**, *10*, 447. [CrossRef]
62. Guasch-Ferré, M.; Hruby, A.; Toledo, E.; Clish, C.B.; Martínez-González, M.A.; Salas-Salvadó, J.; Hu, F.B. Metabolomics in Prediabetes and Diabetes: A Systematic Review and Meta-analysis. *Diabetes Care* **2016**, *39*, 833–846. [CrossRef]
63. Ruiz-Canela, M.; Hruby, A.; Clish, C.B.; Liang, L.; Martínez-González, M.A.; Hu, F.B. Comprehensive Metabolomic Profiling and Incident Cardiovascular Disease: A Systematic Review. *J. Am. Heart Assoc. Cardiovasc. Cerebrovasc. Dis.* **2017**, *6*, e005705. [CrossRef] [PubMed]
64. Loo, R.L.; Zou, X.; Appel, L.J.; Nicholson, J.K.; Holmes, E. Characterization of metabolic responses to healthy diets and association with blood pressure: Application to the Optimal Macronutrient Intake Trial for Heart Health (OmniHeart), a randomized controlled study. *Am. J. Clin. Nutr.* **2018**, *107*, 323–334. [CrossRef] [PubMed]
65. Khakimov, B.; Poulsen, S.K.; Savorani, F.; Acar, E.; Gürdeniz, G.; Larsen, T.M.; Astrup, A.; Dragsted, L.O.; Engelsen, S.B. New Nordic Diet versus Average Danish Diet: A Randomized Controlled Trial Revealed Healthy Long-Term Effects of the New Nordic Diet by GC-MS Blood Plasma Metabolomics. *J. Proteome Res.* **2016**, *15*, 1939–1954. [CrossRef] [PubMed]
66. Guasch-Ferré, M.; Zheng, Y.; Ruiz-Canela, M.; Hruby, A.; Martínez-González, M.A.; Clish, C.B.; Corella, D.; Estruch, R.; Ros, E.; Fitó, M. Plasma acylcarnitines and risk of cardiovascular disease: Effect of Mediterranean diet interventions–3. *Am. J. Clin. Nutr.* **2016**, *103*, 1408–1416. [CrossRef] [PubMed]
67. Guasch-Ferré, M.; Hu, F.B.; Ruiz-Canela, M.; Bulló, M.; Toledo, E.; Wang, D.D.; Corella, D.; Gómez-Gracia, E.; Fiol, M.; Estruch, R. Plasma Metabolites from Choline Pathway and Risk of Cardiovascular Disease in the PREDIMED (Prevention with Mediterranean Diet) Study. *J. Am. Heart Assoc.* **2017**, *6*, e006524. [CrossRef] [PubMed]
68. Yu, E.; Ruiz-Canela, M.; Guasch-Ferré, M.; Zheng, Y.; Toledo, E.; Clish, C.B.; Salas-Salvadó, J.; Liang, L.; Wang, D.D.; Corella, D.; et al. Increases in Plasma Tryptophan Are Inversely Associated with Incident Cardiovascular Disease in the Prevención con Dieta Mediterránea (PREDIMED) Study. *J. Nutr.* **2017**, *147*, 314–332. [CrossRef] [PubMed]
69. Wang, D.D.; Toledo, E.; Hruby, A.; Rosner, B.A.; Willett, W.C.; Sun, Q.; Razquin, C.; Zheng, Y.; Ruiz-Canela, M.; Guasch-Ferré, M.; et al. Plasma Ceramides, Mediterranean Diet, and Incident Cardiovascular Disease in the PREDIMED Trial (Prevención con Dieta Mediterránea) Clinical Perspective. *Circulation* **2017**, *135*, 2028–2040. [CrossRef] [PubMed]
70. Zheng, Y.; Hu, F.B.; Ruiz-Canela, M.; Clish, C.B.; Dennis, C.; Salas-Salvado, J.; Hruby, A.; Liang, L.; Toledo, E.; Corella, D.; et al. Metabolites of Glutamate Metabolism Are Associated with Incident Cardiovascular Events in the PREDIMED PREvención con DIeta MEDiterránea (PREDIMED) Trial. *J. Am. Heart Assoc. Cardiovasc. Cerebrovasc. Dis.* **2016**, *5*, e00375. [CrossRef]
71. Razquin, C.; Liang, L.; Toledo, E.; Clish, C.B.; Ruiz-Canela, M.; Zheng, Y.; Wang, D.D.; Corella, D.; Castaner, O.; Ros, E.; et al. Plasma lipidome patterns associated with cardiovascular risk in the PREDIMED trial: A case-cohort study. *Int. J. Cardiol.* **2018**, *253*, 126–132. [CrossRef]

72. Ruiz-Canela, M.; Guasch-Ferré, M.; Toledo, E.; Clish, C.B.; Razquin, C.; Liang, L.; Wang, D.D.; Corella, D.; Estruch, R.; Hernáez, Á.; et al. Plasma branched chain/aromatic amino acids, enriched Mediterranean diet and risk of type 2 diabetes: Case-cohort study within the PREDIMED Trial. *Diabetologia* **2018**, *61*, 1560–1571. [CrossRef] [PubMed]
73. Yu, E.; Ruiz-Canela, M.; Razquin, C.; Guasch-Ferre, M.; Toledo, E.; Wang, D.D.; Papandreou, C.; Dennis, C.; Clish, C.; Liang, L.; et al. Changes in Arginine are Inversely Associated with Type 2 Diabetes: A Case-Cohort Study in the PREDIMED Trial. *Diabetes Obes. Metab.* **2019**, *21*, 397–401. [CrossRef] [PubMed]
74. Razquin, C.; Toledo, E.; Clish, C.B.; Ruiz-Canela, M.; Dennis, C.; Corella, D.; Papandreou, C.; Ros, E.; Estruch, R.; Guasch-Ferré, M.; et al. Plasma Lipidomic Profiling and Risk of Type 2 Diabetes in the PREDIMED Trial. *Diabetes Care* **2018**, *41*, 2617–2624. [CrossRef] [PubMed]
75. Yu, E.; Papandreou, C.; Ruiz-Canela, M.; Guasch-Ferre, M.; Clish, C.B.; Dennis, C.; Liang, L.; Corella, D.; Fitó, M.; Razquin, C.; et al. Association of Tryptophan Metabolites with Incident Type 2 Diabetes in the PREDIMED Trial: A Case-Cohort Study. *Clin. Chem.* **2018**, *64*, 1211–1220. [CrossRef] [PubMed]
76. Papandreou, C.; Bulló, M.; Zheng, Y.; Ruiz-Canela, M.; Yu, E.; Guasch-Ferré, M.; Toledo, E.; Clish, C.; Corella, D.; Estruch, R.; et al. Plasma trimethylamine-N-oxide and related metabolites are associated with type 2 diabetes risk in the Prevención con Dieta Mediterránea (PREDIMED) trial. *Am. J. Clin. Nutr.* **2018**, *108*, 163–173. [PubMed]
77. Toledo, E.; Wang, D.D.; Ruiz-Canela, M.; Clish, C.B.; Razquin, C.; Zheng, Y.; Guasch-Ferré, M.; Hruby, A.; Corella, D.; Gómez-Gracia, E. Plasma lipidomic profiles and cardiovascular events in a randomized intervention trial with the Mediterranean diet. *Am. J. Clin. Nutr.* **2017**, *106*, 973–983. [PubMed]
78. Ruiz-Canela, M.; Toledo, E.; Clish, C.B.; Hruby, A.; Liang, L.; Salas-Salvadó, J.; Razquin, C.; Corella, D.; Estruch, R.; Ros, E.; et al. Plasma Branched-Chain Amino Acids and Incident Cardiovascular Disease in the PREDIMED Trial. *Clin. Chem.* **2016**, *62*, 582–592. [CrossRef]
79. Guasch-Ferré, M.; Ruiz-Canela, M.; Li, J.; Zheng, Y.; Bulló, M.; Wang, D.D.; Toledo, E.; Clish, C.; Corella, D.; Estruch, R.; et al. Plasma acylcarnitines and risk of type 2 diabetes in a Mediterranean population at high cardiovascular risk. *J. Clin. Endocrinol. Metab.* **2018**. [CrossRef]
80. Turnbaugh, P.J.; Ley, R.E.; Hamady, M.; Fraser-Liggett, C.; Knight, R.; Gordon, J.I. The human microbiome project: Exploring the microbial part of ourselves in a changing world. *Nature* **2007**, *449*, 804–810. [CrossRef]
81. Thomas, S.; Izard, J.; Walsh, E.; Batich, K.; Chongsathidkiet, P.; Clarke, G.; Sela, D.A.; Muller, A.J.; Mullin, J.M.; Albert, K.; et al. The Host Microbiome Regulates and Maintains Human Health: A Primer and Perspective for Non-Microbiologists. *Cancer Res.* **2017**, *77*, 1783–1812. [CrossRef]
82. Lopez-Legarrea, P.; Fuller, N.R.; Zulet, M.A.; Martinez, J.A.; Caterson, I.D. The influence of Mediterranean, carbohydrate and high protein diets on gut microbiota composition in the treatment of obesity and associated inflammatory state. *Asia Pac. J. Clin. Nutr.* **2014**, *23*, 360–368.
83. Marlow, G.; Ellett, S.; Ferguson, I.R.; Zhu, S.; Karunasinghe, N.; Jesuthasan, A.C.; Han, D.Y.; Fraser, A.G.; Ferguson, L.R. Transcriptomics to study the effect of a Mediterranean-inspired diet on inflammation in Crohn's disease patients. *Hum. Genom.* **2013**, *7*, 24. [CrossRef] [PubMed]
84. Del Chierico, F.; Gnani, D.; Vernocchi, P.; Petrucca, A.; Alisi, A.; Dallapiccola, B.; Nobili, V.; Lorenza, P. Meta-Omic Platforms to Assist in the Understanding of NAFLD Gut Microbiota Alterations: Tools and Applications. *Int. J. Mol. Sci.* **2014**, *15*, 684–711. [CrossRef] [PubMed]
85. Tosti, V.; Bertozzi, B.; Fontana, L. Health Benefits of the Mediterranean Diet: Metabolic and Molecular Mechanisms. *J. Gerontol. Ser. A* **2017**, *73*, 318–326. [CrossRef] [PubMed]
86. Bajzer, M.; Seeley, R.J. Physiology: Obesity and gut flora. *Nature* **2006**, *444*, 1009–1010. [CrossRef] [PubMed]
87. Caesar, R.; Fåk, F.; Bäckhed, F. Effects of gut microbiota on obesity and atherosclerosis via modulation of inflammation and lipid metabolism. *J. Intern. Med.* **2010**, *268*, 320–328. [CrossRef] [PubMed]
88. Diamant, M.; Blaak, E.E.; de Vos, W.M. Do nutrient-gut-microbiota interactions play a role in human obesity, insulin resistance and type 2 diabetes? *Obes. Rev.* **2011**, *12*, 272–281. [CrossRef] [PubMed]
89. Iyer, A.; Fairlie, D.P.; Prins, J.B.; Hammock, B.D.; Brown, L. Inflammatory lipid mediators in adipocyte function and obesity. *Nat. Rev. Endocrinol.* **2010**, *6*, 71–82. [CrossRef]
90. Singh, R.K.; Chang, H.-W.; Yan, D.; Lee, K.M.; Ucmak, D.; Wong, K.; Abrouk, M.; Farahnik, B.; Nakamura, M.; Zhu, T.H.; et al. Influence of diet on the gut microbiome and implications for human health. *J. Transl. Med.* **2017**, *15*, 73. [CrossRef]

91. Zhang, C.; Zhang, M.; Wang, S.; Han, R.; Cao, Y.; Hua, W.; Mao, Y.; Zhang, X.; Pang, X.; Wei, C.; et al. Interactions between gut microbiota, host genetics and diet relevant to development of metabolic syndromes in mice. *ISME J.* **2010**, *4*, 232–241. [CrossRef]
92. Gutierrez-Diaz, I.; Fernandez-Navarro, T.; Sanchez, B.; Margolles, A.; Gonzalez, S. Mediterranean diet and faecal microbiota: A transversal study. *Food Funct.* **2016**, *7*, 2347–2356. [CrossRef]
93. Fitó, M.; Guxens, M.; Corella, D.; Sáez, G.; Estruch, R.; de la Torre, R.; Francés, F.; Cabezas, C.; López-Sabater, M.D.C.; Marrugat, J.; et al. Effect of a traditional Mediterranean diet on lipoprotein oxidation: A randomized controlled trial. *Arch. Intern. Med.* **2007**, *167*, 1195–1203. [CrossRef] [PubMed]
94. Queipo-Ortuño, M.I.; Boto-Ordóñez, M.; Murri, M.; Gomez-Zumaquero, J.M.; Clemente-Postigo, M.; Estruch, R.; Cardona Diaz, F.; Andrés-Lacueva, C.; Tinahones, F.J. Influence of red wine polyphenols and ethanol on the gut microbiota ecology and biochemical biomarkers. *Am. J. Clin. Nutr.* **2012**, *95*, 1323–1334. [CrossRef] [PubMed]
95. Vanegas, S.M.; Meydani, M.; Barnett, J.B.; Goldin, B.; Kane, A.; Rasmussen, H.; Brown, C.; Vangay, P.; Knights, D.; Jonnalagadda, S.; et al. Substituting whole grains for refined grains in a 6-wk randomized trial has a modest effect on gut microbiota and immune and inflammatory markers of healthy adults. *Am. J. Clin. Nutr.* **2017**, *105*, 635–650. [CrossRef] [PubMed]
96. Shankar, V.; Gouda, M.; Moncivaiz, J.; Gordon, A.; Reo, N.V.; Hussein, L.; Paliy, O. Differences in Gut Metabolites and Microbial Composition and Functions between Egyptian and U.S. Children Are Consistent with Their Diets. *mSystems* **2017**, *2*, e00169-16. [CrossRef] [PubMed]
97. Wu, G.D.; Chen, J.; Hoffmann, C.; Bittinger, K.; Chen, Y.-Y.; Keilbaugh, S.A.; Bewtra, M.; Knights, D.; Walters, W.A.; Knight, R.; et al. Linking Long-Term Dietary Patterns with Gut Microbial Enterotypes. *Science* **2011**, *334*, 105–108. [CrossRef]
98. Bohn, T.; Desmarchelier, C.; Dragsted, L.O.; Nielsen, C.S.; Stahl, W.; Rühl, R.; Keijer, J.; Borel, P. Host-related factors explaining interindividual variability of carotenoid bioavailability and tissue concentrations in humans. *Mol. Nutr. Food Res.* **2017**, *61*, 1600685. [CrossRef] [PubMed]
99. Sen, A.; Ren, J.; Ruffin, M.T.; Turgeon, D.K.; Brenner, D.E.; Sidahmed, E.; Rapai, M.E.; Cornellier, M.L.; Djuric, Z. Relationships between Serum and Colon Concentrations of Carotenoids and Fatty Acids in Randomized Dietary Intervention Trial. *Cancer Prev. Res.* **2013**, *6*, 558. [CrossRef]
100. Djuric, Z.; Bassis, C.M.; Plegue, M.A.; Ren, J.; Chan, R.; Sidahmed, E.; Turgeon, D.K.; Ruffin, M.T., IV; Kato, I.; Sen, A. Colonic Mucosal Bacteria Are Associated with Inter-Individual Variability in Serum Carotenoid Concentrations. *J. Acad. Nutr. Diet.* **2018**, *118*, 606–616. [CrossRef]
101. De Filippis, F.; Pellegrini, N.; Vannini, L.; Jeffery, I.B.; La Storia, A.; Laghi, L.; Serrazanetti, D.I.; Di Cagno, R.; Ferrocino, I.; Lazzi, C.; et al. High-level adherence to a Mediterranean diet beneficially impacts the gut microbiota and associated metabolome. *Gut* **2016**, *65*, 1812. [CrossRef]
102. Gutiérrez-Díaz, I.; Fernández-Navarro, T.; Salazar, N.; Bartolomé, B.; Moreno-Arribas, M.V.; de Andres-Galiana, E.J.; Fernández-Martínez, J.L.; de los Reyes-Gavilán, C.G.; Gueimonde, M.; González, S. Adherence to a Mediterranean Diet Influences the Fecal Metabolic Profile of Microbial-Derived Phenolics in a Spanish Cohort of Middle-Age and Older People. *J. Agric. Food Chem.* **2017**, *65*, 586–595. [CrossRef]
103. Garcia-Mantrana, I.; Selma-Royo, M.; Alcantara, C.; Collado, M.C. Shifts on Gut Microbiota Associated to Mediterranean Diet Adherence and Specific Dietary Intakes on General Adult Population. *Front. Microbiol.* **2018**, *9*, 890. [CrossRef]
104. Haro, C.; Montes-Borrego, M.; Rangel-Zúñiga, O.A.; Alcalá-Díaz, J.F.; Gómez-Delgado, F.; Pérez-Martínez, P.; Delgado-Lista, J.; Quintana-Navarro, G.M.; Tinahones, F.J.; Landa, B.B.; et al. Two Healthy Diets Modulate Gut Microbial Community Improving Insulin Sensitivity in a Human Obese Population. *J. Clin. Endocrinol. Metab.* **2016**, *101*, 233–242. [CrossRef] [PubMed]
105. Karlsson, F.H.; Tremaroli, V.; Nookaew, I.; Bergström, G.; Behre, C.J.; Fagerberg, B.; Nielsen, J.; Bäckhed, F. Gut metagenome in European women with normal, impaired and diabetic glucose control. *Nature* **2013**, *498*, 99. [CrossRef] [PubMed]
106. Qin, J.; Li, Y.; Cai, Z.; Li, S.; Zhu, J.; Zhang, F.; Liang, S.; Zhang, W.; Guan, Y.; Shen, D.; et al. A metagenome-wide association study of gut microbiota in type 2 diabetes. *Nature* **2012**, *490*, 55. [CrossRef] [PubMed]

107. Haro, C.; García-Carpintero, S.; Rangel-Zúñiga, O.A.; Alcalá-Díaz, J.F.; Landa, B.B.; Clemente, J.C.; Pérez-Martínez, P.; López-Miranda, J.; Pérez-Jiménez, F.; Camargo, A. Consumption of Two Healthy Dietary Patterns Restored Microbiota Dysbiosis in Obese Patients with Metabolic Dysfunctio. *Mol. Nutr. Food Res.* **2017**, *61*, 1700300. [CrossRef] [PubMed]
108. Mitsou, E.K.; Kakali, A.; Antonopoulou, S.; Mountzouris, K.C.; Yannakoulia, M.; Panagiotakos, D.B.; Kyriacou, A. Adherence to the Mediterranean diet is associated with the gut microbiota pattern and gastrointestinal characteristics in an adult population. *Br. J. Nutr.* **2017**, *117*, 1645–1655. [CrossRef]
109. Haro, C.; Garcia-Carpintero, S.; Alcala-Diaz, J.F.; Gomez-Delgado, F.; Delgado-Lista, J.; Perez-Martinez, P.; Rangel Zuñiga, O.A.; Quintana-Navarro, G.M.; Landa, B.B.; Clemente, J.C.; et al. The gut microbial community in metabolic syndrome patients is modified by diet. *J. Nutr. Biochem.* **2016**, *27*, 27–31. [CrossRef]
110. Cani, P.D. Human gut microbiome: Hopes, threats and promises. *Gut* **2018**, *67*, 1716–1725. [CrossRef]
111. UNC. Gut Microbiome, Diet and Health. Available online: https://www.uncnri.org/index.php/gut-microbiome-diet-and-health/ (accessed on 20 January 2019).
112. Zmora, N.; Zeevi, D.; Korem, T.; Segal, E.; Elinav, E. Taking it Personally: Personalized Utilization of the Human Microbiome in Health and Disease. *Cell Host Microbe* **2016**, *19*, 12–20. [CrossRef]
113. Zhao, L.; Zhang, F.; Ding, X.; Wu, G.; Lam, Y.Y.; Wang, X.; Fu, H.; Xue, X.; Lu, C.; Ma, J.; et al. Gut bacteria selectively promoted by dietary fibers alleviate type 2 diabetes. *Science* **2018**, *359*, 1151–1156. [CrossRef]
114. Ottosson, F.; Brunkwall, L.; Ericson, U.; Nilsson, P.M.; Almgren, P.; Fernandez, C.; Melander, O.; Orho-Melander, M. Connection Between BMI-Related Plasma Metabolite Profile and Gut Microbiota. *J. Clin. Endocrinol. Metab.* **2018**, *103*, 1491–1501. [CrossRef] [PubMed]
115. Hadrich, D. Microbiome Research Is Becoming the Key to Better Understanding Health and Nutrition. *Front. Genet.* **2018**, *9*. [CrossRef] [PubMed]

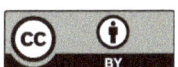

© 2019 by the authors. Licensee MDPI, Basel, Switzerland. This article is an open access article distributed under the terms and conditions of the Creative Commons Attribution (CC BY) license (http://creativecommons.org/licenses/by/4.0/).

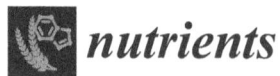

Review

Overview of Human Intervention Studies Evaluating the Impact of the Mediterranean Diet on Markers of DNA Damage

Cristian Del Bo'[1,*], Mirko Marino[1], Daniela Martini[2], Massimiliano Tucci[1], Salvatore Ciappellano[1], Patrizia Riso[1,†] and Marisa Porrini[1,†]

[1] Department of Food, Environmental and Nutritional Sciences (DeFENS), Università degli Studi di Milano, 20122 Milan, Italy; mirko.marino@unimi.it (M.M.); massimiliano.tucci.mt@gmail.com (M.T.); salvatore.ciappellano@unimi.it (S.C.); patrizia.riso@unimi.it (P.R.); marisa.porrini@unimi.it (M.P.)
[2] Human Nutrition Unit, Department of Veterinary Science, University of Parma, 43125 Parma, Italy; daniela.martini@unipr.it
* Correspondence: cristian.delbo@unimi.it; Tel.: +39-025-031-6730
† PR and MP equally contributed to this work.

Received: 29 December 2018; Accepted: 11 February 2019; Published: 13 February 2019

Abstract: The Mediterranean diet (MD) is characterized by high consumption of fruits, vegetables, cereals, potatoes, poultry, beans, nuts, lean fish, dairy products, small quantities of red meat, moderate alcohol consumption, and olive oil. Most of these foods are rich sources of bioactive compounds which may play a role in the protection of oxidative stress including DNA damage. The present review provides a summary of the evidence deriving from human intervention studies aimed at evaluating the impact of Mediterranean diet on markers of DNA damage, DNA repair, and telomere length. The few results available show a general protective effect of MD alone, or in combination with bioactive-rich foods, on DNA damage. In particular, the studies reported a reduction in the levels of 8-hydroxy-2′–deoxyguanosine and a modulation of DNA repair gene expression and telomere length. In conclusion, despite the limited literature available, the results obtained seem to support the beneficial effects of MD dietary pattern in the protection against DNA damage susceptibility. However, further well-controlled interventions are desirable in order to confirm the results obtained and provide evidence-based conclusions.

Keywords: Mediterranean diet; DNA damage; DNA repair; telomere length; dietary intervention study

1. Introduction

Oxidative stress is a condition characterized by an imbalance between formation of reactive oxygen species (ROS) and antioxidant defense mechanisms. Overproduction of ROS can cause oxidative damage to lipids, proteins, and DNA [1]. The integrity and stability of DNA is essential to life and for the maintenance of normal cell functions. The most common types of stressors, apart from oxidative species, include chemical agents, ultraviolet/ionizing radiation, and xenobiotics that can contribute to DNA damage and to formation of base deamination, base alkylation, base dimerization, base oxidation, and single/double strand breakage [1]. The resulting DNA damage, if not properly repaired, can increase risk of mutagenesis and bring to the onset or the development of numerous degenerative diseases including cardiovascular diseases (CVDs), diabetes mellitus, Alzheimer's disease, and cancer [2–4]. Chronic oxidative stress has also been reported as a critical mechanism involved in telomere shortening [5]. Telomeres consist of long stretches of TTAGGG-DNA repeats associated with specific proteins and located at the end of chromosomes. They are involved in the protection of chromosomic stability and have been recognized as potential biomarkers of biological aging [6].

Increasing evidence suggests the crucial role of dietary and lifestyle habits as determinants of DNA oxidative damage [7,8], DNA repair [9], and telomere length [10]. Bioactives and bioactive-rich foods can exert a protective effect against oxidative stress resulting in lower DNA damage. For instance, DNA damage protection has been observed in several human intervention studies following the consumption of tomato [11,12], broccoli [13,14], spinach [15,16], blueberry [17,18], orange juice [19,20], nuts [21,22], green tea [23,24], and coffee [25,26]. Most of these foods are present in the Mediterranean diet (MD) and represent a rich sources of bioactive compounds such as vitamins, carotenoids, glucosinolates, and polyphenols acting as antioxidants or activators of endogenous multiple defense systems [27,28]. In addition, food bioactives have been demonstrated to induce DNA repair activity and to help in maintaining telomere length [10].

The MD has been identified as a sustainable and healthy dietary pattern characterized by a high intake of vegetables, legumes, fruits and nuts, cereals, olive oil, a moderately high intake of fish, a low-to-moderate intake of dairy products, a low intake of meat and poultry, and a regular but moderate intake of alcohol, primarily in the form of wine and generally within meals [29,30]. The adherence to the MD has been recognized to have a favorable effect on blood pressure, insulin sensitivity, lipid profile, inflammation, and oxidative stress, with a consequent decreased risk of numerous non-communicable diseases such as CVDs, cancer, and related deaths [31–33]. The results of PREDIMED (PREvención con DIeta MEDiterránea), a multicenter, randomized, nutritional intervention trial carried out in Spain from 2003 to 2011, demonstrated the protective effect of the traditional MD against CVD in individuals at high cardiovascular risk [34–37].

The exact mechanisms by which MD exerts its protective effects are not yet completely understood since numerous aspects such as lifestyle and environmental factors, characterizing Mediterranean style, can be involved and may interact contributing to the health benefits observed. However, the intake of bioactive compounds with a direct and/or indirect antioxidant action could represent a plausible, even if not the unique, explanation for the apparent benefits. A specific target of this protection could be represented by the defense of DNA from oxidative damage. The present review summarizes the main findings derived from human intervention studies addressing the impact of the MD on DNA protection and telomere length.

2. Materials and Methods

2.1. Search Strategy and Study Selection

PUBMED (http://www.ncbi.nlm.nih.gov/pubmed) and EMBASE (http://www.embase.com/) databases (updated December 2018) were searched to identify pertinent articles. The searches used the combination of the following terms: (Diet, Mediterranean OR Mediterranean diet OR diets, Mediterranean OR Mediterranean diets) AND (DNA damage OR DNA damages OR damage, DNA OR damages, DNA OR DNA injury OR DNA injuries OR injuries, DNA OR injury, DNA OR genotoxic stress OR genotoxic stresses OR stresses, genotoxic OR stress, genotoxic OR telomeric DNA damage OR telomere length). The retrieved papers were also screened for additional papers. The search strategy is summarized in Figure 1.

The search was limited to human intervention studies. No other specific restrictions for the selection of the studies have been used with the exception of the language. Only papers written in English have been considered. Two independent reviewers (MM and DM) conducted the literature search in the scientific databases and assessed and verified the eligibility of the studies based on the title and abstract. Disagreement between reviewers was resolved through consultation with a third independent reviewer (CDB) to reach a consensus.

Data extraction of the papers meeting the inclusion criteria was performed by two reviewers (MM and MT). The following information was reported: (1) first author name and year of publication; (2) the country where the study was performed; (3) study design; (4) subjects' characteristics; (5) characteristics of the control group; (6) characteristics of the intervention group; (7) list of markers of DNA damage; and (8) main findings.

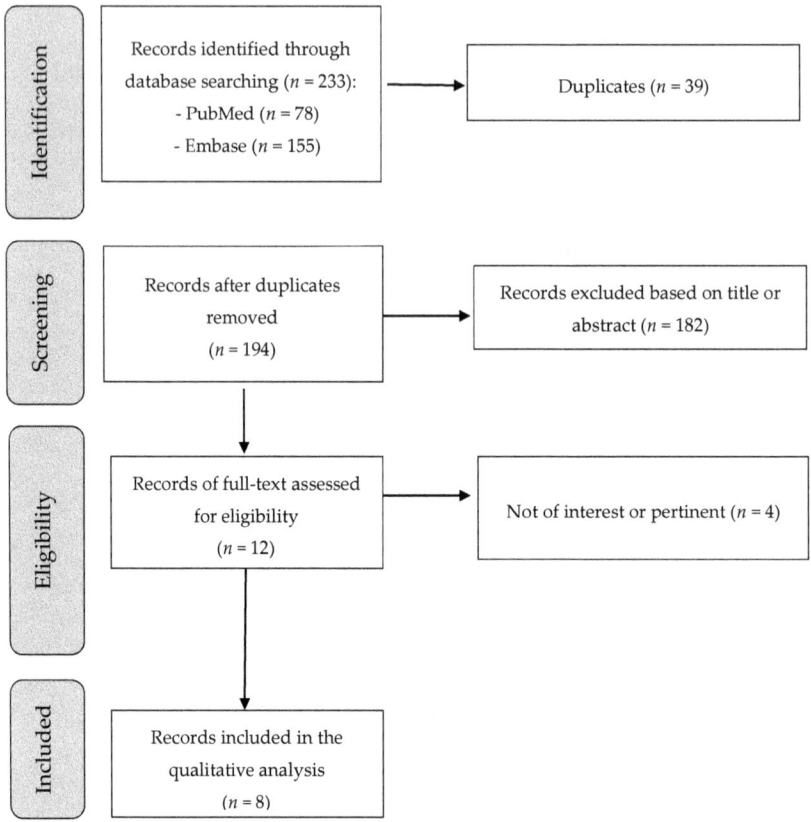

Figure 1. Flowchart of the study selection process.

2.2. Risk of Bias in Individual Studies

Risk of bias in individual studies was assessed independently by two review authors (MM and DM) by considering the following components to produce the resulting scores: (1) Selection Bias—Sequence generation and allocation concealment; (2) Performance Bias—Blinding of participants and personnel; (3) Detection Bias—Blinding of outcome assessment; (4) Attrition Bias—Incomplete outcome data; (5) Reporting Bias—Selective reporting; and (6) Other Bias. Scores were assessed considering three potential bias risks: "Low risk of bias", when the study presented the considered characteristics; "High risk of bias", when the study did not fully highlight the considered characteristics; and "Unclear risk of bias", when it was not possible to attribute one of the two other scores ("Low risk" or "High risk") due to missing information. All disagreements were resolved by consensus with a third reviewer (CDB).

3. Results and Discussion

3.1. Study Selection

A total of 233 records were identified from PubMed and EMBASE database search. After removing 39 duplicate articles, 194 studies were screened and 182 excluded based on title or abstract. The full text of eligible studies ($n = 12$) was read; a total of four records were excluded because not of interest or pertinent. At the end of the selection process a total of 8 human intervention studies were included in the review [38–45].

3.2. Study Characteristics

The main characteristics of the studies included in the review are reported in Table 1. Six out of eight studies were conducted in Spain [39–42,44,45], one in New Zealand [38], and one in Chile [43]. The study population included males and females of different age (young, adults and older subjects), and with different characteristics: healthy subjects [39,41], individuals with high cardiovascular risk [44,45], metabolic syndrome [40], and prostate cancer [38]. All the studies showed a randomized controlled design with the exception of one non-randomized and non-controlled study [38]. The duration of the intervention varied from a minimum of 4 weeks [39,41,43] up to 5 years [44,45]. Most of the investigations did not analyze the effects of MD alone but in combination with olive oil [40,42], nuts [40], wine [43], or MD supplemented with coenzyme Q10 [39,41]. Among the various markers of DNA oxidative damage, 8-hydroxy-2'-deoxyguanosine (8-oxo-dG) was the main evaluated, followed by the expression of DNA repair genes and telomere length. Only one study quantified the levels of strand breaks and oxidatively-induced DNA damage in peripheral blood mononuclear cells (PBMCs) [38].

3.3. Risk of Bias of the Studies

Risks of bias within individual studies are reported in Figures S1 and S2. On the whole, the results show an unclear risk of bias for most of the types of bias. The performance (blinding of participants and personnel) and the selection (i.e., random sequence generation) represent the highest risks of bias.

3.4. Main Findings

The characteristics of the intervention, the type of markers analyzed and the main findings of the studies are reported in Table 2. On the whole, the results obtained show that MD alone or in combination with specific bioactive-rich foods (i.e. olive oil, nuts, red wine) or antioxidant compounds (i.e., coenzyme Q10), may exert a protection against DNA damage and play an important role in the modulation of DNA repair genes (e.g. down-regulation of growth arrest and DNA-damage-inducible alpha, polymerase (DNA directed)). In particular, three studies reported a reduction of the levels of 8-oxo-dG in urine [40], plasma [41], or peripheral blood leukocytes [43] following the intervention with the MD alone or in combination with others foods/dietary components, while one study did not report a significant effect [42]. Conversely, one study showed a significant decrease in the levels of oxidatively-induced, but not endogenous, DNA damage [38]. Regarding DNA repair capacity, two studies showed a significant modulation of the genes involved in this repair pathway activity [39,41], while one study failed to report a significant effect [42]. The effect of MD on telomere length has been investigated within the PREDIMED-NAVARRA study. One paper did not show any effect on telomere length after MD intervention [44], while the other reported a significant increase in telomeres depending on different individual gene variants [45].

Table 1. Characteristics of the studies

Reference	Country	Subject Characteristics	Study Design	Control
Erdrich et al. [38]	New Zealand	Subjects = 20 (F = 0; M = 20) with prostate cancer, Age = 52-74 years; BMI = 23-33 kg/m^2 Non-smokers = 7; former-smokers = 13	One arm intervention	N.A.
Gutierrez-Mariscal et al. [39]	Spain	Subjects = 20 (F = 10; M = 10); Age = > 65 years; BMI = 20-40 kg/m^2 Non-smokers = 20	Randomized, controlled crossover trial	Western diet rich in SFA (6 subjects)
Mitjavila et al. [40]	Spain	Subjects = 110 (F = 110; M = 0) with MetS; Age = 55-80 years; BMI = < 35 kg/m^2 Non-smokers	Multicentric, randomized, controlled, parallel clinical trial PREDIMED	Low-fat diet (37 subjects)
Gutierrez-Mariscal et al. [41]	Spain	Subjects = 20 (F = 10; M = 10); Age = > 65 years; BMI = 20-40 kg/m^2 Non-smokers=20	Randomized, controlled crossover trial	Western diet rich in SFA (6 subjects)
Konstantinidou et al. [42]	Spain	Subjects = 90 (F = 64; M = 26); Age = 20-50 years; BMI = < 30 kg/m^2 Smokers = N.A.	Randomized, parallel, controlled clinical trial	Habitual diet (30 subjects)
Urquiaga et al. [43]	Chile	Subjects = 42 (F = 0; M = 42); Age = 20-27 years; BMI = N.A. Smokers = N.A.	Partially randomized, controlled, trial	Occidental diet (21 subjects)
García-Calzon et al. [44]	Spain	Subjects = 520 (F = 286; M = 234) at high CV risk; Age = 55-80 years; BMI = 25-35 kg/m^2 Non-smokers = 326; former-smokers = 117; smokers = 77	Multicentric, randomized, controlled, parallel clinical trial PREDIMED-NAVARRA	Low-fat diet (140 subjects)
García-Calzon et al. [45]	Spain	Subjects = 521 at high CV risk Pro/pro group = 451 (F = 244; M = 207); Ala carrier group = 70 (F = 64; M = 25) Age = 60-80 years F, 55-80 years M; BMI = 25-35 kg/m^2	Multicentric, randomized, controlled, parallel clinical trial PREDIMED-NAVARRA	Low-fat diet (140 subjects)

Legend: BMI: body mass index; CV: cardiovascular; EVOO: extra virgin olive oil; F: female; M: male; MD: Mediterranean diet; MetS: metabolic syndrome; N.A: not available; PREDIMED: PREvención con DIeta MEDiterránea project; SFA: saturated fatty acid.

Table 2. Main findings about the role of Mediterranean diet in the modulation of markers of DNA damage, DNA repair, and telomere length.

Reference	Intervention	Markers of DNA Damage	Main Findings
Erdrich et al. [38]	Adherence to Mediterranean-style diet consisting of: extra virgin olive oil, fresh frozen salmon (200 g/week), unsweetened pure pomegranate juice (1 L/week) and samples of a variety of canned legumes 3 months	Percentage DNA in the tail	↓cell DNA damage ($p = 0.013$)
Gutierrez-Mariscal et al. [39]	MD supplemented with Q10 (7 subjects) Only MD (7 subjects) 4 weeks Each diet	Gadd45a Ogg1 APE-1/Ref-1 DNA pol β XPC	↓ Gadd45a mRNA levels MD plus Q10 vs. SFA ($p = 0.044$) ↓ nuclear Gadd45a levels MD plus Q10 vs. SFA ($p = 0.023$ and $p = 0.038$, respectively) ↑Ogg1 mRNA levels during postprandial period SFA vs. MD plus Q10 ($p = 0.048$) ↑ nuclear APE-1/ Ref-1 protein level during the postprandial period and long-term consumption SFA vs. MD plus Q10 ($p = 0.038$ and $p = 0.028$, respectively) ↓ DNApolβmRNA levels MD plus Q10 vs. SFA ($p = 0.041$) ↑ nuclear DNApolβ protein levels SFA vs. MD plus Q10 ($p = 0.044$) ↑ XPC mRNA levels during postprandial period SFA vs. MD plus Q10 ($p = 0.019$)
Mitjavila et al. [40]	MD plus EVOO (38 subjects) MD plus nuts (35 subjects) 1 year	8-OH-dG	↓ Urinary 8-OH-dG concentrations MD groups vs. Control ($p < 0.001$)
Gutierrez-Mariscal et al. [41]	MD supplemented Q10 (7 subjects) Only MD (7 subjects) 4 weeks	8-OH-dG P53 p-p53 (Ser20) p53R2	↓ 8-OH-dG plasma concentrations MD and MD plus Q10 vs. SFA ($p < 0.0001$) ↓ 8-OH-dG plasma concentrations MD vs. MD plus Q10 ($p < 0.001$) ↓ postprandial levels of cytoplasmic p53 MD plus Q10 vs. SFA and MD ($p < 0.05$) ↓ nuclear p-p53 (Ser20) postprandial levels MD plus Q10 vs. SFA and MD ($p = 0.0013$). ↑ p53 mRNA levels postprandial and after 2 h SFA vs. MD ($p = 0.047$). ↔ mRNA p53R2 MD plus Q10 vs. SFA vs. MD ($p > 0.05$)
Konstantinidou et al. [42]	MD plus VOO (30 subjects) MD plus WOO (30 subjects) 3 months	8-OH-dG CCNG1 POLK TP53 DCLREIC DNA ERCC5 XRCC5	↓ polymerase (DNA directed)- (POLK) MD vs. control group ($p < 0.05$) ↔ 8-OH-dG, CCNG1, TP53, DCLREIC, ERCC5, XRCC5 MD vs. control group ($p > 0.05$)
Urquiaga et al. [43]	MD (21 subjects) 3 months	8-OH-dG	↓ 8-OH-dG in DNA from peripheral blood leukocytes MD group vs. OD group ($p < 0.008$)
García-Calzón et al. [44]	MD plus EVOO (210 subjects) MD plus nuts (170 subjects) 5 years	Telomere length	↔ telomere length MD plus EVOO vs. Control ↓ telomere length MD plus nuts vs. Control ($p < 0.001$)
García-Calzón et al. [45]	MD plus EVOO (212 subjects) MD plus nuts (169 subjects) 5 years	Telomere length	↑ telomere length Ala carriers group plus MD vs. Pro/pro group plus MD ($p < 0.01$)

Legend: APE-1/Ref-1: Reduction-oxidation factor 1-apurinic/apyrimidinic endonuclease; CCNG1: Cyclin G1; DCLREIC: DNA cross-link repair 1C; DNA pol β: DNA polymerase beta; EVOO: extra virgin olive oil; ERCC5: excision repair cross-complementing rodent repair deficiency, complementation group 5; Gadd45a: growth arrest and DNA-damage-inducible alpha; MD: Mediterranean diet; OD: Occidental diet; Ogg1: 8-oxoguanine DNA glycosylase; P53: protein 53; P-p53 (Ser20): pospho-p53 (serine20); p53R2: p53 inducible ribonucleotide reductase gene; POLK: polymerase (DNA directed); Q10: Coenzyme Q10; SFA: saturated fatty acids; TP53: tumor protein p53; VOO: virgin olive oil; WOO: washed virgin olive oil; XRCC5: X-ray repair complementing defective repair in Chinese hamster cells 5 (double-strand-break rejoining; Ku autoantigen, 80 kDa); XPC: xeroderma pigmentosum, complementation group C; 8-OH-dG: 8-hydroxy-2′-deoxyguanosine.

To the best of our knowledge, this is the first review aimed at providing evidence on the effects of MD in the modulation of DNA damage, DNA repair genes, and telomere length. The availability of data on protection from DNA damage is significant, since it has been reported to play a crucial role in the development of degenerative diseases, while the adherence to MD can represent a protective dietary pattern.

It is noteworthy that most of the studies focused their attention on the dietary fat quality as possible determinant of DNA damage and numerous diseases. In particular, it has been suggested that the amount and quality of dietary fats could be important for the maintenance of DNA stability. Some researchers found that a polyunsaturated fatty acid (PUFA)-rich diet was associated with reduced DNA damage [46], while saturated fatty acid (SFA) intake was demonstrated to increase DNA damage [47]. In this regard, a recent study evaluated the association between fat intake, as part of a modified Mediterranean style dietary intervention study, and several markers of inflammation and oxidative stress including DNA damage [48]. The authors found an inverse correlation between DNA damage and monounsaturated fatty acids (MUFAs), particularly oleic acid, while a positive correlation was observed between DNA damage and the intake of dairy products and red meat (possibly due to SFAs) [48].

The role of MUFAs and PUFAs in the modulation of the levels of DNA damage and DNA repair has been poorly investigated in vivo and results, in particular for PUFA, are quite controversial. For example, Bishop et al. [48] found a positive correlation between DNA damage and circulating levels of omega-6 PUFA. Similar findings were found in other in vivo studies hypothesizing a process of lipid peroxidation as determinant of DNA damage [49–51]. Conversely, numerous other studies have reported a protection of MUFAs and PUFAs against oxidative stress and DNA damage [46, 52,53]. In the present review, the role of olive oil and nuts as food sources of MUFA and PUFAs respectively, but not limited to them, has been evaluated within a context of Mediterranean diet. Mitjavila and colleagues [40] performed a randomized, controlled, parallel clinical trial in which 110 female subjects with metabolic syndrome, recruited within the PREDIMED study, were randomly assigned to three intervention groups: (1) MD *plus* nuts; (2) MD *plus* extra virgin olive oil; and (3) control diet (advice on low-fat diet). The effects of these three interventions on the levels of DNA damage and other parameters related to cardiovascular health were evaluated after 1-year follow-up. The results obtained showed an overall significant improvement of cardiovascular health outcomes and a reduction in the urinary levels of 8-OH-dG in the MD group as compared to the control group. In another study, Konstantinidou and coworkers [42] investigated the effects of the traditional MD, associated with the consumption of two different virgin olive oils, on the expression of atherosclerosis markers and related genes including DNA damage and DNA repair genes. To this aim, the authors performed a randomized, parallel, controlled clinical trial with three different interventions: (1) MD *plus* virgin olive oil; (2) MD *plus* washed virgin olive oil (low content in polyphenols compared to normal virgin olive oil); (3) control diet consisting in the habitual diet of the participants. The impact of the dietary interventions was evaluated in 90 subjects (30 subjects for each arm of intervention) after 3 months. The results have shown an overall general improvement of the MD intervention on the genes and markers related to atherosclerosis, while the effect on the urinary levels of 8-OH-dG was significant only after the intervention with virgin olive oil but not washed virgin olive oil. Conversely, the effect on the modulation of DNA repair genes was significant only when considering the global effect of both the interventions with the MD and olive oil. The results showed a down-regulation of polymerase (DNA directed) k (POLK) gene expression, suggesting a protective role of the MD on DNA oxidation and damage. In fact, POLK is a specialized DNA polymerase that catalyzes the translesion DNA synthesis, which allows DNA replication in the presence of lesions. The authors attributed the beneficial effects of the intervention to presence of MUFAs and other components (i.e. polyphenols) provided by olive oil and the MD.

SFAs may promote cell transformation by negatively regulating the DNA damage response pathway [49]. Gutierrez-Mariscal et al. [41] evaluated the impact of a 4-week intervention with MD and MD *plus* coenzyme Q10 (a fat-soluble bioactive with antioxidant activity), compared to a SFA-rich diet, on different markers of DNA damage and DNA repair in a group of elderly subjects. The authors found a significant decrease in p53 protein levels (a transcription factor which mediates the cellular response to DNA damage), as well as plasma circulating 8-OH-dG levels (as marker of DNA damage), following both the Mediterranean dietary approaches but not with the diet rich in SFAs. The authors also demonstrated, in the same population, that the adherence to MD was able to control the expression of DNA repair genes, while the intervention with the SFA diet triggered the p53-dependent DNA repair machinery, as defense mechanism in response to a stress condition [26]. Similarly, Urquiaga et al. [43] investigated the effect of a 3-month MD intervention versus an Occidental diet (OD, resembling a Western or U.S. diet) richer in fat, in particular SFAs, in a group of young healthy subjects. During the first and the third month, subjects received the prepared diets alone, while during the second month they were asked also to add 240 mL of red wine (corresponding to 2 glasses per day). Subjects on MD, compared to those on OD (higher in SFAs), had reduced levels of 8-OH-dG in peripheral blood leucocytes. However, since both the diets included a moderate consumption of red wine for a period of 30 days, a positive or negative contribution of this product in the results obtained cannot be excluded.

DNA damage has been positively associated with cancer risk. In fact, it has been clearly documented that DNA lesions can alter the primary structure of the double helix thereby affecting transcription and replication [53]. Moreover, erroneous DNA repair of lesions can lead to mutations or chromosomal aberrations affecting oncogenes and tumor suppressor genes; the effect is that cells undergo malignant transformation resulting in cancerous growth with deleterious consequences for individual's health [53]. Several epidemiological studies reported an inverse association between MD adherence and neoplastic diseases [54–56] at the level of different sites such as breast [57], colorectal [58], bladder [59], and prostate cancer [60]. In the present review, we included a dietary intervention study performed on 20 subjects with prostate cancer in which the effect of a modified Mediterranean-style diet, consisting in extra-virgin olive oil, fresh frozen salmon, unsweetened pure pomegranate juice and canned legumes, was evaluated [38]. The intervention was a 3-month non-randomized controlled trial in which the levels of DNA damage in individual cells were evaluated by the comet assay [61,62]. The authors documented that dietary changes towards a modified Mediterranean-style pattern could have beneficial effects in terms of reduction of oxidatively-induced DNA damage in this specific target group [38]. This effect was attributed to an undeterminable synergistic effect of dietary components provided through the MD intervention.

Some observational and ex-vivo studies have shown that a greater adherence to MD was associated not only with an improvement of health status, but also with longer telomeres and higher telomerase activity in the elderly [63–66]. Garcia-Calzón and colleagues [44] found that a higher baseline adherence to the MD was associated with longer telomerases in women, but not in men, from the PREDIMED-NAVARRA study. After the 5-year intervention, the results obtained showed that the MD failed to prevent telomere shortening in this target group of older subjects. However, further data elaboration, by considering some gene variants (i.e., Pro/Ala polymorphisms of the peroxisome proliferator-activated receptor γ2), showed that subjects with Ala carrier variant had increased telomeres length following MD intervention [45]. Moreover, the research team documented that the adherence to MD intervention improved obesity parameters [67] and dietary inflammatory index [68], likely slowing down telomere shortening.

4. Conclusions

Undoubtedly, the MD represents a balanced and healthy dietary pattern associated with a reduced risk of major chronic diseases. However, the role of the MD in the modulation of DNA damage, as potential contributor in disease onset, is poorly investigated. Apart from PREDIMED, most of the studies did not focus on the role of the MD as such, but in combination with specific bioactives and/or bioactive-rich foods; thus, specific contributions are difficult to discern. Although preliminary, the papers reviewed seem to strengthen the hypothesis of a potential role of MD in the protection of

DNA damage and in the modulation of DNA repair genes and telomere length. However, the studies show several limitations due to the numerous bias and confounding factors apparently present in the experimental designs. For these reasons, the results in the present review can represent a starting point for further well-controlled intervention studies targeted on the specific effects of traditional and/or revised MD pattern in the modulation of DNA damage. These studies will be useful to provide more evidence-based proof of MD protective activity and to reveal the molecular mechanisms at the base of the protection observed.

Supplementary Materials: The following are available online at http://www.mdpi.com/2072-6643/11/2/391/s1, Figure S1: Risk of bias graph: review authors' judgements about each risk of bias item presented as percentages across all included studies, Figure S2: Risk of bias summary: review authors' judgements about each risk of bias item for each included study.

Author Contributions: M.M., D.M. and M.T. made the literature search, reviewed the abstracts of the studies selected, performed the analysis of risk o bias and prepared the tables; C.D.B. acted as a third independent reviewer and wrote the first draft of the manuscript. S.C. improved the quality of the manuscript. P.R. and M.P. critically revised the scientific contents of the manuscript and improved the quality of the manuscript.

Funding: This research received no external funding.

Acknowledgments: This work was supported by the European Cooperation for Science and Technology (CA COST Action CA15132, The comet assay as a human biomonitoring tool (hCOMET)). The authors are grateful for support granted by Ministero delle Politiche Agricole, Alimentari, Forestali e del Turismo (MIPAAFT) and the work was performed within the framework of the European Joint Programming Initiative "A Healthy Diet for a Healthy Life" (JPI HDHL) MaPLE. We thank Donato Angelino for its help in the management of risk of bias.

Conflicts of Interest: The authors declare no conflict of interest.

References

1. Thanan, R.; Oikawa, S.; Hiraku, Y.; Ohnishi, S.; Ma, N.; Pinlaor, S.; Yongvanit, P.; Kawanishi, S.; Murata, M. Oxidative stress and its significant roles in neurodegenerative diseases and cancer. *Int. J. Mol. Sci.* **2014**, *16*, 193–217. [CrossRef] [PubMed]
2. Mahat, R.K.; Singh, N.; Gupta, A.; Rathore, V. Oxidative DNA damage and carotid intima media thickness as predictors of cardiovascular disease in pre-diabetic subjects. *J. Cardiovasc. Dev. Dis.* **2018**, *5*, 15. [CrossRef] [PubMed]
3. Basu, A.K. DNA damage, mutagenesis and cancer. *Int. J. Mol. Sci.* **2018**, *19*, 970. [CrossRef] [PubMed]
4. Blasiak, J.; Arabski, M.; Krupa, R.; Wozniak, K.; Zadrozny, M.; Kasznicki, J.; Zurawska, M.; Drzewoski, J. DNA damage and repair in type 2 diabetes mellitus. *Mutat. Res.* **2004**, *554*, 297–304. [CrossRef] [PubMed]
5. Coluzzi, E.; Colamartino, M.; Cozzi, R.; Leone, S.; Meneghini, C.; O'Callaghan, N.; Sgura, A. Oxidative stress induces persistent telomeric DNA damage responsible for nuclear morphology change in mammalian cells. *PLoS ONE* **2014**, *9*, e110963. [CrossRef] [PubMed]
6. Prasad, K.N.; Wu, M.; Bondy, S.C. Telomere shortening during aging: Attenuation by antioxidants and anti-inflammatory agents. *Mech. Ageing Dev.* **2017**, *164*, 61–66. [CrossRef] [PubMed]
7. Giovannelli, L.; Saieva, C.; Masala, G.; Testa, G.; Salvini, S.; Pitozzi, V.; Riboli, E.; Dolara, P.; Palli, D. Nutritional and lifestyle determinants of DNA oxidative damage: A study in a Mediterranean population. *Carcinogenesis* **2002**, *23*, 1483–1489. [CrossRef] [PubMed]
8. Fenech, M.; Bonassi, S. The effect of age, gender, diet and lifestyle on DNA damage measured using micronucleus frequency in human peripheral blood lymphocytes. *Mutagenesis* **2011**, *26*, 43–49. [CrossRef] [PubMed]
9. Prado, R.P.; dos Santos, B.F.; Pinto, C.L.; de Assis, K.R.; Salvadori, D.M.; Ladeira, M.S. Influence of diet on oxidative DNA damage, uracil misincorporation and DNA repair capability. *Mutagenesis* **2010**, *25*, 483–487. [CrossRef]
10. Freitas-Simoes, T.M.; Ros, E.; Sala-Vila, A. Nutrients, foods, dietary patterns and telomere length: Update of epidemiological studies and randomized trials. *Metabolism* **2016**, *65*, 406–415. [CrossRef]
11. Riso, P.; Pinder, A.; Santangelo, A.; Porrini, M. Does tomato consumption effectively increase the resistance of lymphocyte DNA to oxidative damage? *Am. J. Clin. Nutr.* **1999**, *69*, 712–718. [CrossRef] [PubMed]

12. Chen, L.; Stacewicz-Sapuntzakis, M.; Duncan, C.; Sharifi, R.; Ghosh, L.; van Breemen, R.; Ashton, D.; Bowen, P.E. Oxidative DNA damage in prostate cancer patients consuming tomato sauce-based entrees as a whole-food intervention. *J. Natl. Cancer Inst.* **2001**, *93*, 1872–1879. [CrossRef]
13. Riso, P.; Martini, D.; Møller, P.; Loft, S.; Bonacina, G.; Moro, M.; Porrini, M. DNA damage and repair activity after broccoli intake in young healthy smokers. *Mutagenesis* **2010**, *25*, 595–602. [CrossRef] [PubMed]
14. Riso, P.; Martini, D.; Visioli, F.; Martinetti, A.; Porrini, M. Effect of broccoli intake on markers related to oxidative stress and cancer risk in healthy smokers and nonsmokers. *Nutr. Cancer* **2009**, *61*, 232–237. [CrossRef] [PubMed]
15. Porrini, M.; Riso, P.; Oriani, G. Spinach and tomato consumption increases lymphocyte DNA resistance to oxidative stress but this is not related to cell carotenoid concentrations. *Eur. J. Nutr.* **2002**, *41*, 95–100. [CrossRef] [PubMed]
16. Moser, B.; Szekeres, T.; Bieglmayer, C.; Wagner, K.H.; Mišík, M.; Kundi, M.; Zakerska, O.; Nersesyan, A.; Kager, N.; Zahrl, J.; et al. Impact of spinach consumption on DNA stability in peripheral lymphocytes and on biochemical blood parameters: Results of a human intervention trial. *Eur. J. Nutr.* **2011**, *50*, 587–589. [CrossRef] [PubMed]
17. Riso, P.; Klimis-Zacas, D.; Del Bo', C.; Martini, D.; Campolo, J.; Vendrame, S.; Møller, P.; Loft, S.; De Maria, R.; Porrini, M. Effect of a wild blueberry (*Vaccinium angustifolium*) drink intervention on markers of oxidative stress, inflammation and endothelial function in humans with cardiovascular risk factors. *Eur. J. Nutr.* **2013**, *52*, 949–961. [CrossRef] [PubMed]
18. Del Bo', C.; Riso, P.; Campolo, J.; Møller, P.; Loft, S.; Klimis-Zacas, D.; Brambilla, A.; Rizzolo, A.; Porrini, M. A single portion of blueberry (*Vaccinium corymbosum* L) improves protection against DNA damage but not vascular function in healthy male volunteers. *Nutr. Res.* **2013**, *33*, 220–227. [CrossRef] [PubMed]
19. Guarnieri, S.; Riso, P.; Porrini, M. Orange juice vs vitamin C: Effect on hydrogen peroxide-induced DNA damage in mononuclear blood cells. *Br. J. Nutr.* **2007**, *97*, 639–643. [CrossRef]
20. Rangel-Huerta, O.D.; Aguilera, C.M.; Martin, M.V.; Soto, M.J.; Rico, M.C.; Vallejo, F.; Tomas-Barberan, F.; Perez-de-la-Cruz, A.J.; Gil, A.; Mesa, M.D. Normal or high polyphenol concentration in orange juice affects antioxidant activity, blood pressure, and body weight in obese or overweight adults. *J. Nutr.* **2015**, *145*, 1808–1816. [CrossRef]
21. Guaraldi, F.; Deon, V.; Del Bo', C.; Vendrame, S.; Porrini, M.; Riso, P.; Guardamagna, O. Effect of short-term hazelnut consumption on DNA damage and oxidized LDL in children and adolescents with primary hyperlipidemia: A randomized controlled trial. *J. Nutr. Biochem.* **2018**, *57*, 206–211. [CrossRef] [PubMed]
22. López-Uriarte, P.; Nogués, R.; Saez, G.; Bulló, M.; Romeu, M.; Masana, L.; Tormos, C.; Casas-Agustench, P.; Salas-Salvadó, J. Effect of nut consumption on oxidative stress and the endothelial function in metabolic syndrome. *Clin. Nutr.* **2010**, *29*, 373–380. [CrossRef]
23. Erba, D.; Riso, P.; Bordoni, A.; Foti, P.; Biagi, P.L.; Testolin, G. Effectiveness of moderate green tea consumption on antioxidative status and plasma lipid profile in humans. *J. Nutr. Biochem.* **2005**, *16*, 144–149. [CrossRef] [PubMed]
24. Ho, C.K.; Choi, S.W.; Siu, P.M.; Benzie, I.F. Effects of single dose and regular intake of green tea (*Camellia sinensis*) on DNA damage, DNA repair, and heme oxygenase-1 expression in a randomized controlled human supplementation study. *Mol. Nutr. Food Res.* **2014**, *58*, 1379–1383. [CrossRef] [PubMed]
25. Bakuradze, T.; Lang, R.; Hofmann, T.; Schipp, D.; Galan, J.; Eisenbrand, G.; Richling, E. Coffee consumption rapidly reduces background DNA strand breaks in healthy humans: Results of a short-term repeated uptake intervention study. *Mol. Nutr. Food Res.* **2016**, *60*, 682–686. [CrossRef] [PubMed]
26. Bakuradze, T.; Lang, R.; Hofmann, T.; Eisenbrand, G.; Schipp, D.; Galan, J.; Richling, E. Consumption of a dark roast coffee decreases the level of spontaneous DNA strand breaks: A randomized controlled trial. *Eur. J. Nutr.* **2015**, *54*, 149–156. [CrossRef] [PubMed]
27. Kiokias, S.; Proestos, C.; Oreopoulou, V. Effect of natural food antioxidants against LDL and DNA oxidative changes. *Antioxidants* **2018**, *7*, 133. [CrossRef] [PubMed]
28. Azqueta, A.; Collins, A. Polyphenols and DNA damage: A mixed blessing. *Nutrients* **2016**, *8*, 785. [CrossRef] [PubMed]
29. Willett, W.C.; Sacks, F.; Trichopoulou, A.; Drescher, G.; Ferro-Luzzi, A.; Helsing, E.; Trichopoulos, D. Mediterranean diet pyramid: A cultural model for healthy eating. *Am. J. Clin. Nutr.* **1995**, *61* (Suppl. 6), S1402–S1406. [CrossRef] [PubMed]

30. Bach-Faig, A.; Berry, E.M.; Lairon, D.; Reguant, J.; Trichopoulou, A.; Dernini, S.; Medina, F.X.; Battino, M.; Belahsen, R.; Miranda, G.; et al. Mediterranean Diet Foundation Expert Group. Mediterranean diet pyramid today. Science and cultural updates. *Public Health Nutr.* **2011**, *14*, 2274–2284. [CrossRef] [PubMed]
31. Koloverou, E.; Panagiotakos, D.B.; Pitsavos, C.; Chrysohoou, C.; Georgousopoulou, E.N.; Grekas, A.; Christou, A.; Chatzigeorgiou, M.; Skoumas, I.; Tousoulis, D.; et al. ATTICA Study Group. Adherence to Mediterranean diet and 10-year incidence (2002-2012) of diabetes: Correlations with inflammatory and oxidative stress biomarkers in the ATTICA cohort study. *Diabetes Metab. Res. Rev.* **2016**, *32*, 73–81. [CrossRef] [PubMed]
32. Dinu, M.; Pagliai, G.; Casini, A.; Sofi, F. Mediterranean diet and multiple health outcomes: An umbrella review of meta-analyses of observational studies and randomised trials. *Eur. J. Clin. Nutr.* **2018**, *72*, 30–43. [CrossRef] [PubMed]
33. Bonaccio, M.; Di Castelnuovo, A.; Costanzo, S.; Gialluisi, A.; Persichillo, M.; Cerletti, C.; Donati, M.B.; de Gaetano, G.; Iacoviello, L. Mediterranean diet and mortality in the elderly: A prospective cohort study and a meta-analysis. *Br. J. Nutr.* **2018**, *120*, 841–854. [CrossRef] [PubMed]
34. Buil-Cosiales, P.; Toledo, E.; Salas-Salvadó, J.; Zazpe, I.; Farràs, M.; Basterra-Gortari, F.J.; Diez-Espino, J.; Estruch, R.; Corella, D.; Ros, E.; et al. Association between dietary fibre intake and fruit, vegetable or whole-grain consumption and the risk of CVD: Results from the PREvención con DIeta MEDiterránea (PREDIMED) trial. *Br. J. Nutr.* **2016**, *116*, 534–546. [CrossRef] [PubMed]
35. Garcia-Arellano, A.; Ramallal, R.; Ruiz-Canela, M.; Salas-Salvadó, J.; Corella, D.; Shivappa, N.; Schröder, H.; Hébert, J.R.; Ros, E.; Gómez-Garcia, E.; et al. Dietary Inflammatory Index and incidence of cardiovascular disease in the PREDIMED Study. *Nutrients* **2015**, *7*, 4124–4138. [CrossRef]
36. Martínez-González, M.A.; Salas-Salvadó, J.; Estruch, R.; Corella, D.; Fitó, M.; Ros, E.; PREDIMED Investigators. Benefits of the Mediterranean Diet: Insights from the PREDIMED Study. *Prog. Cardiovasc. Dis.* **2015**, *58*, 50–60.
37. Guasch-Ferré, M.; Salas-Salvadó, J.; Ros, E.; Estruch, R.; Corella, D.; Fitó, M.; Martínez-González, M.A.; PREDIMED Investigators. The PREDIMED trial, Mediterranean diet and health outcomes: How strong is the evidence? *Nutr. Metab. Cardiovasc. Dis.* **2017**, *27*, 624–632.
38. Erdrich, S.; Bishop, K.S.; Karunasinghe, N.; Han, D.Y.; Ferguson, L.R. A pilot study to investigate if New Zealand men with prostate cancer benefit from a Mediterranean-style diet. *PeerJ* **2015**, *3*, e1080. [CrossRef]
39. Gutierrez-Mariscal, F.M.; Yubero-Serrano, E.M.; Rangel-Zúñiga, O.A.; Marín, C.; García-Rios, A.; Perez-Martinez, P.; Delgado-Lista, J.; Malagón, M.M.; Tinahones, F.J.; Pérez-Jimenez, F.; et al. Postprandial activation of p53-dependent DNA repair is modified by Mediterranean diet supplemented with coenzyme Q10 in elderly subjects. *J. Gerontol. A Biol. Sci. Med. Sci.* **2014**, *69*, 886–893. [CrossRef] [PubMed]
40. Mitjavila, M.T.; Fandos, M.; Salas-Salvadó, J.; Covas, M.I.; Borrego, S.; Estruch, R.; Lamuela-Raventós, R.; Corella, D.; Martínez-Gonzalez, M.Á.; Sánchez, J.M.; et al. The Mediterranean diet improves the systemic lipid and DNA oxidative damage in metabolic syndrome individuals. A randomized, controlled, trial. *Clin. Nutr.* **2013**, *32*, 172–178. [CrossRef]
41. Gutierrez-Mariscal, F.M.; Perez-Martinez, P.; Delgado-Lista, J.; Yubero-Serrano, E.M.; Camargo, A.; Delgado-Casado, N.; Cruz-Teno, C.; Santos-Gonzalez, M.; Rodriguez-Cantalejo, F.; Castaño, J.P.; et al. Mediterranean diet supplemented with coenzyme Q10 induces postprandial changes in p53 in response to oxidative DNA damage in elderly subjects. *Age* **2012**, *34*, 389–403. [CrossRef] [PubMed]
42. Konstantinidou, V.; Covas, M.I.; Muñoz-Aguayo, D.; Khymenets, O.; de la Torre, R.; Saez, G.; del Carmen Tormos, M.; Toledo, E.; Marti, A.; Ruiz-Gutiérrez, V.; et al. In vivo nutrigenomic effects of virgin olive oil polyphenols within the frame of the Mediterranean diet: A randomized controlled trial. *FASEB J.* **2010**, *24*, 2546–2557. [CrossRef] [PubMed]
43. Urquiaga, I.; Strobel, P.; Perez, D.; Martinez, C.; Cuevas, A.; Castillo, O.; Marshall, G.; Rozowski, J.; Leighton, F. Mediterranean diet and red wine protect against oxidative damage in young volunteers. *Atherosclerosis* **2010**, *211*, 694–699. [CrossRef] [PubMed]
44. García-Calzón, S.; Martínez-González, M.A.; Razquin, C.; Arós, F.; Lapetra, J.; Martínez, J.A.; Zalba, G.; Marti, A. Mediterranean diet and telomere length in high cardiovascular risk subjects from the PREDIMED-NAVARRA study. *Clin. Nutr.* **2016**, *35*, 1399–1405. [CrossRef] [PubMed]
45. García-Calzón, S.; Martínez-González, M.A.; Razquin, C.; Corella, D.; Salas-Salvadó, J.; Martínez, J.A.; Zalba, G.; Marti, A. Pro12Ala polymorphism of the PPARγ2 gene interacts with a mediterranean diet to

prevent telomere shortening in the PREDIMED-NAVARRA randomized trial. *Circ. Cardiovasc. Genet.* **2015**, *8*, 91–99. [CrossRef]
46. Müllner, E.; Brath, H.; Pleifer, S.; Schiermayr, C.; Baierl, A.; Wallner, M.; Fastian, T.; Millner, Y.; Paller, K.; Henriksen, T.; et al. Vegetables and PUFA-rich plant oil reduce DNA strand breaks in individuals with type 2 diabetes. *Mol. Nutr Food Res.* **2013**, *57*, 328–338. [CrossRef] [PubMed]
47. Zeng, L.; Wu, G.Z.; Goh, K.J.; Lee, Y.M.; Ng, C.C.; You, A.B.; Wang, J.; Jia, D.; Hao, A.; Yu, Q.; et al. Saturated fatty acids modulate cell response to DNA damage: Implication for their role in tumorigenesis. *PLoS ONE* **2008**, *3*, e2329. [CrossRef] [PubMed]
48. Bishop, K.S.; Erdrich, S.; Karunasinghe, N.; Han, D.Y.; Zhu, S.; Jesuthasan, A.; Ferguson, L.R. An investigation into the association between DNA damage and dietary fatty acid in men with prostate cancer. *Nutrients* **2015**, *7*, 405–422. [CrossRef]
49. Jenkinson, A.; Franklin, M.F.; Wahle, K.; Duthie, G.G. Dietary intakes of polyunsaturated fatty acids and indices of oxidative stress in human volunteers. *Eur. J. Clin. Nutr.* **1999**, *53*, 523–528. [CrossRef]
50. Kimura, Y.; Sato, M.; Kurotani, K.; Nanri, A.; Kawai, K.; Kasai, H.; Imaizumi, K.; Mizoue, T. PUFAs in serum cholesterol ester and oxidative DNA damage in Japanese men and women. *Am. J. Clin. Nutr.* **2012**, *95*, 1209–1214. [CrossRef]
51. Sakai, C.; Ishida, M.; Ohba, H.; Yamashita, H.; Uchida, H.; Yoshizumi, M.; Ishida, T. Fish oil omega-3 polyunsaturated fatty acids attenuate oxidative stress-induced DNA damage in vascular endothelial cells. *PLoS ONE* **2017**, *12*, e0187934. [CrossRef] [PubMed]
52. Kikugawa, K.; Yasuhara, Y.; Ando, K.; Koyama, K.; Hiramoto, K.; Suzuki, M. Protective effect of supplementation of fish oil with high n-3 polyunsaturated fatty acids against oxidative stress-induced DNA damage of rat liver in vivo. *J. Agric. Food Chem.* **2003**, *51*, 6073–6079. [CrossRef] [PubMed]
53. Dizdaroglu, M. Oxidatively induced DNA damage and its repair in cancer. *Mutat. Res. Rev. Mutat. Res.* **2015**, *763*, 212–245. [CrossRef] [PubMed]
54. Grosso, G.; Buscemi, S.; Galvano, F.; Mistretta, A.; Marventano, S.; La Vela, V.; Drago, F.; Gangi, S.; Basile, F.; Biondi, A. Mediterranean diet and cancer: Epidemiological evidence and mechanism of selected aspects. *BMC Surg.* **2013**, *13* (Suppl. 2), S14. [CrossRef] [PubMed]
55. Schwingshackl, L.; Schwedhelm, C.; Galbete, C.; Hoffmann, G. Adherence to Mediterranean diet and risk of cancer: An updated systematic review and meta-analysis. *Nutrients* **2017**, *9*, 1063. [CrossRef] [PubMed]
56. Giacosa, A.; Barale, R.; Bavaresco, L.; Gatenby, P.; Gerbi, V.; Janssens, J.; Johnston, B.; Kas, K.; La Vecchia, C.; Mainguet, P.; et al. Cancer prevention in Europe: The Mediterranean diet as a protective choice. *Eur. J. Cancer Prev.* **2013**, *22*, 90–95. [CrossRef] [PubMed]
57. Turati, F.; Carioli, G.; Bravi, F.; Ferraroni, M.; Serraino, D.; Montella, M.; Giacosa, A.; Toffolutti, F.; Negri, E.; Levi, F.; et al. Mediterranean diet and breast cancer risk. *Nutrients* **2018**, *10*, 326. [CrossRef]
58. Grosso, G.; Biondi, A.; Galvano, F.; Mistretta, A.; Marventano, S.; Buscemi, S.; Drago, F.; Basile, F. Factors associated with colorectal cancer in the context of the Mediterranean diet: A case-control study. *Nutr. Cancer* **2014**, *66*, 558–565. [CrossRef]
59. Bravi, F.; Spei, M.E.; Polesel, J.; Di Maso, M.; Montella, M.; Ferraroni, M.; Serraino, D.; Libra, M.; Negri, E.; La Vecchia, C.; et al. Mediterranean diet and bladder cancer risk in Italy. *Nutrients* **2018**, *10*, 1061. [CrossRef]
60. Russo, G.I.; Solinas, T.; Urzì, D.; Privitera, S.; Campisi, D.; Cocci, A.; Carini, M.; Madonia, M.; Cimino, S.; Morgia, G. Adherence to Mediterranean diet and prostate cancer risk in Sicily: Population-based case-control study. *Int. J. Impot. Res.* **2018**. [CrossRef]
61. Collins, A.R. Measuring oxidative damage to DNA and its repair with the comet assay. *Biochim. Biophys. Acta* **2014**, *1840*, 794–800. [CrossRef] [PubMed]
62. Møller, P. The comet assay: Ready for 30 more years. *Mutagenesis* **2018**, *33*, 1–7. [CrossRef] [PubMed]
63. Boccardi, V.; Esposito, A.; Rizzo, M.R.; Marfella, R.; Barbieri, M.; Paolisso, G. Mediterranean diet, telomere maintenance and health status among elderly. *PLoS ONE* **2013**, *8*, e62781. [CrossRef] [PubMed]
64. Crous-Bou, M.; Fung, T.T.; Prescott, J.; Julin, B.; Du, M.; Sun, Q.; Rexrode, K.M.; Hu, F.B.; De Vivo, I. Mediterranean diet and telomere length in nurses' health study: Population based cohort study. *BMJ* **2014**, *349*, g6674. [CrossRef] [PubMed]
65. Gu, Y.; Honig, L.S.; Schupf, N.; Lee, J.H.; Luchsinger, J.A.; Stern, Y.; Scarmeas, N. Mediterranean diet and leukocyte telomere length in a multi-ethnic elderly population. *Age* **2015**, *37*, 24. [CrossRef] [PubMed]

66. Marin, C.; Delgado-Lista, J.; Ramirez, R.; Carracedo, J.; Caballero, J.; Perez-Martinez, P.; Gutierrez-Mariscal, F.M.; Garcia-Rios, A.; Delgado-Casado, N.; Cruz-Teno, C.; et al. Mediterranean diet reduces senescence-associated stress in endothelial cells. *Age* **2012**, *34*, 1309–1316. [CrossRef] [PubMed]
67. García-Calzón, S.; Gea, A.; Razquin, C.; Corella, D.; Lamuela-Raventós, R.M.; Martínez, J.A.; Martínez-González, M.A.; Zalba, G.; Marti, A. Longitudinal association of telomere length and obesity indices in an intervention study with a Mediterranean diet: The PREDIMED-NAVARRA trial. *Int. J. Obes.* **2014**, *38*, 177–182. [CrossRef] [PubMed]
68. García-Calzón, S.; Zalba, G.; Ruiz-Canela, M.; Shivappa, N.; Hébert, J.R.; Martínez, J.A.; Fitó, M.; Gómez-Gracia, E.; Martínez-González, M.A.; Marti, A. Dietary inflammatory index and telomere length in subjects with a high cardiovascular disease risk from the PREDIMED-NAVARRA study: Cross-sectional and longitudinal analyses over 5 y. *Am. J. Clin. Nutr.* **2015**, *102*, 897–904. [CrossRef] [PubMed]

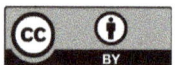

© 2019 by the authors. Licensee MDPI, Basel, Switzerland. This article is an open access article distributed under the terms and conditions of the Creative Commons Attribution (CC BY) license (http://creativecommons.org/licenses/by/4.0/).

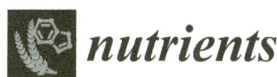

Article

Adherence to the Mediterranean Diet is Associated with Better Sleep Quality in Italian Adults

Justyna Godos [1], Raffaele Ferri [2], Filippo Caraci [2,3], Filomena Irene Ilaria Cosentino [2], Sabrina Castellano [4], Fabio Galvano [1,†] and Giuseppe Grosso [1,*,†]

1. Department of Biomedical and Biotechnological Sciences, University of Catania, 95123 Catania, Italy; justyna.godos@student.uj.edu.pl (J.G.); fgalvano@unict.it (F.G.)
2. Oasi Research Institute - IRCCS, 94018 Troina, Italy; rferri@oasi.en.it (R.F.); carafil@hotmail.com (F.C.); fcosentino@oasi.en.it (F.I.I.C.)
3. Department of Drug Sciences, University of Catania, 95125 Catania, Italy
4. Department of Educational Sciences, University of Catania, 95124 Catania, Italy; sabrinacastellano@hotmail.it
* Correspondence: giuseppe.grosso@unict.it; Tel.: +39-0954-781-187
† These authors contributed equally to this work.

Received: 20 February 2019; Accepted: 25 April 2019; Published: 28 April 2019

Abstract: Background: Sleep quality has been associated with human health and diseases, including cognitive decline and dementia; however major determinants of sleep disorders are largely unknown. The aim of this study was to evaluate the association between sleep quality and adherence to the Mediterranean dietary pattern in a sample of Italian adults. Methods: A total of 1936 individuals were recruited in the urban area of Catania during 2014–2015 through random sampling. A food frequency questionnaire and validated instruments were used to assess the adherence to the Mediterranean diet and sleep quality (Pittsburg sleep quality index). Multivariate logistic regressions were performed to determine the association between exposure and outcome. Results: A total of 1314 individuals (67.9% of the cohort) reported adequate sleep quality: for each point increase of the Mediterranean diet score, individuals were 10% more likely to have adequate sleep quality. In an additional analysis stratifying the sample by weight status, the association between sleep quality and high adherence to the Mediterranean diet was observed only among normal/overweight individuals but not in obese participants. Conclusions: high adherence to a Mediterranean diet is associated with better sleep quality either toward direct effect on health or indirect effects through improvement of weight status.

Keywords: Mediterranean diet; sleep quality; cognitive decline; dementia; weight status; mental health; obesity; cohort; Italy

---

1. Introduction

Epidemiological evidence suggests that sleeping habits might be related to human health, including cardio-metabolic and mental health outcomes [1,2]. Most of existing evidence focuses on sleep duration, suggesting that lack of sleep may exert negative effects on a variety of systems [3]. The mechanisms mediating the relation between sleep and health status are not entirely clear, but are likely to be multifactorial, involving hormonal disruption, metabolic impairment, and inflammatory processes [4,5]. Although short term sleep deprivation is associated to decrements in the psychomotor vigilance task, the most consistent finding animal studies showed that chronic unhealthy sleeping behaviors may impact central nervous system structural plasticity in different ways, including reduction of spine density and attenuation of synaptic efficacy in the hippocampus [6]. Long-term changes in sleep quality and architecture have been related to cognitive impairment; while the incidence of sleep disorders may increase with normal aging, further impairment of sleep-dependent memory consolidation has been observed in relation with neurodegenerative diseases, including dementias and Alzheimer's disease [7].

It is not clear whether sleep disturbances occur with higher rate in individuals having cognitive impairment or dementia, or they may also represent an independent risk factor for such pathological conditions. However, sleep disorders and cognitive decline seem to be somehow connected at the pathophysiological level [8]. Therefore, it is potentially important to identify determinants of sleep disorders in middle-aged and older adults as a strategy to prevent cognitive decline and dementia.

Among the many factors studied, diet has been the focus of recent attention due to the potential relation with both sleep quality and its related health outcomes [9]. The Mediterranean dietary pattern has gained popularity over recent decades due to its palatable taste and a strong evidence of benefits for health [10]. Despite a single definition of Mediterranean diet cannot be achieved, it refers to the traditional diet of Southern Italian people explored in the 60s by Ancel Keys, characterized by certain peculiarities including high consumption of plant-based foods (such as fruit, vegetable, legumes and nuts), preference for whole-grain cereals, fish (whenever available) and dairy products instead of other sources of refined carbohydrates and animal proteins, respectively; other characteristics were the daily consumption of olive oil and moderate intake of alcohol (mostly red wine) during meals [11]. A combination of these features has been further investigated in several studies, leading to the development of a number of adherence scores ideally optimized for type of population (i.e., geographical localization), diet parameters availability (i.e., completeness of dietary questionnaires), and generalizability of results (i.e., use of comparable scores) [12]. High adherence to the Mediterranean diet has been associated with a number of cardio-metabolic health outcomes [13,14], including lower risk of cardiovascular-related disorders [15,16], diabetes [17], metabolic syndromes [18,19], and non-alcoholic fatty liver disease [20,21]. These beneficial effects are ascribed to various mechanisms, mostly involving a high content in antioxidants and healthy dietary fats, which in turn may improve insulin sensitivity, reduce vascular inflammation and improve endothelial dysfunction [22]. Lately, a large body of literature has also shown that adherence to a Mediterranean dietary pattern may exert benefits also toward mental health and neurological outcomes, including stroke, cognitive impairment, depression, and dementia [23–28]. Recent evidence shows a relation between adherence to the Mediterranean diet and sleep duration and quality in adults [29–31], but only few studies have been performed and more research is warranted to better investigate such a relation. The aim of this study was to evaluate the association between sleep quality and adherence to the Mediterranean dietary pattern in a sample of Italian adults.

2. Materials and Methods

2.1. Study Population

The Mediterranean healthy Eating, Aging, and Lifestyles (MEAL) study is cross-sectional study aimed to explore the relation between nutritional and lifestyle behaviors characterizing individuals living in the Mediterranean area. The detailed study protocol with the rationale, design, and methods has been described in detail elsewhere [32]. Briefly, the cohort consisted of a random sample of men and women (age 18+ years) registered in the records of local general practitioners in the urban area of Catania, one of the largest cities in the east coast of Sicily, southern Italy, during 2014–2015. The sampling technique included stratification by municipality area, age, and sex of inhabitants, and randomization into subgroups, with randomly selected general practitioners being the sampling units, and individuals registered to them comprising the final sample units. Pregnant women were not considered in this study. Participants randomly selected for recruitment were stratified by sex and 10-year age groups. The theoretical sample size was set at 1500 individuals to provide a specific relative precision of 5% (Type I error, 0.05; Type II error, 0.10), taking into account an anticipated 70% participation rate. Out of 2405 individuals invited, the final sample size was 2044 participants (response rate of 85%). All the study procedures were carried out in accordance with the Declaration of Helsinki (1989) of the World Medical Association. Participants provided written informed consent and the study protocol was approved by the ethics committee of the referent health authority.

2.2. Data Collection

Data regarding demographic (i.e., age, sex, educational and occupational level) and lifestyle characteristics (i.e., physical activity, smoking and drinking habits) were collected. Educational level was categorized as: (i) low (primary/secondary), (ii) medium (high school), and (iii) high (university). Occupational level was classified as: (i) unemployed, (ii) low (unskilled workers), (iii) medium (partially skilled workers), and (iv) high (skilled workers). Physical activity level was assessed using International Physical Activity Questionnaires (IPAQs) [33], which are comprised a set of questionnaires (5 domains) on time spent being physically active in the last 7 days that allow categorization of physical activity as: (i) low, (ii) moderate, and (iii) high. Smoking status was classified as: (i) non-smoker, (ii) ex-smoker, and (iii) current smoker. Alcohol consumption was categorized as (i) none, (ii) moderate drinker (0.1-12 g/d) and (iii) regular drinker (>12 g/d). Anthropometric measurements were performed according to standardized methods [34]. Height was measured to the nearest 0.5 cm without shoes, with the back square against the wall tape, eyes looking straight ahead, with a right-angle triangle resting on the scalp and against the wall. Body mass index (BMI) was calculated, and patients were categorized as under/normal weight (BMI <25 kg/m^2), overweight (BMI 25 to 29.9 kg/m^2), and obese (BMI ≥30 kg/m^2) [35].

2.3. Dietary Assessment

Dietary data was collected using long and short food frequency questionnaires (FFQs), developed and previously validated for the Sicilian population [36,37]. The FFQs consisted of 110 food and drink items representative of the diet during the previous 6 months. Participants of the study were asked how often, on average, they had consumed foods and drinks included in the FFQ, with nine responses ranging from "never" to "4–5 times per day". Intake of food items characterized by seasonality referred to consumption during the period in which the food was available and then adjusted by its proportional intake over one year. After exclusion of 107 entries with unreliable intakes (<1000 or >6000 kcal/d, controlled case by case and validated due to missing food items or unreliable answers), a total of 1936 individuals were included in the analyses for the present study.

2.4. Adherence to the Mediterranean Diet

Mediterranean diet adherence was assessed using the score developed by Sofi et al. [15]. Briefly, a scoring system (the MEDI-LITE score) was built based on existing literature weighting all the median (or mean) values for the sample size of each study population and then calculating a mean value of all the weighted medians; hence, two standard deviations were used to determine three different categories of consumption for each food group. For food groups, typical of the Mediterranean diet (fruit, vegetables, cereals, legumes and fish), two points were given to the highest category of consumption, one point for the middle category and zero points for the lowest category of intake. Contrariwise, for food groups not typical of the Mediterranean diet (meat and meat-based products, dairy products), two points were given for the lowest category, one point for the middle category and zero points for the highest category of consumption. Regarding alcohol, categories related to the alcohol unit (one alcohol unit = 12 g of alcohol) were used by giving two points to the middle category (1–2 alcohol units/d), one point to the lowest category (>1 alcohol unit/d) and zero points to the highest category of consumption (>2 alcohol units/d). The final score comprised nine food categories (including olive oil) with a score ranging from zero points (lowest adherence) to 18 points (highest adherence).

2.5. Sleep Quality

The Pittsburg sleep quality index (PSQI) [38] was used to assess participants' sleep quality and disturbances in the past six month. It consists of 19 items which are rated on a four-point scale (0–3) and grouped into seven components (sleep quality, sleep latency, sleep duration, habitual sleep efficiency, sleep disturbance, use of sleeping medications, and daytime dysfunction). The item scores in each component were summed and converted to component scores ranging from 0 (better) to 3 (worse) based on guidelines. Total PSQI scores were calculated as the summation of seven component scores ranging from zero to 21, where higher score indicates worse condition. A total global PSQI score of <5 is indicative of adequate sleep quality.

2.6. Statistical Analysis

Categorical variables are presented as frequencies of occurrence and percentages differences between groups were tested using a Chi-squared test. First, the difference between distribution of background variables by sleep quality (adequate vs. inadequate) was tested. Second, differences in distribution of sleep-related characteristics between groups of individuals divided into quartiles of Mediterranean diet adherence score (Q1 had the lowest adherence, Q4 had the highest adherence) was tested. The relation between adherence to the Mediterranean diet and sleep-related outcomes was tested through multivariate logistic regression analysis adjusted for baseline characteristics (age, sex, marital, educational and occupational status, smoking and alcohol drinking habits, and physical activity level) comparing individuals grouped into quartiles or estimating the association by 1-point increase of the Mediterranean diet adherence score. A sensitivity analysis excluding, one at a time, each individual component of the Mediterranean diet adherence score was performed. Finally, a subgroup analysis by weight status categorization (normal/overweight and obese individuals) has been performed to test stability of results. All reported p values were based on two-sided tests and compared to a significance level of 5%. SPSS 17 (SPSS Inc., Chicago, IL, USA) software was used for all the statistical analysis.

3. Results

A total of 1314 individuals (67.9% of the sample) reported an overall adequate sleep quality according to the PSQI score. The distribution of the baseline characteristics of the study participants by sleep quality revealed that there were no significant differences between groups with the exception of occupational level, as there was a significantly higher proportion of individuals with adequate quality of sleep in the highest category than in the lower. However, the distribution was not linear, and a high proportion of individuals with adequate quality of sleep were present also in the lowest category (Table 1).

Table 1. Baseline characteristics of the study participants by sleep quality. n indicates the number of individuals that satisfy each condition within the total sample; % indicates the percentages of individuals that satisfy each condition within the total sample.

	Sleep Quality		p-Value
	Inadequate ($n = 622$)	Adequate ($n = 1314$)	
Sex, n (%)			0.052
Men	278 (44.7)	526 (40.0)	
Women	344 (55.3)	788 (60.0)	
Age groups, n (%)			0.161
<30	124 (19.9)	226 (17.2)	
30–49	218 (35.0)	485 (36.9)	
50–69	209 (33.6)	416 (31.7)	
≥70	71 (11.4)	187 (14.2)	
Educational status, n (%)			0.119
Low	224 (36.0)	473 (36.0)	
Medium	248 (39.9)	472 (35.9)	
High	150 (24.1)	369 (28.1)	
Occupational status, n (%)			0.011
Unemployed	131 (24.8)	330 (29.2)	
Low	84 (15.9)	181 (16.1)	
Medium	167 (31.6)	273 (24.2)	
High	146 (27.7)	345 (30.5)	

Table 1. Cont.

	Sleep Quality		p-Value
	Inadequate (n = 622)	Adequate (n = 1314)	
Smoking status, n (%)			0.595
Never smoker	375 (60.3)	820 (62.4)	
Former smoker	89 (14.3)	187 (14.2)	
Current smoker	158 (25.4)	307 (23.4)	
Physical activity level, n (%)			0.169
Low	93 (16.6)	236 (20.2)	
Moderate	291 (52.0)	565 (48.4)	
High	176 (31.4)	367 (31.4)	
Health status, n (%)			
Hypertension	292 (46.9)	684 (52.1)	0.036
Type-2 diabetes	45 (7.2)	101 (7.7)	0.725
Dyslipidemias	118 (19.0)	238 (18.1)	0.649
Cardiovascular disease	57 (9.3)	97 (7.6)	0.198
Cancer	19 (3.1)	59 (4.5)	0.134
Weight status, n (%)			0.372
Normal	267 (47.6)	584 (47.2)	
Overweight	205 (36.5)	425 (34.4)	
Obese	89 (15.9)	228 (18.4)	

The relation between specific indicators of sleep quality of the study participants by quartiles of the Mediterranean diet adherence score are reported in Table 2. Among participants more adherent to the dietary pattern (the highest quartile, Q4) there was a higher proportion of individuals with overall better sleep quality compared to the less adherent (the lowest quartile, Q1; 72.4% vs. 58.9%; P <0.001); among specific domains of the PSQI, significantly lower occurrences of shorter sleep durations, longer sleep latency, day dysfunction due to sleepiness, very low sleep efficiency and self-reported sleep quality occurred among participants in the highest quartile of the Mediterranean diet adherence score.

Table 2. Overall sleep quality and sleep-related characteristics of the study participants by quartiles of Mediterranean diet adherence score. n indicates the number of individuals that satisfy each condition within the total sample; % indicates the percentages of individuals that satisfy each condition within the total sample.

	Mediterranean Diet Adherence Score *				p-Value
	Q1	Q2	Q3	Q4	
Overall sleep quality, n (%)					<0.001
Adequate	272 (58.9)	403 (68.0)	440 (72.6)	199 (72.4)	
Inadequate	190 (41.1)	190 (32.0)	166 (27.4)	76 (27.6)	
Sleep duration, n (%)					<0.001
>7 h	246 (53.2)	371 (62.6)	376 (62.0)	171 (62.2)	
6–7 h	111 (24.0)	130 (21.9)	137 (22.6)	57 (20.7)	
5–6 h	65 (14.1)	58 (9.8)	74 (12.2)	33 (12.0)	
<5 h	40 (8.7)	34 (5.7)	19 (3.1)	14 (5.1)	
Sleep disturbance, n (%)					0.311
None	53 (11.5)	54 (9.1)	74 (12.2)	35 (12.7)	
Low	335 (72.5)	444 (74.9)	451 (74.4)	207 (75.3)	
Medium	74 (16.0)	95 (16.0)	81 (13.4)	33 (12.0)	
High	0	0	0	0	
Sleep latency, n (%)					0.003
Very short	172 (37.2)	253 (42.7)	298 (49.2)	135 (49.1)	
Short	153 (33.1)	210 (35.4)	181 (29.9)	85 (30.9)	
Medium	101 (21.9)	94 (15.9)	97 (16.0)	41 (14.9)	
Long	36 (7.8)	36 (6.1)	30 (5.0)	14 (5.1)	
Day dysfunction, n (%)					<0.001
None	296 (64.1)	433 (73.0)	440 (72.6)	201 (73.1)	
Low	75 (16.2)	91 (15.3)	93 (15.3)	30 (10.9)	
Medium	35 (7.6)	28 (4.7)	27 (4.5)	23 (8.4)	
High	56 (12.1)	41 (6.9)	46 (7.6)	21 (7.6)	

Table 2. Cont.

	Mediterranean Diet Adherence Score *				
	Q1	Q2	Q3	Q4	p-Value
Sleep efficiency, n (%)					<0.001
High	296 (64.1)	433 (73.0)	440 (72.6)	201 (73.1)	
Medium	75 (16.2)	91 (15.3)	93 (15.3)	30 (10.9)	
Low	35 (7.6)	28 (4.7)	27 (4.5)	23 (8.4)	
Very low	56 (12.1)	41 (6.9)	46 (7.6)	21 (7.6)	
Self-rated sleep quality, n (%)					0.043
Very low	14 (3.0)	29 (4.9)	15 (2.5)	13 (4.7)	
Low	17 (3.7)	15 (2.5)	15 (2.5)	0 (0)	
Medium	17 (3.7)	26 (4.4)	20 (3.3)	11 (4.0)	
High	414 (89.6)	523 (88.2)	556 (91.7)	251 (91.3)	
Need medication to sleep, n (%)	48 (10.4)	70 (11.8)	50 (8.3)	24 (8.7)	0.187

* Groups represent individuals divided into quartiles.

Among the whole sample, a higher adherence to the Mediterranean diet was associated with a higher likelihood of adequate overall sleep quality (highest vs. lowest quartile, OR = 1.82, 95% CI: 1.32, 2.52; Table 3). However, among the specific indicators of sleep quality, only sleep latency was significantly associated with higher adherence to the dietary pattern, while no day dysfunction due to sleepiness was associated with the third quartile of the Mediterranean diet adherence score, but not with the highest. When considering the relation with 1-point increase of the Mediterranean diet adherence score, the multivariate regression analysis revealed that individuals were 10% more likely to have an overall adequate sleep quality, while among individual components of the PSQI score, 1-point increase of the dietary adherence score was significantly associated with having adequate sleep duration, latency, and efficiency (Table 3).

Table 3. Association between overall and individual domains of sleep quality and adherence and quartiles of the Mediterranean diet adherence score. Odds ratios indicate the probability that a subject was an adequate sleeper to the probability that the subject was not, between subjects included in each quartile, compared to those included in the lowest.

	Mediterranean Diet Adherence Score				
	Q1	Q2	Q3	Q4	1-Point Increment
	OR (95% CI) *				
Adequate sleep quality	1	1.48 (1.15, 1.90) §	1.85 (1.43, 2.39) §	1.82 (1.32, 2.52) §	1.10 (1.05, 1.16) §
Sleep duration	1	1.39 (1.04, 1.86) §	1.29 (0.97, 1.71)	1.35 (0.94, 1.92)	1.07 (1.02, 1.12) §
Sleep disturbance	1	0.81 (0.51, 1.30)	1.26 (0.82, 1.95)	1.31 (0.77, 2.21)	1.04 (0.97, 1.12)
Sleep latency	1	1.12 (0.84, 1.50)	1.64 (1.23, 2.17) §	1.52 (1.07, 2.16)	1.07 (1.02, 1.12) §
Day dysfunction	1	1.12 (0.85, 1.49)	1.42 (1.07, 1.88) #	1.25 (0.88, 1.77)	1.04 (1.00, 1.09) #
Sleep efficiency	1	1.36 (1.00, 1.84) #	1.33 (0.98, 1.80)	1.40 (0.95, 2.05)	1.06 (1.01, 1.12) #
Need medication to sleep	1	0.67 (0.42, 1.07)	1.34 (0.80, 2.25)	1.05 (0.57, 1.93)	1.03 (0.95, 1.11)
Self-rated sleep quality	1	1.04 (0.73, 1.48)	1.16 (0.83, 1.64)	1.30 (0.86, 1.98)	1.04 (0.98, 1.09)

* adjusted for age (continuous), sex (male/female), BMI (<25 kg/m^2, 25–30 kg/m^2, >30 kg/m^2), physical activity (low/medium/high), educational status (low/medium/high), occupational status (unemployed/low/medium/high), smoking status (current/former/never), alcohol consumption (no/moderate/regular), health status (presence of hypertension, type-2 diabetes, dyslipidaemias, cardiovascular disease, cancer), and total energy intake. # indicates $p < 0.05$. § indicates $p < 0.001$.

An alternative analysis by excluding one at the time each individual component of the Mediterranean diet adherence score was performed in order to test whether any of these could explain alone the association of the score (Table 4). The results show that the association was robust, as the association with overall sleep quality was significant in all alternative scores; moreover, exclusion of no individual component, besides olive oil, showed significant association with the aforementioned aspects of sleep quality, including sleep duration, latency, and efficacy, suggesting that olive oil may play an independent role in sleep quality.

Table 4. Association between overall and individual domains of sleep quality and alternative Mediterranean diet adherence scores with exclusion of each individual component one at the time. Odds ratios indicate the probability that a subject was an adequate sleeper to the probability that the subject was not, between subjects included in each 1-point score, compared to those having 1 unit lower.

	Mediterranean Diet Adherence Score, 1-Point Increment Recalculated Excluding:								
	Fruit	Vegetable	Legume	Dairy	Whole-grain	Fish	Meat	Olive oil	Alcohol
					OR (95% CI) *				
Overall sleep quality	1.12 (1.06, 1.18) §	1.11 (1.06, 1.17) §	1.10 (1.05, 1.17) §	1.13 (1.07, 1.19) §	1.09 (1.04, 1.15) #	1.11 (1.06, 1.17) §	1.10 (1.05, 1.15) §	1.09 (1.03, 1.14) #	1.10 (1.05, 1.15) §
Sleep duration	1.08 (1.02, 1.14) #	1.07 (1.02, 1.12) #	1.08 (1.03, 1.14) #	1.08 (1.03, 1.14) #	1.06 (1.01, 1.11) #	1.07 (1.02, 1.13) #	1.07 (1.02, 1.13) #	1.04 (0.99, 1.09)	1.06 (1.01, 1.11) #
Sleep disturbance	1.03 (0.95, 1.11)	1.03 (0.95, 1.11)	1.06 (0.98, 1.15)	1.07 (0.99, 1.16)	1.05 (0.97, 1.13)	1.06 (0.98, 1.14)	1.03 (0.96, 1.11)	1.03 (0.96, 1.11)	1.04 (0.97, 1.12)
Sleep latency	1.08 (1.03, 1.14) #	1.09 (1.03, 1.14) #	1.07 (1.02, 1.13) #	1.07 (1.02, 1.12) #	1.06 (1.01, 1.11) #	1.08 (1.03, 1.14) #	1.08 (1.03, 1.13) #	1.06 (1.01, 1.11) #	1.07 (1.02, 1.12) #
Day dysfunction	1.04 (0.99, 1.09)	1.04 (0.99, 1.10)	1.04 (0.99, 1.10)	1.06 (1.01, 1.11) #	1.05 (1.00, 1.10) #	1.05 (1.00, 1.10) #	1.05 (1.00, 1.10)#	1.04 (0.99, 1.09)	1.04 (0.99, 1.09)
Sleep efficiency	1.06 (1.00, 1.12) #	1.07 (1.01, 1.12) #	1.06 (1.01, 1.12) #	1.09 (1.03, 1.15) #	1.06 (1.01, 1.11) #	1.06 (1.01, 1.12) #	1.06 (1.01, 1.12) #	1.05 (1.00, 1.11) #	1.07 (1.02, 1.12) #
Need medication to sleep	1.04 (0.96, 1.14)	1.03 (0.95, 1.12)	1.03 (0.94, 1.12)	1.02 (0.94, 1.10)	1.03 (0.96, 1.12)	1.04 (0.96, 1.13)	1.04 (0.96, 1.12)	1.02 (0.94, 1.10)	1.02 (0.95, 1.10)
Self-rated sleep quality	1.03 (0.96, 1.09)	1.04 (0.98, 1.10)	1.04 (0.98, 1.11)	1.04 (0.98, 1.11)	1.05 (0.99, 1.11)	1.04 (0.98, 1.10)	1.04 (0.98, 1.10)	1.03 (0.97, 1.10)	1.04 (0.98, 1.10)

* adjusted for age (continuous), sex (male/female), BMI (<25 kg/m², 25–30 kg/m², >30 kg/m²), physical activity (low/medium/high), educational status (low/medium/high), occupational status (unemployed/low/medium/high), smoking status (current/former/never), alcohol consumption (no/moderate/regular), health status (presence of hypertension, type-2 diabetes, dyslipidaemias, cardiovascular disease, cancer), and total energy intake. # indicates $p < 0.05$. § indicates $p < 0.001$.

Table 5 summarizes the results of a supplementary analysis, in which the associations of all endpoints were tested separately according to body weight status of study participants, leading to some differences: Specifically, the association between adequate sleep quality and higher adherence to the Mediterranean diet was observed only among normal/overweight individuals (highest vs. lowest quartile, OR = 2.30, 95% CI: 1.49, 3.54; 1-point increase, OR = 1.10, 95% CI: 1.04, 1.16), while this was not found in obese participants. Among the specific indicators of sleep quality, only sleep latency was associated with the diet score in the former group, but not in the latter (Table 5).

Table 5. Association between overall and individual domains of sleep quality and adherence and quartiles of the Mediterranean diet adherence score by weight status. Odds ratios indicate the probability that a subject was an adequate sleeper to the probability that the subject was not, between subjects included in each 1-point score, compared to those having 1 unit lower.

	Mediterranean Diet Adherence Score				
	Q1	Q2	Q3	Q4	1-Point Increment
	OR (95% CI) *				
Normal/overweight					
Overall sleep quality	1	1.22 (0.87, 1.71)	1.79 (1.27, 2.54) §	2.30 (1.49, 3.54) §	1.10 (1.04, 1.16) §
Sleep duration	1	1.32 (0.94, 1.83)	1.29 (0.92, 1.79)	1.32 (0.89, 1.97)	1.06 (1.01, 1.12) #
Sleep disturbance	1	0.82 (0.47, 1.40)	1.28 (0.77, 2.13)	1.22 (0.67, 2.22)	1.03 (0.95, 1.12)
Sleep latency	1	1.08 (0.77, 1.51)	1.96 (1.40, 2.74) §	1.62 (1.09, 2.41) §	1.09 (1.03, 1.15) #
Day dysfunction	1	1.26 (0.91, 1.74)	1.51 (1.09, 2.10) §	1.27 (0.86, 1.88)	1.03 (0.97, 1.08)
Sleep efficiency	1	1.32 (0.92, 1.88)	1.29 (0.90, 1.84)	1.48 (0.96, 2.28)	1.04 (0.99, 1.10)
Need medication to sleep	1	0.62 (0.37, 1.04)	1.24 (0.69, 2.23)	0.97 (0.50, 1.89)	1.01 (0.92, 1.10)
Self-rated sleep quality	1	0.97 (0.65, 1.46)	1.27 (0.85, 1.89)	1.31 (0.82, 2.08)	1.04 (0.98, 1.11)
Obese					
Overall sleep quality	1	0.91 (0.39, 2.15)	1.11 (0.49, 2.50)	1.12 (0.33, 3.79)	1.12 (0.95, 1.32)
Sleep duration	1	1.67 (0.75, 3.73)	1.58 (0.75, 3.36)	2.68 (0.80, 8.96)	1.09 (0.94, 1.26)
Sleep disturbance	1	1.38 (0.42, 4.54)	1.71 (0.59, 4.92)	3.41 (0.81, 14.36)	1.20 (0.98, 1.49)
Sleep latency	1	1.08 (0.49, 2.36)	0.69 (0.33, 1.43)	0.65 (0.21, 2.01)	0.89 (0.77, 1.03)
Day dysfunction	1	0.69 (0.32, 1.49)	1.06 (0.52, 2.19)	1.22 (0.39, 3.79)	1.07 (0.93, 1.23)
Sleep efficiency	1	1.91 (0.81, 4.50)	1.32 (0.61, 2.87)	1.46 (0.44, 4.81)	1.13 (0.97, 1.33)
Need medication to sleep	1	0.48 (0.09, 2.40)	1.36 (0.24, 7.59)	1.57 (0.40, 5.92)	1.21 (0.87, 1.69)
Self-rated sleep quality	1	1.28 (0.54, 3.00)	0.87 (0.38, 1.97)	0.92 (0.25, 3.30)	0.95 (0.81, 1.11)

* adjusted for age (continuous), sex (male/female), BMI (<25 kg/m^2, 25–30 kg/m^2, >30 kg/m^2), physical activity (low/medium/high), educational status (low/medium/high), occupational status (unemployed/low/medium/high), smoking status (current/former/never), alcohol consumption (no/moderate/regular), health status (presence of hypertension, type-2 diabetes, dyslipidaemia, cardiovascular disease, cancer), and total energy intake. # indicates $p < 0.05$. § indicates $p < 0.001$.

4. Discussion

In the present study, a relation between sleep quality and adherence to the Mediterranean dietary pattern has been reported in a cohort of Southern Italian adults. Among the main domains investigated, only sleep latency resulted in being independently associated with higher adherence to this dietary pattern, suggesting that the overall sleep quality rather than specific aspects are associated with a healthier diet. Considering the impact of sleep-related habits toward adverse health outcomes, it is crucial to investigate and identify potential dietary determinants of sleep quality.

To our knowledge, only two studies previously investigated the association between adherence to the Mediterranean diet and sleep parameters in adults [29,30]. One study was conducted on about 1500 older adults living in Spain followed up for 2.8 years and monitored for their sleep duration and indicators of poor sleep quality. The authors found that individuals more adherent to the Mediterranean dietary pattern had a lower risk of a variation (increase or decrease) in sleep duration of more than 2 h and were also at lower risk of poor sleep quality [29]. Another study investigated the relation between adherence to the Mediterranean diet and specific aspects of sleeping, such as insomnia symptoms, finding a positive effect with adherence to a Mediterranean dietary pattern [30]. Some studies investigated the association between sleep duration and overall diet quality [39,40], while others also explored the relation between sleep patterns and eating behaviors, such as unbalanced food variety, irregular meal times, snacking between meals, eating out, and other potentially unhealthy eating habits [41,42]. Concerning our specific findings on sleep latency, intervention studies suggest a causal association between higher fat and carbohydrate intake close to bedtime and high sleep latency [43], thus confirming our results. In general, a consistent relation between dietary behaviors, nutrition quality, and sleep-related habits has been reported in most of the aforementioned studies. However, the direction of the association is debatable, whether better dietary habits might lead to better sleeping patterns or the other way around. In fact, experimental studies demonstrated both ways of association: on one side, it has been demonstrated that a high-quality diet improved sleep duration; on the other, it has been shown that sleep deprivation may increase appetite for high-calorie foods [44].

The Mediterranean dietary pattern may assure an adequate nutritional profile, including high consumption of fruit, vegetable, fish, whole-grains, olive oil, and limited amounts of meat, dairy and alcohol [45]. Previous reports from the cohort investigated in this study showed a significant inverse relation between higher adherence to the Mediterranean diet and likelihood of being obese [46], hypertensive [47] or suffer from dyslipidemia [48]. However, no individual component of the Mediterranean diet has been shown to be responsible alone for such associations, while some evidence on consumption of certain classes of polyphenols (such as flavonoids, phenolic acids and phytoestrogens) may explain, at least in part, these previous findings [49,50]. Similar considerations have been drafted while examining the association between higher adherence to the Mediterranean diet and mental health, which in turn might be associated with improved sleep patterns [51,52]. Richness of the Mediterranean diet in bioactive compounds with beneficial effects, such as antioxidant or anti-inflammatory properties, may exert neuroprotection and reduce oxidative damage and cerebral ischemia [53]. In fact, impaired antioxidant defense responses, such as increased rate of oxidative processes in several organs, including heart, liver and brain, have been reported during sleep deprivation while increased neuro-inflammation has been postulated to contribute to poor sleep quality [54,55]. Further evidence also shows that sleep duration and quality may be mediated by C-reactive protein (CRP), γ-glutamyl transferase (GGT), carotenoids, uric acid, and some vitamins, including vitamin C and D [56,57]. The high content of the Mediterranean diet in polyunsaturated fatty acids (PUFA) and phytochemicals, such as polyphenols, have been demonstrated to have an impact on inflammatory biomarkers [58]. Cohort studies have shown an inverse association between dietary PUFA [59,60] and polyphenols with better mental health (i.e., depressive symptoms, cognitive impairment, etc.) [61–63]. A variety of neuroprotective activities have been described, including anti-amyloidogenic efficacy, neuroprotection via modulation of neural mediators, and modulation of different signaling pathways [64,65]. Moreover, environmental stimuli (including exercise, but also sleep and dietary patterns) have been linked to hippocampal neurogenesis, a phenomenon occurring also in human adults, that seems to be linked to a number of pathological conditions, including stress, anxiety and depression, and cognitive impairment [66]. The resulting benefits of high adherence to the Mediterranean diet on sleep, cognition, mood, and Alzheimer's disease may, thus, also depend on the enhancement of structural and functional brain plasticity mediated by components of this dietary pattern, such as PUFA and polyphenols [67,68].

In addition to the aforementioned potential mechanisms, in this study we also hypothesized that the association between adherence to the Mediterranean diet and sleep quality might somehow mediate the effects of obesity on sleep quality; this relation has been reported in previous papers [69], but rarely investigated in light of dietary factors associated with weight status. In a sub-analysis of the present study we found that adherence to the Mediterranean diet was significant in normal and overweight individuals, but was not evident in the obese. Prospective cohort studies showed evidence of a causal relation between short sleep duration and occurrence of obesity at later age [70]. The most studied mechanism relating sleep and body weight regards the balance between leptin and ghrelin, two hormones involved in food intake and energy balance which have been demonstrated to be altered following sleep disturbances [71]. Leptin is an adipocyte-derived hormone that suppresses hunger and stimulates energy expenditure while ghrelin is stomach-derived peptide that stimulates appetite and fat production. Some studies showed that short sleep and sleep deprivation may decrease circulating leptin and increase ghrelin levels [72], despite findings not being univocal [73,74]. Among other hormones potentially involved in the relation between sleep quality and body weight, some studies showed that sleep disturbances may increase morning cortisol levels, inhibit insulin sensitivity and growth hormone secretion [75,76]. The relation between poor sleep and obesity has been widely demonstrated, and also the other way around, where excess body weight may favor the occurrence of sleep apnea, which in turn causes scarce sleep quality [77]. Most important, recent evidence shows that obstructive sleep apnea may have an impact on the structure and function of blood vessels, adversely affecting cognition in addition to culminating in mortality and morbidity [78]. Hypoxia, hypertension, hypo-perfusion, endothelial dysfunction, inflammation, and oxidative stress noted in obstructive sleep apnea patients also occur in Alzheimer's disease patients, suggesting a pathological commonality that may relate both conditions [79]. In this context, higher adherence to a Mediterranean dietary pattern has been proven to provide advantages on metabolic profiles and long-term weight status maintenance [80,81]. Also in this regard, Mediterranean dietary polyphenols have been hypothesized to potentially play a role in weight management through a number of mechanisms, including activation of β-oxidation; a prebiotic effect for gut microbiota; induction of satiety; stimulation of energy expenditure by inducing thermogenesis in brown adipose tissue; modulation of adipose tissue inhibiting adipocyte differentiation; promotion of adipocyte apoptosis and increasing lipolysis [82,83]. Thus, it may be possible that the association between adherence to the Mediterranean diet and sleep quality retrieved in our study may, in fact, be mediated by a better weight status. This hypothesis will need further exploration in future studies.

The findings of this study should be considered in light of some limitations. First, the real direction of the associations retrieved cannot be identified through cross-section studies and reverse causation should be taken into account as potential explanation of the results presented. It is noteworthy to emphasize that even with a prospective study design, the possibility that sleep and dietary patterns are part of an overall healthier or unhealthier lifestyle pattern cannot be ruled out, and that only further research into mechanistic and experimental studies would clarify the nature of the association. Second, the use of self-reported FFQs and sleep quality tools may be affected by recall and social desirability biases. However, the tools used in this study are well-established instruments to investigate the research question proposed and methods are comparable to the existing literature. Third, given the variety of Mediterranean adherence scores used in the literature, results may not be directly comparable with studies using other instruments. However, the adherence score used in the present study is based on the summary of scientific literature providing evidence of association between the Mediterranean diet and health outcomes, suggesting the robustness of the instrument. Forth, despite controlling for occupational status, we were unable to test the role of financial allowance in the study participants, which might play a role in adherence to the Mediterranean diet and could be further investigated. Moreover, within the same category of occupational status we had no data for jobs that possibly required night shifts or had characteristics that might have influenced sleeping patterns. However, assuming a random distribution for such types of jobs (meaning not associated with adherence to the Mediterranean diet), this potential bias should be non-differential among exposure groups.

5. Conclusions

In conclusion, high adherence to a Mediterranean dietary pattern is associated with better sleep quality, either toward a direct effect on health or indirect effects through improvement of weight status. Further research should explore whether investigating sleep quality within the context of adherence to the Mediterranean diet might be part of an overall healthier lifestyle pattern, and should investigate the topic with a prospective and longitudinal study design. Future experimental studies are needed to test the impact of sleep quality on health and dietary intake allowing to investigate on causality and mechanisms. Finally, the potential mediating effect of weight status on the relation between Mediterranean diet and sleep quality requires further investigation.

Author Contributions: J.G. conceived the study, performed the analysis, interpreted the data and wrote the manuscript. R.F. and F.C. contributed to the drafting of the manuscript and provided expertise for the interpretation of the results and clinical aspects. F.I.I.C. and S.C. critically revised the manuscript and provided expertise in clinical aspects. G.G. and F.G. provided the data and reviewed the draft, equally contributing to the paper. All authors read and approved the final version of manuscript.

Funding: This study was partially supported by a fund from the Italian Ministry of Health "Ricerca Corrente" (RC n. 2751594) (Drs. Ferri, Caraci and Cosentino).

Acknowledgments: J.G. is a PhD student in the International PhD Program in Neuroscience at the University of Catania.

Conflicts of Interest: The authors declare no conflict of interest.

References

1. Matricciani, L.; Bin, Y.S.; Lallukka, T.; Kronholm, E.; Dumuid, D.; Paquet, C.; Olds, T. Past, present, and future: trends in sleep duration and implications for public health. *Sleep Heal.* **2017**, *3*, 317–323. [CrossRef]
2. Zhao, C.; Noble, J.M.; Marder, K.; Hartman, J.S.; Gu, Y.; Scarmeas, N. Dietary Patterns, Physical Activity, Sleep, and Risk for Dementia and Cognitive Decline. *Nutr. Rep.* **2018**, *7*, 1–11. [CrossRef] [PubMed]
3. Itani, O.; Jike, M.; Watanabe, N.; Kaneita, Y. Short sleep duration and health outcomes: a systematic review, meta-analysis, and meta-regression. *Sleep Med.* **2017**, *32*, 246–256. [CrossRef]
4. Atkinson, G.; Davenne, D. Relationships between sleep, physical activity and human health. *Physiol. Behav.* **2007**, *90*, 229–235. [PubMed]
5. Irwin, M.R. Why sleep is important for health: A psychoneuroimmunology perspective. *Annu. Rev. Psychol.* **2015**, *66*, 143–172. [CrossRef]
6. Raven, F.; Van Der Zee, E.A.; Meerlo, P.; Havekes, R. The role of sleep in regulating structural plasticity and synaptic strength: Implications for memory and cognitive function. *Sleep Med. Rev.* **2018**, *39*, 3–11. [CrossRef] [PubMed]
7. Pace-Schott, E.F.; Spencer, R.M. Sleep-dependent memory consolidation in healthy aging and mild cognitive impairment. *Curr. Top. Behav. Neurosci.* **2015**, *25*, 307–330.
8. Wu, M.N.; Rosenberg, P.B.; Spira, A.P.; Wennberg, A.M. Sleep Disturbance, Cognitive Decline, and Dementia: A Review. *Semin. Neurol.* **2017**, *37*, 395–406. [CrossRef]
9. Jansen, E.C.; Dunietz, G.L.; Tsimpanouli, M.-E.; Guyer, H.M.; Shannon, C.; Hershner, S.D.; O'Brien, L.M.; Baylin, A. Sleep, Diet, and Cardiometabolic Health Investigations: a Systematic Review of Analytic Strategies. *Nutr. Rep.* **2018**, *7*, 235–258. [CrossRef]
10. Martinez-Lacoba, R.; Pardo-Garcia, I.; Amo-Saus, E.; Escribano-Sotos, F. Mediterranean diet and health outcomes: A systematic meta-review. *Eur. J. Public Health* **2018**, *28*, 955–961. [CrossRef]
11. Villani, A.; Sultana, J.; Doecke, J.; Mantzioris, E. Differences in the interpretation of a modernized Mediterranean diet prescribed in intervention studies for the management of type 2 diabetes: how closely does this align with a traditional Mediterranean diet? *Eur. J. Nutr.* **2018**, 1–12. [CrossRef] [PubMed]
12. Zaragoza-Martí, A.; Cabañero-Martínez, M.; Hurtado-Sánchez, J.; Laguna-Pérez, A.; Ferrer-Cascales, R. Evaluation of Mediterranean diet adherence scores: a systematic review. *BMJ Open* **2018**, *8*, e019033. [CrossRef] [PubMed]
13. Huo, R.; Du, T.; Xu, Y.; Xu, W.; Chen, X.; Sun, K.; Yu, X. Effects of mediterranean-style diet on glycemic control, weight loss and cardiovascular risk factors among type 2 diabetes individuals: A meta-analysis. *Eur. J. Clin. Nutr.* **2015**, *69*, 1200–1208. [CrossRef] [PubMed]
14. Mocciaro, G.; Ziauddeen, N.; Godos, J.; Marranzano, M.; Chan, M.-Y.; Ray, S. Does a Mediterranean-type dietary pattern exert a cardio-protective effect outside the Mediterranean region? A review of current evidence. *Int. J. Food. Sci. Nutr.* **2018**, *69*, 524–535. [CrossRef] [PubMed]
15. Sofi, F.; Macchi, C.; Abbate, R.; Gensini, G.F.; Casini, A. Mediterranean diet and health status: An updated meta-analysis and a proposal for a literature-based adherence score. *Public Health Nutr.* **2014**, *17*, 2769–2782. [CrossRef]
16. Grosso, G.; Marventano, S.; Yang, J.; Micek, A.; Pajak, A.; Scalfi, L.; Galvano, F.; Kales, S.N. A comprehensive meta-analysis on evidence of mediterranean diet and cardiovascular disease: Are individual components equal? *Crit. Rev. Food Sci. Nutr.* **2017**, *57*, 3218–3232. [CrossRef]

17. Schwingshackl, L.; Missbach, B.; Konig, J.; Hoffmann, G. Adherence to a mediterranean diet and risk of diabetes: A systematic review and meta-analysis. *Public Health Nutr.* **2015**, *18*, 1292–1299. [CrossRef]
18. Kastorini, C.M.; Milionis, H.J.; Esposito, K.; Giugliano, D.; Goudevenos, J.A.; Panagiotakos, D.B. The effect of mediterranean diet on metabolic syndrome and its components: A meta-analysis of 50 studies and 534,906 individuals. *J. Am. Coll. Cardiol.* **2011**, *57*, 1299–1313. [CrossRef]
19. Godos, J.; Zappala, G.; Bernardini, S.; Giambini, I.; Bes-Rastrollo, M.; Martinez-Gonzalez, M. Adherence to the mediterranean diet is inversely associated with metabolic syndrome occurrence: A meta-analysis of observational studies. *Int. J. Food Sci. Nutr.* **2017**, *68*, 138–148. [CrossRef] [PubMed]
20. Sofi, F.; Casini, A. Mediterranean diet and non-alcoholic fatty liver disease: New therapeutic option around the corner? *World J. Gastroenterol.* **2014**, *20*, 7339–7346. [CrossRef] [PubMed]
21. Godos, J.; Federico, A.; Dallio, M.; Scazzina, F. Mediterranean diet and nonalcoholic fatty liver disease: Molecular mechanisms of protection. *Int. J. Food Sci. Nutr.* **2017**, *68*, 18–27. [CrossRef] [PubMed]
22. Grosso, G.; Mistretta, A.; Marventano, S.; Purrello, A.; Vitaglione, P.; Calabrese, G.; Drago, F.; Galvano, F. Beneficial effects of the Mediterranean diet on metabolic syndrome. *Curr. Pharm. Des.* **2014**, *20*, 5039–5044. [CrossRef] [PubMed]
23. Lakkur, S.; Judd, S.E. Diet and stroke: Recent evidence supporting a Mediterranean style diet and food in the primary prevention of stroke. *Stroke* **2015**, *46*, 2007–2011. [CrossRef]
24. Petersson, S.D.; Philippou, E. Mediterranean Diet, Cognitive Function, and Dementia: A Systematic Review of the Evidence123. *Adv. Nutr. Int. J.* **2016**, *7*, 889–904. [CrossRef]
25. Psaltopoulou, T.; Sergentanis, T.N.; Panagiotakos, D.B.; Sergentanis, I.N.; Kosti, R.; Scarmeas, N. Mediterranean diet, stroke, cognitive impairment, and depression: A meta-analysis. *Ann. Neurol.* **2013**, *74*, 580–591. [CrossRef] [PubMed]
26. Safouris, A.; Tsivgoulis, G.; Sergentanis, T.; Psaltopoulou, T. Mediterranean Diet and Risk of Dementia. *Curr. Res.* **2015**, *12*, 736–744. [CrossRef]
27. Valls-Pedret, C.; Sala-Vila, A.; Serra-Mir, M.; Corella, D.; de la Torre, R.; Martinez-Gonzalez, M.A.; Martinez-Lapiscina, E.H.; Fito, M.; Perez-Heras, A.; Salas-Salvado, J.; et al. Mediterranean diet and age-related cognitive decline: A randomized clinical trial. *JAMA Intern. Med.* **2015**, *175*, 1094–1103. [CrossRef]
28. Aridi, Y.S.; Walker, J.L.; Wright, O.R.L. The Association between the Mediterranean Dietary Pattern and Cognitive Health: A Systematic Review. *Nutrients* **2017**, *9*, 674. [CrossRef]
29. Campanini, M.Z.; Guallar-Castillon, P.; Rodriguez-Artalejo, F.; Lopez-Garcia, E. Mediterranean diet and changes in sleep duration and indicators of sleep quality in older adults. *Sleep* **2017**, *40*. [CrossRef] [PubMed]
30. Jaussent, I.; Dauvilliers, Y.; Ancelin, M.-L.; Dartigues, J.-F.; Tavernier, B.; Touchon, J.; Ritchie, K.; Besset, A. Insomnia symptoms in older adults: associated factors and gender differences. *Am. J. Geriatr. Psychiatry* **2011**, *19*, 88–97. [CrossRef]
31. Castro-Diehl, C.; Wood, A.C.; Redline, S.; Reid, M.; A Johnson, D.; E Maras, J.; Jacobs, D.R.; Shea, S.; Crawford, A.; St-Onge, M.-P.; et al. Mediterranean diet pattern and sleep duration and insomnia symptoms in the Multi-Ethnic Study of Atherosclerosis. *Sleep* **2018**, *41*, 41. [CrossRef] [PubMed]
32. Grosso, G.; Marventano, S.; D'Urso, M.; Mistretta, A.; Galvano, F. The mediterranean healthy eating, ageing, and lifestyle (meal) study: Rationale and study design. *Int. J. Food Sci. Nutr.* **2017**, *68*, 577–586. [CrossRef] [PubMed]
33. Craig, C.L.; Marshall, A.L.; Sjostrom, M.; Bauman, A.E.; Booth, M.L.; Ainsworth, B.E.; Pratt, M.; Ekelund, U.; Yngve, A.; Sallis, J.F.; et al. International physical activity questionnaire: 12-country reliability and validity. *Med. Sci. Sports Exerc.* **2003**, *35*, 1381–1395. [CrossRef] [PubMed]
34. Mistretta, A.; Marventano, S.; Platania, A.; Godos, J.; Grosso, G.; Galvano, F. Metabolic profile of the Mediterranean healthy Eating, Lifestyle and Aging (MEAL) study cohort. *Mediterr. J. Nutr. Metab.* **2017**, *10*, 131–140. [CrossRef]
35. World Health Organization. *Obesity: Preventing and managing the global epidemic. Report of a who consultation presented at the world health organization*; World Health Organization: Geneva, Switzerland, 1997; Volume Publication WHO/NUT/NCD/98.1.
36. Marventano, S.; Mistretta, A.; Platania, A.; Galvano, F.; Grosso, G. Reliability and relative validity of a food frequency questionnaire for Italian adults living in Sicily, Southern Italy. *Int. J. Food Sci. Nutr.* **2016**, *67*, 857–864. [CrossRef]

37. Buscemi, S.; Rosafio, G.; Vasto, S.; Massenti, F.M.; Grosso, G.; Galvano, F.; Rini, N.; Barile, A.M.; Maniaci, V.; Cosentino, L.; et al. Validation of a food frequency questionnaire for use in Italian adults living in Sicily. *Int. J. Food Sci. Nutr.* **2015**, *66*, 426–438. [CrossRef] [PubMed]
38. Buysse, D.J.; Reynolds, C.F., 3rd; Monk, T.H.; Berman, S.R.; Kupfer, D.J. The pittsburgh sleep quality index: A new instrument for psychiatric practice and research. *Psychiatry Res.* **1989**, *28*, 193–213. [CrossRef]
39. Stern, J.H.; Grant, A.S.; Thomson, C.A.; Tinker, L.; Hale, L.; Brennan, K.M.; Woods, N.F.; Chen, Z. Short sleep duration is associated with decreased serum leptin, increased energy intake, and decreased diet quality in postmenopausal women. *Obesity* **2014**, *22*, E55–E61. [CrossRef]
40. Haghighatdoost, F.; Karimi, G.; Esmaillzadeh, A.; Azadbakht, L. Sleep deprivation is associated with lower diet quality indices and higher rate of general and central obesity among young female students in Iran. *Nutrition* **2012**, *28*, 1146–1150. [CrossRef]
41. Kant, A.K.; Graubard, B.I. Association of self-reported sleep duration with eating behaviors of american adults: Nhanes 2005-2010. *Am. J. Clin. Nutr.* **2014**, *100*, 938–947. [CrossRef]
42. Kim, S.; DeRoo, L.A.; Sandler, D.P. Eating patterns and nutritional characteristics associated with sleep duration. *Public Health Nutr.* **2011**, *14*, 889–895. [CrossRef] [PubMed]
43. Crispim, C.A.; Zimberg, I.Z.; Dos Reis, B.G.; Diniz, R.M.; Tufik, S.; De Mello, M.T. Relationship between Food Intake and Sleep Pattern in Healthy Individuals. *J. Clin. Sleep Med.* **2011**, *7*, 659–664. [CrossRef]
44. St-Onge, M.P.; Mikic, A.; Pietrolungo, C.E. Effects of diet on sleep quality. *Adv. Nutr.* **2016**, *7*, 938–949. [CrossRef] [PubMed]
45. D'Alessandro, A.; De Pergola, G. The Mediterranean Diet: its definition and evaluation of a priori dietary indexes in primary cardiovascular prevention. *Int. J. Food Sci. Nutr.* **2018**, *69*, 647–659. [CrossRef] [PubMed]
46. Zappala, G.; Buscemi, S.; Mule, S.; La Verde, M.; D'Urso, M.; Corleo, D.; Marranzano, M. High adherence to mediterranean diet, but not individual foods or nutrients, is associated with lower likelihood of being obese in a mediterranean cohort. *Eat. Weight Disord.* **2017**, *23*, 605–614. [CrossRef] [PubMed]
47. La Verde, M.; Mule, S.; Zappala, G.; Privitera, G.; Maugeri, G.; Pecora, F.; Marranzano, M. Higher adherence to the mediterranean diet is inversely associated with having hypertension: Is low salt intake a mediating factor? *Int. J. Food Sci. Nutr.* **2018**, *69*, 235–244. [CrossRef] [PubMed]
48. Platania, A.; Zappala, G.; Mirabella, M.U.; Gullo, C.; Mellini, G.; Beneventano, G.; Maugeri, G.; Marranzano, M. Association between Mediterranean diet adherence and dyslipidaemia in a cohort of adults living in the Mediterranean area. *Int. J. Food Sci. Nutr.* **2017**, *69*, 608–618. [CrossRef] [PubMed]
49. Godos, J.; Sinatra, D.; Blanco, I.; Mulè, S.; La Verde, M.; Marranzano, M. Association between Dietary Phenolic Acids and Hypertension in a Mediterranean Cohort. *Nutrients* **2017**, *9*, 1069. [CrossRef]
50. Godos, J.; Bergante, S.; Satriano, A.; Pluchinotta, F.R.; Marranzano, M. Dietary Phytoestrogen Intake is Inversely Associated with Hypertension in a Cohort of Adults Living in the Mediterranean Area. *Molecules* **2018**, *23*, 368. [CrossRef]
51. Huhn, S.; Masouleh, S.K.; Stumvoll, M.; Villringer, A.; Witte, A.V. Components of a Mediterranean diet and their impact on cognitive functions in aging. *Front. Aging Neurosci.* **2015**, *7*, 132. [CrossRef]
52. Knight, A.; Bryan, J.; Murphy, K. Is the Mediterranean diet a feasible approach to preserving cognitive function and reducing risk of dementia for older adults in Western countries? New insights and future directions. *Ageing Res. Rev.* **2016**, *25*, 85–101. [CrossRef] [PubMed]
53. Ayuso, M.I.; Gonzalo-Gobernado, R.; Montaner, J. Neuroprotective diets for stroke. *Neurochem. Int.* **2017**, *107*, 4–10. [CrossRef]
54. A Clark, I.; Vissel, B. Inflammation-sleep interface in brain disease: TNF, insulin, orexin. *J. Neuroinflammation* **2014**, *11*, 51. [CrossRef]
55. Everson, C.A.; Laatsch, C.D.; Hogg, N. Antioxidant defense responses to sleep loss and sleep recovery. *Am. J. Physiol. Integr. Comp. Physiol.* **2005**, *288*, R374–R383. [CrossRef]
56. Kanagasabai, T.; Ardern, C.I. Inflammation, Oxidative Stress, and Antioxidants Contribute to Selected Sleep Quality and Cardiometabolic Health Relationships: A Cross-Sectional Study. *Mediat. Inflamm.* **2015**, *2015*, 1–11. [CrossRef] [PubMed]
57. Kanagasabai, T.; Ardern, C.I. Contribution of Inflammation, Oxidative Stress, and Antioxidants to the Relationship between Sleep Duration and Cardiometabolic Health. *Sleep* **2015**, *38*, 1905–1912. [CrossRef]
58. Ricker, M.A.; Haas, W.C. Anti-Inflammatory Diet in Clinical Practice: A Review. *Nutr. Clin. Pr.* **2017**, *32*, 318–325. [CrossRef] [PubMed]

59. Grosso, G.; Micek, A.; Marventano, S.; Castellano, S.; Mistretta, A.; Pajak, A.; Galvano, F. Dietary n-3 PUFA, fish consumption and depression: A systematic review and meta-analysis of observational studies. *J. Affect. Disord.* **2016**, *205*, 269–281. [CrossRef] [PubMed]
60. Zhang, Y.; Chen, J.; Qiu, J.; Li, Y.; Wang, J.; Jiao, J. Intakes of fish and polyunsaturated fatty acids and mild-to-severe cognitive impairment risks: A dose-response meta-analysis of 21 cohort studies. *Am. J. Clin. Nutr.* **2016**, *103*, 330–340. [CrossRef] [PubMed]
61. Godos, J.; Castellano, S.; Ray, S.; Grosso, G.; Galvano, F. Dietary Polyphenol Intake and Depression: Results from the Mediterranean Healthy Eating, Lifestyle and Aging (MEAL) Study. *Molecules* **2018**, *23*, 999. [CrossRef] [PubMed]
62. Chang, S.-C.; Cassidy, A.; Willett, W.C.; Rimm, E.B.; O'Reilly, E.J.; I Okereke, O. Dietary flavonoid intake and risk of incident depression in midlife and older women123. *Am. J. Clin. Nutr.* **2016**, *104*, 704–714. [CrossRef]
63. Potì, F.; Santi, D.; Spaggiari, G.; Zimetti, F.; Zanotti, I. Polyphenol Health Effects on Cardiovascular and Neurodegenerative Disorders: A Review and Meta-Analysis. *Int. J. Mol. Sci.* **2019**, *20*, 351. [CrossRef]
64. Hornedo-Ortega, R.; Cerezo, A.B.; De Pablos, R.M.; Krisa, S.; Richard, T.; García-Parrilla, M.C.; Troncoso, A.M. Phenolic Compounds Characteristic of the Mediterranean Diet in Mitigating Microglia-Mediated Neuroinflammation. *Front. Cell. Neurosci.* **2018**, *12*, 373. [CrossRef]
65. Grosso, G.; Galvano, F.; Marventano, S.; Malaguarnera, M.; Bucolo, C.; Drago, F.; Caraci, F. Omega-3 Fatty Acids and Depression: Scientific Evidence and Biological Mechanisms. *Oxidative Med. Cell. Longev.* **2014**, *2014*, 1–16. [CrossRef] [PubMed]
66. Dias, G.P.; Cavegn, N.; Nix, A.; do Nascimento Bevilaqua, M.C.; Stangl, D.; Zainuddin, M.S.; Nardi, A.E.; Gardino, P.F.; Thuret, S. The role of dietary polyphenols on adult hippocampal neurogenesis: Molecular mechanisms and behavioural effects on depression and anxiety. *Oxid. Med. Cell. Longev.* **2012**, *541971*. [CrossRef]
67. Maruszak, A.; Pilarski, A.; Murphy, T.; Branch, N.; Thuret, S. Hippocampal neurogenesis in alzheimer's disease: Is there a role for dietary modulation? *J. Alzheimers Dis.* **2014**, *38*, 11–38. [CrossRef] [PubMed]
68. Murphy, T.; Dias, G.P.; Thuret, S. Effects of Diet on Brain Plasticity in Animal and Human Studies: Mind the Gap. *Neural Plast.* **2014**, *2014*, 1–32. [CrossRef]
69. Wu, Y.; Zhai, L.; Zhang, D. Sleep duration and obesity among adults: a meta-analysis of prospective studies. *Sleep Med.* **2014**, *15*, 1456–1462. [CrossRef] [PubMed]
70. Fatima, Y.; Doi, S.A.R.; Mamun, A.A. Longitudinal impact of sleep on overweight and obesity in children and adolescents: A systematic review and bias-adjusted meta-analysis. *Obes. Rev.* **2015**, *16*, 137–149. [CrossRef] [PubMed]
71. Bodosi, B.; Gardi, J.; Hajdu, I.; Szentirmai, E.; Obal, F., Jr.; Krueger, J.M. Rhythms of ghrelin, leptin, and sleep in rats: Effects of the normal diurnal cycle, restricted feeding, and sleep deprivation. *Am. J. Physiol. Regul. Integr. Comp. Physiol.* **2004**, *287*, R1071–R1079. [CrossRef] [PubMed]
72. Taheri, S.; Lin, L.; Austin, D.; Young, T.; Mignot, E. Short sleep duration is associated with reduced leptin, elevated ghrelin, and increased body mass index. *PLoS Med.* **2004**, *1*, e62. [CrossRef] [PubMed]
73. Littman, A.J.; Vitiello, M.V.; Foster-Schubert, K.; Ulrich, C.M.; Tworoger, S.S.; Potter, J.D.; Weigle, D.S.; McTiernan, A. Sleep, ghrelin, leptin and changes in body weight during a 1-year moderate-intensity physical activity intervention. *Int. J. Obes. (Lond).* **2007**, *31*, 466–475. [CrossRef] [PubMed]
74. St-Onge, M.-P.; O'Keeffe, M.; Roberts, A.L.; Roychoudhury, A.; Laferrere, B. Short Sleep Duration, Glucose Dysregulation and Hormonal Regulation of Appetite in Men and Women. *Sleep* **2012**, *35*, 1503–1510. [CrossRef] [PubMed]
75. Lanfranco, F.; Motta, G.; Minetto, M.A.; Ghigo, E.; Maccario, M. Growth hormone/insulin-like growth factor-I axis in obstructive sleep apnea syndrome: An update. *J. Endocrinol. Investig.* **2010**, *33*, 192–196. [CrossRef] [PubMed]
76. Garcia-Garcia, F.; Juárez-Aguilar, E.; Santiago-García, J.; Cardinali, D.P. Ghrelin and its interactions with growth hormone, leptin and orexins: Implications for the sleep–wake cycle and metabolism. *Sleep Med. Rev.* **2014**, *18*, 89–97. [CrossRef]
77. Fatima, Y.; Doi, S.A.; Mamun, A.A. Sleep quality and obesity in young subjects: a meta-analysis. *Obes. Rev.* **2016**, *17*, 1154–1166. [CrossRef]
78. Stranks, E.K.; Crowe, S.F. The Cognitive Effects of Obstructive Sleep Apnea: An Updated Meta-analysis. *Arch. Clin. Neuropsychol.* **2016**, *31*, 186–193. [CrossRef] [PubMed]

79. Daulatzai, M.A. Evidence of neurodegeneration in obstructive sleep apnea: Relationship between obstructive sleep apnea and cognitive dysfunction in the elderly. *J. Neurosci.* **2015**, *93*, 1778–1794. [CrossRef]
80. Mancini, J.G.; Filion, K.B.; Atallah, R.; Eisenberg, M.J. Systematic Review of the Mediterranean Diet for Long-Term Weight Loss. *Am. J. Med.* **2016**, *129*, 407–415.e4. [CrossRef]
81. Ros, E.; Martinez-Gonzalez, M.A.; Estruch, R.; Salas-Salvadó, J.; Fitó, M.; Martínez, J.A.; Corella, D. Mediterranean Diet and Cardiovascular Health: Teachings of the PREDIMED Study123. *Adv. Nutr. Int. J.* **2014**, *5*, 330S–336S. [CrossRef]
82. Castro-Barquero, S.; Lamuela-Raventós, R.M.; Doménech, M.; Estruch, R. Relationship between Mediterranean Dietary Polyphenol Intake and Obesity. *Nutrients* **2018**, *10*, 1523. [CrossRef] [PubMed]
83. Marranzano, M.; Ray, S.; Godos, J.; Galvano, F. Association between dietary flavonoids intake and obesity in a cohort of adults living in the Mediterranean area. *Int. J. Food Sci. Nutr.* **2018**, *69*, 1020–1029. [CrossRef] [PubMed]

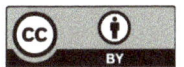

© 2019 by the authors. Licensee MDPI, Basel, Switzerland. This article is an open access article distributed under the terms and conditions of the Creative Commons Attribution (CC BY) license (http://creativecommons.org/licenses/by/4.0/).

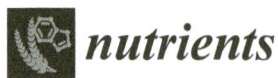

Article

Adherence to a Mediterranean Dietary Pattern Is Associated with Higher Quality of Life in a Cohort of Italian Adults

Justyna Godos [1,†], Sabrina Castellano [2,†] and Marina Marranzano [1,*]

1. Department of Medical and Surgical Sciences and Advanced Technologies "G.F. Ingrassia", University of Catania, 95123 Catania, Italy; justyna.godos@student.uj.edu.pl
2. Department of Educational Sciences, University of Catania, 95124 Catania, Italy; sabrinacastellano@hotmail.it
* Correspondence: marranz@unict.it; Tel.: +39-095-378-2180
† These authors contributed equally to this work.

Received: 30 March 2019; Accepted: 28 April 2019; Published: 29 April 2019

Abstract: Background: The observed rise in non-communicable diseases may be attributed to the ongoing changes of urban environment and society, as well as greater awareness of health-related issues and subsequent higher rates of diagnosis, which all contribute to the overall quality of life. The aim of the study was to test the association between adherence to the Mediterranean dietary pattern and self-reported quality of life in a cohort of Italian adults. Methods: The demographic and dietary characteristics of 2044 adults living in southern Italy were analyzed. Food frequency questionnaires (FFQs) and a Mediterranean diet adherence score were used to assess dietary intake. The Manchester Short Appraisal (MANSA) was used to assess self-rated quality of life. Multivariate logistic regression analyses were used to test the associations. Results: A significant linear trend of association was found for the overall quality of life and adherence to Mediterranean diet score. All of the components of the MANSA, with the exception of self-rated mental health, were individually associated with higher adherence to this dietary pattern. Conclusions: Adherence to a healthy dietary pattern is associated with the measures of better overall perceived quality of life.

Keywords: Mediterranean diet; quality of life; mental health; fruit; vegetable; dairy; nuts; fish; whole-grain; food groups

---

1. Introduction

Modern society and "Westernized" lifestyle has been negatively associated with the mental and physical health of the population. The observed rise in non-communicable diseases may depend on ongoing changes of urban environment and society, as well as a greater awareness of health-related issues and subsequent higher rates of diagnosis [1]. Quality of life has been generally used as an outcome of interest to evaluate the general condition of health and well-being of a person [2]. Self-perceived health status may obviously depend on current health conditions; more importantly, it has been found to be a close predictor of mortality [3–5]. In this context, factors that influence health-related quality of life of general population have paramount importance for their potential preventive role in improving health. Among major risk factors, poor nutrition has been considered as the main contributor to non-communicable diseases, including mental disorders [6]. There are indirect links between dietary patterns and mental disorders, including socioeconomic circumstances, obesity, and occurrence of conditions that might be associated with, or drivers of, chronic conditions (i.e., cardiovascular disease) [7]. However, investigating the relation between the risk factors that affect self-perceived health might be helpful to provide proof for potential underlying mechanisms.

The Mediterranean diet appears to be protective against cardio-metabolic diseases [8–10], neurodegenerative disorders [11,12], and certain cancers [13] amongst the most studied dietary patterns. The Mediterranean dietary pattern does not stand for a unique pattern of foods; rather, refer to the consumption of foods that characterize the dietary habits of the individuals living in the Mediterranean coasts [14,15]. The higher consumption of majority of plant-derived foods, such as fruit, vegetable, legume, and whole-grains, using olive oil as main source of fat, moderate alcohol consumption, moderate intake of fish and dairy products, and limited intake of meat and highly processed foods [16] represent the key features of this dietary pattern. Moreover, the beneficial effects of Mediterranean diet may relay on the high content in antioxidants and anti-inflammatory compounds, which have been hypothesized to play a role in the prevention of both physical and mental disorders [17]. Such findings suggest that adherence to the Mediterranean diet may be associated with better health and, consequently, better perceived health. In fact, previous observational studies showed that a higher adherence to the Mediterranean diet was associated with a better health-related quality of life [18–22]. Aspects that are related not only to physical health, but also to mental and psychosocial health, have underlined the importance of engagement in social activities as the potential determinant of better collective well-being [23,24]. Individuals living in the Mediterranean area may benefit of a characteristic way of living, in particular, through better social interactions with their next of kin and their community, including the frequency of contacts [25], network size [26], and relationships that are derived from personal choice [27], which is associated with positive outcomes and higher quality of life [28]. However, the number of studies investigating the association between Mediterranean diet and quality of life is limited and the topic may have further application for public health purposes, is therefore worth further examination. Thus, this study aimed to test the association between self-reported quality of life and the adherence to the Mediterranean dietary pattern in a cohort of Italian adults.

2. Materials and Methods

2.1. Study Population

The study sample was constituted of participants of the Mediterranean healthy Eating, Aging, and Lifestyles (MEAL) study, an observational investigation that is primarily focused on nutritional habits and their relation with a cluster of lifestyle behaviors that characterize the classical Mediterranean lifestyle. The study protocol with the rationale, design, and methods have been described in detail elsewhere [29]. Briefly, the cohort consisted of 2044 men and women older than 18 years old (mean and standard deviation 48.1 ± 17.5 years) that were recruited in the urban area of Catania, which is one of the largest cities in the east coast of Sicily, southern Italy during 2014–2015. A random sample of individuals registered in the records of local general practitioners was invited to participate. The sampling technique included stratification by municipality area, age, and sex of inhabitants, and randomization into subgroups, with randomly selected general practitioners being the sampling units, and the individuals registered to them comprising the final sample units. Out of the 2405 individuals invited, the final sample size was 2044 participants (response rate of 85%). All of the study procedures were carried out in accordance with the Declaration of Helsinki (1989) of the World Medical Association. Participants provided written informed consent and the ethics committee of the referent health authority approved the study protocol.

2.2. Data Collection

Data regarding demographic (i.e., age, sex, educational and occupational level) and lifestyle characteristics (i.e., physical activity, smoking and drinking habits) were collected. The educational level was categorized as (i) low (primary/secondary), (ii) medium (high school), and (iii) high (university), while occupational level was categorized as (i) unemployed, (ii) low (unskilled workers), (iii) medium (partially skilled workers), and (iv) high (skilled workers). Physical activity level was evaluated through the International Physical Activity Questionnaires (IPAQ) [30], which comprised a set of questionnaires (five domains) on time that is spent being physically active in the last seven days that allow for categorizing physical activity as (i) low, (ii) moderate, and (iii) high. Smoking status was categorized as (i) non-smoker, (ii) former smoker, and (iii) current smoker. Alcohol consumption was categorized as (i) none, (ii) moderate drinker (0.1–12 g/day), and (iii) regular drinker (>12 g/day). Anthropometric measurements were collected using standardized methods [31]. Standing height was measured through a scale stadiometer to the nearest 0.5 cm and weight to the nearest 0.1 kg without shoes, with the back square against the wall tape, eyes looking straight ahead, and with a right-angle triangle resting on the scalp and against the wall. Body mass index (BMI) was calculated, and the patients were categorized as under/normal weight (BMI < 25 kg/m^2), overweight (BMI 25 to 29.9 kg/m^2), and obese (BMI > 30 kg/m^2) [32]. Information from measurements was integrated with general practitioners computerized records in order to ascertain the cases of hypertension, diabetes, dyslipidemia, previous cardiovascular disease event, and cancer (all diagnoses were confirmed by a specialist before being registered).

2.3. Dietary Assessment

Long and short food frequency questionnaires (FFQs) specifically developed and validated for the Sicilian population were used to collect dietary data [33,34]. The FFQs consisted of 110 food and drink items that were representative of the diet during the last six months. The participants were asked how often, on average, they had consumed foods and drinks included in the FFQ, with nine responses ranging from "never" to "4–5 times per day". The intake of food items characterized by seasonality referred to consumption during the period in which the food was available and then adjusted by its proportional intake in one year. A total of 1937 individuals were included in the analyses for the present study after the exclusion of 107 entries with unreliable intakes (<1000 or >6000 kcal/day, controlled case by case, and being validated due to missing food items or unreliable answers).

2.4. Adherence to the Mediterranean Diet

A score derived from the literature assessed the Mediterranean diet adherence: briefly, a scoring system (the MEDI-LITE score) was built while taking into consideration median (or mean) values that were reported in selected studies and two standard deviations to determine three different categories of consumption for each food group [35,36]. For food groups that typically characterize the Mediterranean diet (fruit, vegetables, cereals, legumes, and fish), two points were given to the highest category of consumption, one point for the middle category, and 0 point for the lowest category. Conversely, for food groups that are not typical of the Mediterranean diet (meat and meat products, dairy products), two points were given for the lowest category, one point for the middle category, and 0 point for the highest category of consumption. For alcohol, categories that are related to the alcohol unit (1 alcohol unit = 12 g of alcohol) were used by giving two points to the middle category (1–2 alcohol units/day), one point to the lowest category (>1 alcohol unit/day), and 0 point to the highest category of consumption (>2 alcohol units/day). The final score comprised nine food categories (including olive oil), with a score ranging from 0 point (lowest adherence) to 18 points (highest adherence).

2.5. Quality of Life Assessment

The Manchester Short Assessment of Quality of Life (MANSA) [37], an instrument that consists of 12 subjective items with a seven-point Likert scale (from "could not be worse" to "could not be better") and four yes/no questions related to objective aspects of social life, assessed quality of life. The instrument assesses satisfaction with life as a whole and across several specific domains (including employment, financial situation, friendships, leisure activities, accommodation, personal safety, people living in household/living alone, sex life, relationship with family, and physical and mental health). An overall satisfaction with overall quality of life was arbitrarily defined as being in the highest quartile of the MANSA score (>70 points).

2.6. Statistical Analysis

The variables were examined for normality and skewness using the Kolmogorov–Smirnov test. The categorical variables are presented as frequencies of occurrence and percentages; differences between groups were tested using the Chi-squared test. The differences in background characteristics across participants grouped into quartiles of the MANSA score were tested. The relation between adherence to the Mediterranean diet and quality of life was tested through multivariate logistic regression analysis (when considering quartiles of the Mediterranean diet adherence score) adjusted for baseline characteristics (age, sex, marital, educational and occupational status, smoking and alcohol drinking habits, physical activity level, health status, and energy intake). All of the reported P values were based on two-sided tests and compared to a significance level of 5%. SPSS 17 (SPSS Inc., Chicago, IL, USA) software was used for all of the statistical calculations.

3. Results

Table 1 presents the main characteristics of the study participants by groups of quality of life score. There were no significant differences in background characteristics by groups of quality of life score, with the exception of age, as, among participants scoring lower points in the quality of life score, there were a higher proportion of younger individuals (Table 1). Regarding the distribution of comorbidities, only prevalence of hypertension was significantly distributed differently across groups of quality of life score, with a slightly lower occurrence among individuals in the second quartile of quality of life (Table 1).

Table 1. Baseline characteristics of the study participants by groups * of quality of life score.

	MANSA Score				
	Group 1	Group 2	Group 3	Group 4	p-value
Sex					0.814
Men	200 (42.4)	196 (39.9)	222 (41.3)	186 (42.8)	
Women	272 (57.6)	295 (60.1)	316 (58.7)	249 (57.2)	
Age groups n, (%)					0.002
<39	172 (36.4)	206 (42.0)	169 (31.4)	136 (31.3)	
40–59	167 (35.4)	161 (32.8)	184 (34.2)	169 (38.9)	
>60	133 (28.2)	124 (25.3)	185 (34.4)	130 (29.9)	
Educational status					0.578
Low	179 (37.9)	162 (33.0)	203 (37.7)	153 (35.2)	
Medium	166 (35.2)	186 (37.9)	201 (37.4)	167 (38.4)	
High	127 (26.9)	143 (29.1)	134 (24.9)	115 (26.4)	
Occupational status					0.442
Unemployed	111 (26.2)	121 (30.0)	132 (29.5)	97 (25.3)	
Low	73 (17.2)	55 (13.6)	75 (16.8)	63 (16.4)	
Medium	126 (29.7)	103 (25.5)	111 (24.8)	100 (26.1)	
High	114 (26.9)	125 (30.9)	129 (28.9)	123 (32.1)	
Smoking status					0.775
Never smoker	284 (60.2)	314 (64.0)	337 (62.6)	260 (59.8)	
Former smoker	115 (24.4)	116 (23.6)	124 (23.0)	110 (25.3)	
Current smoker	73 (15.5)	61 (12.4)	77 (14.3)	65 (14.9)	
Physical activity level					0.104
Low	82 (19.4)	87 (19.8)	89 (18.6)	71 (18.3)	
Moderate	227 (53.7)	226 (51.4)	222 (46.4)	181 (46.8)	
High	114 (27.0)	127 (28.9)	167 (34.9)	135 (34.9)	

Table 1. Cont.

	MANSA Score				
	Group 1	Group 2	Group 3	Group 4	p-value
Comorbidities					
Hypertension, n (%)	238 (50.4)	223 (45.4)	278 (51.7)	237 (54.5)	0.043
Diabetes, n (%)	30 (6.4)	34 (6.9)	43 (8.0)	39 (9.0)	0.450
Dyslipidemia, n (%)	87 (18.4)	87 (17.7)	98 (18.2)	84 (19.3)	0.939
Cardiovascular diseases, n (%)	38 (8.2)	37 (7.8)	41 (7.9)	38 (8.9)	0.921
Cancer, n (%)	21 (4.4)	11 (2.2)	30 (5.6)	16 (3.7)	0.052
Obesity, n (%)	68 (16.2)	82 (18.0)	101 (20.0)	66 (15.9)	0.332

* Groups were defined as quartiles of MANSA.

Table 2 shows the frequency distribution and association between quartiles of Mediterranean diet adherence score and the overall and individual domains of quality of life. A significant linear trend of association was found for overall quality of life (for the highest vs. the lowest quartile, OR = 10.01, 95% CI: 6.53, 15.33) and most of the domains besides satisfaction for "mental health" and "people with whom individual lives", for which the association was stronger in the third quartile of the Mediterranean diet adherence score.

Table 2. Distribution and association between overall quality of life and individual domain satisfaction of the study participants and Mediterranean diet adherence score (participants were grouped into quartiles of the score).

	Mediterranean Diet Score, OR (95% CI)				
	Q1	Q2	Q3	Q4	P for trend
Overall QoL *	52 (11.3)	36 (6.1)	190 (31.4)	157 (57.1)	
OR (95% CI) #	1	0.42 (0.24, 0.71)	3.66 (2.52, 5.30)	10.01 (6.53, 15.33)	<0.001
Life as a whole, n (%) §	94 (20.3)	172 (29.0)	333 (55.0)	143 (52.0)	
OR (95% CI) #	1	1.53 (1.09, 2.13)	5.04 (3.67, 6.93)	4.14 (2.83, 6.06)	0.142
Job (when having one), n (%) §	71 (15.4)	140 (23.6)	234 (38.6)	120 (43.6)	
OR (95% CI) #	1	1.52 (1.06, 2.19)	3.40 (2.42, 4.76)	4.37 (2.94, 6.49)	<0.001
Financial situation, n (%) §	71 (15.4)	102 (17.2)	140 (23.1)	91 (33.1)	
OR (95% CI) #	1	1.13 (0.77, 1.64)	1.65 (1.16, 2.35)	2.83 (1.89, 4.25)	<0.001
Amount and quality of friends, n (%) §	143 (31.0)	224 (37.8)	329 (54.3)	149 (54.2)	
OR (95% CI) #	1	1.23 (0.91, 1.66)	2.39 (1.79, 3.19)	2.40 (1.68, 3.43)	0.056
Leisure activities, n (%) §	96 (20.8)	131 (22.1)	229 (37.8)	98 (35.6)	
OR (95% CI) #	1	0.91 (0.64, 1.29)	2.00 (1.46, 2.75)	1.74 (1.18, 2.57)	<0.001
Housing, n (%) §	168 (36.4)	291 (49.1)	336 (55.4)	154 (56.0)	
OR (95% CI) #	1	1.94 (1.45, 2.59)	2.27 (1.70, 3.02)	2.34 (1.64, 3.34)	<0.001
Personal safety, n (%) §	170 (36.8)	190 (32.0)	296 (48.8)	163 (59.3)	
OR (95% CI) #	1	0.74 (0.55, 1.00)	1.65 (1.24, 2.19)	2.37 (1.66, 3.37)	<0.001
People with whom individual lives, n (%) §	21 (45.9)	400 (67.5)	494 (81.5)	173 (62.9)	
OR (95% CI) #	1	2.64 (1.96, 3.54)	5.59 (4.05, 7.72)	1.98 (1.39, 2.84)	0.293
Sex life, n (%) §	124 (26.8)	231 (39.0)	325 (53.6)	132 (48.0)	
OR (95% CI) #	1	1.89 (1.38, 2.57)	3.51 (2.59, 4.75)	2.79 (1.93, 4.03)	0.254
Relationship with family, n (%) §	237 (51.3)	434 (73.2)	467 (77.1)	171 (62.2)	
OR (95% CI) #	1	2.87 (2.11, 3.89)	3.14 (2.32, 4.26)	1.62 (1.13, 2.32)	0.178
Physical health, n (%) §	146 (31.6)	191 (32.2)	335 (55.3)	138 (50.2)	
OR (95% CI) #	1	0.86 (0.63, 1.17)	2.62 (1.96, 3.51)	2.13 (1.49, 3.05)	0.652
Mental health, n (%) §	233 (50.4)	382 (64.4)	514 (84.8)	161 (58.5)	
OR (95% CI) #	1	1.87 (1.40, 2.50)	5.31 (3.82, 7.37)	1.36 (0.95, 1.93)	0.542

* an overall satisfaction with overall quality of life was arbitrarily defined as being in the highest quartile of the MANSA score (>70 points); § answers reflecting satisfaction of the domains were "pleased" and "couldn't be better"; # adjusted for age (continuous), sex (male/female), BMI (<25 kg/m^2, 25-30 kg/m^2, >30 kg/m^2), physical activity (low/medium/high), educational status (low/medium/high), occupational status (unemployed/low/medium/high), smoking status (current/former/never), alcohol consumption (no/moderate/regular), health status (presence of hypertension, type-2 diabetes, dyslipidaemias, cardiovascular disease, cancer), and total energy intake.

Table 3 shows the association between individual components of the Mediterranean diet adherence score and the overall and individual domains of quality of life score. All of the components were associated with overall quality of life, despite only fruit, vegetable, and legume being associated with nearly all domains of quality of life, while other components only partially.

Table 3. Association between overall quality of life and individual domain satisfaction § of the study participants and individual components of the Mediterranean diet score.

	Mediterranean Diet Score Components, OR (95% CI)							
	Fruit	Vegetable	Legume	Dairy	Whole-grain	Fish	Meat	Olive oil	Alcohol
Overall QoL *	1.99 (1.54, 2.57)	2.14 (1.66, 2.75)	2.53 (1.92, 3.33)	1.90 (1.47, 2.47)	1.66 (1.29, 2.13)	1.80 (1.38, 2.35)	1.50 (1.13, 1.97)	1.53 (1.19, 1.98)	1.82 (1.23, 2.69)
Life as a whole	1.81 (1.46, 2.26)	1.52 (1.22, 1.89)	2.01 (1.60, 2.52)	1.40 (1.13, 1.75)	1.39 (1.11, 1.73)	1.45 (1.16, 1.80)	1.13 (0.89, 1.43)	1.28 (1.03, 1.59)	1.44 (1.00, 2.09)
Job (when having one)	1.61 (1.28, 2.03)	1.46 (1.16, 1.84)	1.53 (1.21, 1.95)	1.33 (1.05, 1.68)	1.29 (1.02, 1.63)	1.43 (1.13, 1.81)	1.31 (1.02, 1.69)	1.61 (1.28, 2.04)	2.05 (1.41, 2.97)
Financial situation	1.67 (1.29, 2.16)	1.21 (0.94, 1.56)	1.58 (1.21, 2.06)	1.19 (0.92, 1.54)	1.04 (0.80, 1.35)	1.11 (0.85, 1.43)	1.18 (0.89, 1.55)	1.22 (0.94, 1.57)	1.46 (0.97, 2.20)
Amount and quality of friends	1.19 (0.96, 1.46)	1.47 (1.19, 1.82)	1.38 (1.12, 1.72)	1.19 (0.97, 1.48)	1.13 (0.91, 1.41)	1.44 (1.16, 1.79)	1.19 (0.95, 1.50)	1.12 (0.91, 1.38)	1.60 (1.11, 2.31)
Leisure activities	1.30 (1.02, 1.64)	1.44 (1.14, 1.82)	1.22 (0.96, 1.55)	1.33 (1.05, 1.69)	1.03 (0.81, 1.31)	1.10 (0.86, 1.39)	1.06 (0.83, 1.37)	1.04 (0.82, 1.31)	1.54 (1.05, 2.27)
Housing	1.25 (1.02, 1.54)	1.21 (0.98, 1.49)	1.57 (1.27, 1.94)	1.20 (0.97, 1.48)	1.12 (0.90, 1.38)	1.50 (1.21, 1.85)	0.96 (0.77, 1.20)	1.16 (0.94, 1.43)	1.41 (0.97, 2.04)
Personal safety	1.26 (1.02, 1.56)	1.17 (0.94, 1.44)	1.54 (1.24, 1.92)	1.30 (1.05, 1.61)	1.18 (0.95, 1.46)	1.27 (1.03, 1.58)	1.30 (1.03, 1.63)	0.99 (0.80, 1.22)	1.16 (0.81, 1.68)
People with whom individual lives	1.70 (1.36, 2.13)	1.37 (1.10, 1.72)	1.98 (1.58, 2.48)	1.18 (0.95, 1.48)	1.05 (0.84, 1.32)	1.38 (1.11, 1.73)	1.01 (0.80, 1.28)	1.09 (0.87, 1.36)	2.34 (1.47, 3.71)
Sex life	1.46 (1.18, 1.81)	1.43 (1.16, 1.77)	1.74 (1.40, 2.17)	1.11 (0.89, 1.37)	1.25 (1.01, 1.56)	1.51 (1.21, 1.88)	1.09 (0.86, 1.37)	1.26 (1.02, 1.56)	1.24 (0.86, 1.79)
Relationship with family	1.36 (1.09, 1.70)	1.34 (1.07, 1.67)	1.60 (1.28, 2.00)	1.09 (0.87, 1.36)	1.06 (0.85, 1.34)	1.16 (0.93, 1.46)	1.09 (0.86, 1.38)	1.29 (1.03, 1.62)	1.66 (1.08, 2.55)
Physical health	1.47 (1.18, 1.81)	1.35 (1.09, 1.67)	1.44 (1.16, 1.79)	1.34 (1.08, 1.66)	1.22 (0.98, 1.52)	1.16 (0.93, 1.44)	1.27 (1.01, 1.59)	1.18 (0.95, 1.46)	1.09 (0.75, 1.58)
Mental health	1.34 (1.08, 1.68)	1.44 (1.15, 1.79)	1.46 (1.17, 1.82)	1.01 (0.81, 1.26)	0.99 (0.79, 1.24)	1.17 (0.94, 1.47)	1.16 (0.91, 1.46)	1.45 (1.16, 1.81)	1.24 (0.83, 1.85)

§ answers reflecting satisfaction of the domains were "pleased" and "couldn't be better". * an overall satisfaction with overall quality of life was arbitrarily defined as being in the highest quartile of the MANSA score (>70 points).

4. Discussion

In this study, we reported a direct association between the adherence to the Mediterranean diet and quality of life measured with a multi-domain instrument. However, another component of the MANSA score result was significantly associated with a higher adherence to the Mediterranean diet. The results are generally in line with previously published studies [18,20–22,38,39], which reinforces the assumption that diet and overall wellbeing (measured as quality of life) are strictly related. When separately considering physical and mental health, we found an association for the physical component of the MANSA score, while no significant results were reported for mental health. These results in line with a study that was conducted in two cohorts of older adults, for which adherence to this dietary pattern was not associated with clinically relevant mental component summaries of the quality of life score used [21]. In contrast, other studies reported an association with mental, rather than physical, health [18]. Despite being unable to perform a direct quantitative comparison between existing evidence due to the differences in study design and methodology that are used to calculate either the adherence to the Mediterranean diet and the quality of life, it is important to identify at least whether a relation does exist, the potential determinants, and the possible mechanisms that underlie it.

High adherence to a Mediterranean dietary pattern has been associated with a longer lifespan and decreased risk of numerous non-communicable diseases, including cardio-metabolic disorders and certain cancers [13]. Previous findings from this cohort showed that individuals that are highly adherent to this dietary pattern were less likely to suffer from obesity [40], hypertension [41], and dyslipidemias [42]; however, in this study, we found that, also after adjustment for clinical status, a high adherence to the Mediterranean diet was associated with a better quality of life when compared to low adherence. Regarding elderly individuals, the Mediterranean diet has also been reported to exert benefits toward depression [11], neurocognitive disorders, and cognitive decline [12], leading to an overall better mental health. In line with this, a number of studies have reported that, not only Mediterranean diet being understood as dietary pattern, but also individual components of the Mediterranean diet, might be associated with better physical and mental health. Specifically, there is a large number of studies reporting a decreased risk of non-communicable diseases associated with higher intake of fish, olive oil [43], fruit and vegetable [44], nuts and seeds [45], as well as with limited consumption of animal proteins and excessive alcohol consumption [46,47]. In addition, some evidence explored the association between fruit and vegetable [48], fish [49], and nuts [50], and specifically quality of life in the general population, despite that results being contrasting and the overall body of literature being focused on this outcome remaining scarce. Moreover, individual clinical trials that specifically focus on one aspect (i.e., low fat diets) did not lead to significant results, suggesting that the prescription of restrictive diets in patients may be interpreted as a different experience with potential detrimental effects [51]. Thus, it is auspicial that dietary interventions on qualitative outcomes, such as quality of life, would benefit from healthy and palatable alternatives, especially those that are a part of the traditional dietary patterns and cultural heritage of a population.

From a mechanistic point of view, interactions between various foods and nutrients occur in the real-world nutrition and the overall variety of a diet might affect the health of individuals through a synergistic action of all its components. Antioxidant micro-nutrients and phytochemicals, such as polyphenols, which are highly contained in the Mediterranean diet, have been hypothesized to exert, at least in part, the potential beneficial effects on physical and mental health of individuals, leading to an overall better quality of life. There is evidence that the Mediterranean diet may also protect from depressive disorders and improve mental health through mechanisms that are related to inflammation, besides the aforementioned association with cardio-metabolic diseases and cancers. The most studied compounds that potentially mediate such effects are omega-3 polyunsaturated fatty acids (mainly derived from fish), monounsaturated fatty acids (mainly derived from olive oil), antioxidant vitamins including, but are not limited to, B-vitamins, vitamin D, vitamin A, and vitamin E (mainly derived from fruit and vegetable) and fiber (also derived from whole-grains), which have been reported to reduce the low-grade inflammatory status and improve the endothelial function and the profile of coagulation and inflammation biomarkers. Finally, results of recent research showed that a number of phytochemical compounds, such as polyphenols, have been associated with various health outcomes, such as a decreased risk of cardiovascular diseases [52], diabetes, hypertension, and metabolic disorders [53–55], depression [56], certain cancers [57], and overall prolonged lifespan [58]. Some evidence of the potentially beneficial effects of some polyphenol classes, such as flavonoids, phenolic acids, and phytoestrogens, have been reported in the same population that was included in this study [8,59]. However, further research is needed to better understand whether these phytochemicals may play a role in the overall health and quality of life of individuals.

Besides the biological connection between the dietary patterns and health, a demonstration of the association between adherence to the Mediterranean diet and quality of life may be part of better cultural background or economic allowance that may lead to a cluster of factors that characterize a healthier lifestyle [60]. On one side, there is evidence that higher adherence to the Mediterranean diet is associated with higher socio-economic status and better income, even in Mediterranean countries [61–63]. On the other, this association is not consistent over the whole Italian territory and other evidence showed that the adherence to this dietary pattern is rather associated with higher cultural status, suggesting that, in certain areas (including the same population on which was conducted the present study), the adherence to the Mediterranean diet is a matter that is related to the cultural heritage rather than economical allowance [64–66]. Besides, in this study, we did not find any significant association between educational and occupational status and quality of life, suggesting that such variables are rather not confounding the association with the dietary factors investigated. Thus, we hypothesize that other aspects that are related to quality of life may be affected by strong bond with cultural heritage characteristic of the Mediterranean area: psychosocial aspects of lifestyle should be addressed, such as family and community support, engagement in social activities, and conviviality are directly linked with health [67]. Some studies have shown evidence regarding the association of socialization (in terms of social networks and social engagement) and cardiovascular [68] and cognitive health [69]. Those individuals that are more adherent to the Mediterranean diet may have also social interactions, such as mealtime conversations, family leisure activities, or other forms of social engagement, which in turn resulted in better quality of life.

The results of this study should be considered in light of some limitations. The most important issue that is common to all studies investigating quality of life, as outcome is the potential reverse causation. Indeed, the cross-sectional nature of the study does not allow for identifying a causal relationship. Among other limitations, even though a trained healthcare worker collects dietary information (either medical doctor, nurse, or nutritionist), data from a FFQ may be subjected to recall bias.

5. Conclusions

In conclusion, higher adherence to the Mediterranean diet was associated with a higher quality of life in adults living in Southern Italy. The results from this study support further investigation that examines the relation between dietary factors and quality of life with better methodological design (i.e., prospective studies). Further evidence is needed to better understand the relation between such life aspects and to plan educational programs that are to improve both dietary aspects and the quality of life of the general population.

Author Contributions: Author contributions: study conceive and design (J.G., M.M.), data management and analysis (J.G., S.C.), data evaluation and results (J.G., S.C.), manuscript drafting (J.G., S.C., M.M.), critical review of the manuscript (M.M.). All authors revised and approved the final version of the manuscript.

Funding: This research was supported by the Department of Medical and Surgical Sciences and Advanced Technologies "G.F. Ingrassia," University of Catania, Italy (Piano Triennale di Sviluppo delle Attivita' di Ricerca Scientifica del Dipartimento 2016–2018).

Conflicts of Interest: The authors declare no conflict of interest.

References

1. Penkalla, A.M.; Kohler, S. Urbanicity and Mental Health in Europe: A Systematic Review. *Eur. J. Health* **2014**, *9*, 163–177. [CrossRef]
2. Evans, S.; Huxley, P. Studies of quality of life in the general population. *Int. Rev. Psychiatr.* **2002**, *14*, 203–211. [CrossRef]
3. Kroenke, C.H.; Kubzansky, L.D.; Adler, N.; Kawachi, I. Prospective Change in Health-Related Quality of Life and Subsequent Mortality among Middle-Aged and Older Women. *Am. J. Public Health* **2008**, *98*, 2085–2091. [CrossRef]
4. Otero-Rodriguez, A.; Leon-Munoz, L.M.; Balboa-Castillo, T.; Banegas, J.R.; Rodriguez-Artalejo, F.; Guallar-Castillon, P. Change in health-related quality of life as a predictor of mortality in the older adults. *Qual. Life Res.* **2010**, *19*, 15–23. [CrossRef] [PubMed]
5. Tsai, S.-Y.; Chi, L.-Y.; Lee, C.-H.; Chou, P. Health-related quality of life as a predictor of mortality among community-dwelling older persons. *Eur. J. Epidemiol.* **2007**, *22*, 19–26. [CrossRef]
6. Logan, A.C.; Jacka, F.N. Nutritional psychiatry research: An emerging discipline and its intersection with global urbanization, environmental challenges and the evolutionary mismatch. *J. Physiol. Anthr.* **2014**, *33*, 22. [CrossRef]
7. Zhang, Y.; Chen, Y.; Ma, L. Depression and cardiovascular disease in elderly: Current understanding. *J. Clin. Neurosci.* **2018**, *47*, 1–5. [CrossRef]
8. Godos, J.; Sinatra, D.; Blanco, I.; Mulè, S.; La Verde, M.; Marranzano, M. Association between Dietary Phenolic Acids and Hypertension in a Mediterranean Cohort. *Nutrients* **2017**, *9*, 1069. [CrossRef]
9. Grosso, G.; Marventano, S.; Yang, J.; Micek, A.; Pajak, A.; Scalfi, L.; Galvano, F.; Kales, S.N. A comprehensive meta-analysis on evidence of Mediterranean diet and cardiovascular disease: Are individual components equal? *Crit. Rev. Food Sci. Nutr.* **2017**, *57*, 3218–3232. [CrossRef]
10. Godos, J.; Zappala, G.; Bernardini, S.; Giambini, I.; Bes-Rastrollo, M.; Martinez-Gonzalez, M. Adherence to the Mediterranean diet is inversely associated with metabolic syndrome occurrence: A meta-analysis of observational studies. *Int. J. Food Sci. Nutr.* **2017**, *68*, 138–148. [CrossRef] [PubMed]
11. Psaltopoulou, T.; Sergentanis, T.N.; Panagiotakos, D.B.; Sergentanis, I.N.; Kosti, R.; Scarmeas, N. Mediterranean diet, stroke, cognitive impairment, and depression: A meta-analysis. *Ann. Neurol.* **2013**, *74*, 580–591. [CrossRef]
12. Loughrey, D.G.; Lavecchia, S.; Brennan, S.; Lawlor, B.A.; Kelly, M.E. The Impact of the Mediterranean Diet on the Cognitive Functioning of Healthy Older Adults: A Systematic Review and Meta-Analysis. *Adv. Nutr.* **2017**, *8*, 571–586. [PubMed]
13. Schwingshackl, L.; Schwedhelm, C.; Galbete, C.; Hoffmann, G. Adherence to Mediterranean Diet and Risk of Cancer: An Updated Systematic Review and Meta-Analysis. *Nutrients* **2017**, *9*, 1063. [CrossRef]
14. Mocciaro, G.; Ziauddeen, N.; Godos, J.; Marranzano, M.; Chan, M.Y.; Ray, S. Does a Mediterranean-type dietary pattern exert a cardio-protective effect outside the Mediterranean region? A review of current evidence. *Int. J. Food Sci. Nutr.* **2018**, *69*, 524–535. [CrossRef]
15. Grosso, G.; Mistretta, A.; Marventano, S.; Purrello, A.; Vitaglione, P.; Calabrese, G.; Drago, F.; Galvano, F. Beneficial effects of the Mediterranean diet on metabolic syndrome. *Curr. Pharm. Des.* **2014**, *20*, 5039–5044. [CrossRef]
16. D'Alessandro, A.; De Pergola, G. The Mediterranean Diet: Its definition and evaluation of a priori dietary indexes in primary cardiovascular prevention. *Int. J. Food Sci. Nutr.* **2018**, *69*, 647–659. [CrossRef]
17. Galbete, C.; Schwingshackl, L.; Schwedhelm, C.; Boeing, H.; Schulze, M.B. Evaluating Mediterranean diet and risk of chronic disease in cohort studies: An umbrella review of meta-analyses. *Eur. J. Epidemiol.* **2018**, *33*, 909–931. [CrossRef] [PubMed]
18. Bonaccio, M.; Di Castelnuovo, A.; Bonanni, A.; Costanzo, S.; De Lucia, F.; Pounis, G.; Zito, F.; Donati, M.B.; De Gaetano, G.; Iacoviello, L. Adherence to a Mediterranean diet is associated with a better health-related quality of life: A possible role of high dietary antioxidant content. *BMJ Open* **2013**, *3*, e003003. [CrossRef] [PubMed]
19. Galilea-Zabalza, I.; Buil-Cosiales, P.; Salas-Salvadó, J.; Toledo, E.; Ortega-Azorin, C.; Diez-Espino, J.; Vázquez-Ruiz, Z.; Zomeño, M.D.; Vioque, J.; Martínez, J.A.; et al. Mediterranean diet and quality of life: Baseline cross-sectional analysis of the PREDIMED-PLUS trial. *PLoS ONE* **2018**, *13*, e0198974. [CrossRef]

20. Henriquez, S.P.; Ruano, C.; de Irala, J.; Ruiz-Canela, M.; Martinez-Gonzalez, M.A.; Sanchez-Villegas, A. Adherence to the Mediterranean diet and quality of life in the SUN Project. *Eur. J. Clin. Nutr.* **2012**, *66*, 360–368. [CrossRef]
21. Pérez-Tasigchana, R.F.; León-Muñoz, L.M.; Lopez-Garcia, E.; Banegas, J.R.; Rodríguez-Artalejo, F.; Guallar-Castillón, P. Mediterranean Diet and Health-Related Quality of Life in Two Cohorts of Community-Dwelling Older Adults. *PLoS ONE* **2016**, *11*, e0151596.
22. Zaragoza-Martí, A.; Ferrer-Cascales, R.; Hurtado-Sánchez, J.A.; Laguna-Pérez, A.; Cabañero-Martínez, M.J. Relationship Between Adherence to the Mediterranean Diet and Health-Related Quality of Life and Life Satisfaction Among Older Adults. *J. Nutr. Health Ageing* **2018**, *22*, 89–96. [CrossRef]
23. Oishi, S. The Psychology of Residential Mobility: Implications for the Self, Social Relationships, and Well-Being. *Perspect. Psychol. Sci.* **2010**, *5*, 5–21. [CrossRef] [PubMed]
24. Litwin, H. Social networks and well-being: A comparison of older people in Mediterranean and non-Mediterranean countries. *J. Gerontol. B. Psychol. Sci. Soc. Sci.* **2010**, *65*, 599–608. [CrossRef] [PubMed]
25. Zunzunegui, M.-V.; Alvarado, B.E.; Del Ser, T.; Otero, A. Social Networks, Social Integration, and Social Engagement Determine Cognitive Decline in Community-Dwelling Spanish Older Adults. *J. Gerontol. Ser. B Psychol. Sci. Soc. Sci.* **2003**, *58*, S93–S100. [CrossRef]
26. Fung, H.H.; Carstensen, L.L.; Lang, F.R. Age-Related Patterns in Social Networks among European Americans and African Americans: Implications for Socioemotional Selectivity across the Life Span. *Int. J. Ageing Hum. Dev.* **2001**, *52*, 185–206. [CrossRef] [PubMed]
27. Litwin, H. What really matters in the social network-mortality as- sociation? A multivariate examination among older Jewish-Israelis. *Eur. J. Ageing* **2007**, *4*, 71–82. [CrossRef] [PubMed]
28. De Belvis, A.G.; Avolio, M.; Spagnolo, A.; Damiani, G.; Sicuro, L.; Cicchetti, A.; Ricciardi, W.; Rosano, A. Factors associated with health-related quality of life: The role of social relationships among the elderly in an Italian region. *Public Health* **2008**, *122*, 784–793. [CrossRef] [PubMed]
29. Grosso, G.; Marventano, S.; D'Urso, M.; Mistretta, A.; Galvano, F. The Mediterranean healthy eating, ageing, and lifestyle (MEAL) study: Rationale and study design. *Int. J. Food Sci. Nutr.* **2017**, *68*, 577–586. [CrossRef]
30. Craig, C.L.; Marshall, A.L.; Sjöström, M.; Bauman, A.E.; Booth, M.L.; Ainsworth, B.E.; Pratt, M.; Ekelund, U.; Yngve, A.; Sallis, J.F.; et al. International Physical Activity Questionnaire: 12-Country Reliability and Validity. *Med. Sci. Sports Exerc.* **2003**, *35*, 1381–1395. [CrossRef]
31. Mistretta, A.; Marventano, S.; Platania, A.; Godos, J.; Grosso, G.; Galvano, F. Metabolic profile of the Mediterranean healthy Eating, Lifestyle and Aging (MEAL) study cohort. *Mediterr. J. Nutr. Metab.* **2017**, *10*, 131–140. [CrossRef]
32. World Health Organization. *Obesity: Preventing and Managing the Global Epidemic. Report of a WHO Consultation*; World Health Organization: Geneva, Switzerland, 1997.
33. Buscemi, S.; Rosafio, G.; Vasto, S.; Massenti, F.M.; Grosso, G.; Galvano, F.; Rini, N.; Barile, A.M.; Maniaci, V.; Cosentino, L.; et al. Validation of a food frequency questionnaire for use in Italian adults living in Sicily. *Int. J. Food Sci. Nutr.* **2015**, *66*, 1–13. [CrossRef] [PubMed]
34. Marventano, S.; Mistretta, A.; Platania, A.; Galvano, F.; Grosso, G. Reliability and relative validity of a food frequency questionnaire for Italian adults living in Sicily, Southern Italy. *Int. J. Food Sci. Nutr.* **2016**, *67*, 857–864. [CrossRef]
35. Marventano, S.; Godos, J.; Platania, A.; Galvano, F.; Mistretta, A.; Grosso, G. Mediterranean diet adherence in the Mediterranean healthy eating, aging and lifestyle (MEAL) study cohort. *Int. J. Food Sci. Nutr.* **2018**, *69*, 100–107. [CrossRef] [PubMed]
36. Sofi, F.; Dinu, M.; Pagliai, G.; Marcucci, R.; Casini, A. Validation of a literature-based adherence score to Mediterranean diet: The MEDI-LITE score. *Int. J. Food Sci. Nutr.* **2017**, *68*, 1–6. [CrossRef]
37. Priebe, S.; Huxley, P.; Knight, S.; Evans, S. Application and Results of the Manchester Short Assessment of Quality of Life (Mansa). *Int. J. Soc. Psychiatry* **1999**, *45*, 7–12. [CrossRef] [PubMed]
38. Munoz, M.A.; Fito, M.; Marrugat, J.; Covas, M.I.; Schroder, H. Adherence to the Mediterranean diet is associated with better mental and physical health. *Br. J. Nutr.* **2009**, *101*, 1821–1827. [CrossRef]
39. Milte, C.M.; Thorpe, M.G.; Crawford, D.; Ball, K.; McNaughton, S.A. Associations of diet quality with health-related quality of life in older Australian men and women. *Exp. Gerontol.* **2015**, *64*, 8–16. [CrossRef] [PubMed]

40. Zappalà, G.; Buscemi, S.; Mulè, S.; La Verde, M.; D'Urso, M.; Corleo, D.; Marranzano, M. High adherence to Mediterranean diet, but not individual foods or nutrients, is associated with lower likelihood of being obese in a Mediterranean cohort. *Eat. Disord. -Stud. Anorex. Bulim. Obes.* **2017**, *23*, 605–614.
41. La Verde, M.; Mule, S.; Zappala, G.; Privitera, G.; Maugeri, G.; Pecora, F.; Marranzano, M. Higher adherence to the Mediterranean diet is inversely associated with having hypertension: Is low salt intake a mediating factor? *Int. J. Food Sci. Nutr.* **2018**, *69*, 235–244. [CrossRef]
42. Platania, A.; Zappala, G.; Mirabella, M.U.; Gullo, C.; Mellini, G.; Beneventano, G.; Maugeri, G.; Marranzano, M. Association between Mediterranean diet adherence and dyslipidaemia in a cohort of adults living in the Mediterranean area. *Int. J. Food Sci. Nutr.* **2018**, *69*, 608–618. [CrossRef]
43. Lopez-Miranda, J.; Perez-Jimenez, F.; Ros, E.; De Caterina, R.; Badimon, L.; Covas, M.I.; Escrich, E.; Ordovás, J.M.; Soriguer, F.; Abiá, R.; et al. Olive oil and health: Summary of the II international conference on olive oil and health consensus report, Jaen and Cordoba (Spain) 2008. *Nutr. Metab. Cardiovasc. Dis.* **2010**, *20*, 284–294. [CrossRef] [PubMed]
44. Rooney, C.; McKinley, M.C.; Woodside, J.V. The potential role of fruit and vegetables in aspects of psychological well-being: A review of the literature and future directions. *Proc. Nutr. Soc.* **2013**, *72*, 420–432. [CrossRef]
45. Grosso, G.; Estruch, R. Nut consumption and age-related disease. *Maturitas* **2016**, *84*, 11–16. [CrossRef]
46. Kouvari, M.; Tyrovolas, S.; Panagiotakos, D.B. Red meat consumption and healthy ageing: A review. *Maturitas* **2016**, *84*, 17–24. [CrossRef] [PubMed]
47. Fragopoulou, E.; Choleva, M.; Antonopoulou, S.; Demopoulos, C.A. Wine and its metabolic effects. A comprehensive review of Clinical Trials. *Metabolism* **2018**, *83*, 102–119. [CrossRef] [PubMed]
48. Steptoe, A.; Perkins-Porras, L.; Hilton, S.; Rink, E.; Cappuccio, F.P. Quality of life and self-rated health in relation to changes in fruit and vegetable intake and in plasma vitamins C and E in a randomised trial of behavioural and nutritional education counselling. *Br. J. Nutr.* **2004**, *92*, 177–184. [CrossRef]
49. Van de Rest, O.; Geleijnse, J.M.; Kok, F.J.; van Staveren, W.A.; Olderikkert, M.G.; Beekman, A.T.; de Groot, L.C. Effect of fish oil supplementation on quality of life in a general population of older Dutch subjects: A randomized, double-blind, placebo-controlled trial. *J. Am. Geriatr. Soc.* **2009**, *57*, 1481–1486. [CrossRef] [PubMed]
50. Van der Valk, J.P.; Gerth van Wijk, R.; Flokstra-de Blok, B.M.; van der Velde, J.L.; de Groot, H.; Wichers, H.J.; Dubois, A.E.; de Jong, N.W. No difference in health-related quality of life, after a food challenge with cashew nut in children participating in a clinical trial. *Pediatr. Allergy Immunol.* **2016**, *27*, 812–817. [CrossRef] [PubMed]
51. Lee, C.; Longo, V. Dietary restriction with and without caloric restriction for healthy aging. *F1000Research* **2016**, *5*. [CrossRef]
52. Hooper, L.; Kroon, P.A.; Rimm, E.B.; Cohn, J.S.; Harvey, I.; Le Cornu, K.A.; Ryder, J.J.; Hall, W.L.; Cassidy, A. Flavonoids, flavonoid-rich foods, and cardiovascular risk: A meta-analysis of randomized controlled trials. *Am. J. Clin. Nutr.* **2008**, *88*, 38–50. [CrossRef]
53. Liu, Y.-J.; Zhan, J.; Liu, X.-L.; Wang, Y.; Ji, J.; He, Q.-Q. Dietary flavonoids intake and risk of type 2 diabetes: A meta-analysis of prospective cohort studies. *Clin. Nutr.* **2014**, *33*, 59–63. [CrossRef]
54. Guasch-Ferre, M.; Merino, J.; Sun, Q.; Fito, M.; Salas-Salvado, J. Dietary Polyphenols, Mediterranean Diet, Prediabetes, and Type 2 Diabetes: A Narrative Review of the Evidence. *Oxid. Med. Cell. Longev.* **2017**, *2017*, 6723931. [CrossRef]
55. Amiot, M.J.; Riva, C.; Vinet, A. Effects of dietary polyphenols on metabolic syndrome features in humans: A systematic review. *Obes. Rev.* **2016**, *17*, 573–586. [CrossRef]
56. Chang, S.-C.; Cassidy, A.; Willett, W.C.; Rimm, E.B.; O'Reilly, E.J.; Okereke, O.I. Dietary flavonoid intake and risk of incident depression in midlife and older women123. *Am. J. Clin. Nutr.* **2016**, *104*, 704–714. [CrossRef]
57. Grosso, G.; Godos, J.; Lamuela-Raventos, R.; Ray, S.; Micek, A.; Pajak, A.; Sciacca, S.; D'Orazio, N.; Del Rio, D.; Galvano, F.; et al. A comprehensive meta-analysis on dietary flavonoid and lignan intake and cancer risk: Level of evidence and limitations. *Mol. Nutr. Food Res.* **2017**, *61*, 1600930. [CrossRef]
58. Grosso, G.; Micek, A.; Godos, J.; Pajak, A.; Sciacca, S.; Galvano, F.; Giovannucci, E.L. Dietary Flavonoid and Lignan Intake and Mortality in Prospective Cohort Studies: Systematic Review and Dose-Response Meta-Analysis. *Am. J. Epidemiol.* **2017**, *185*, 1304–1316. [CrossRef]

59. Godos, J.; Bergante, S.; Satriano, A.; Pluchinotta, F.R.; Marranzano, M. Dietary Phytoestrogen Intake is Inversely Associated with Hypertension in a Cohort of Adults Living in the Mediterranean Area. *Molecules* **2018**, *23*, 368. [CrossRef]
60. Moreiras, O.; Cuadrado, C. Mediterranean Diet and Lifestyle: Special Aspects of Spain. *Int. J. Vitam. Nutr.* **2001**, *71*, 154–158. [CrossRef]
61. Bonaccio, M.; Bes-Rastrollo, M.; De Gaetano, G.; Iacoviello, L. Challenges to the Mediterranean diet at a time of economic crisis. *Nutr. Metab. Cardiovasc. Dis.* **2016**, *26*, 1057–1063. [CrossRef]
62. Bonaccio, M.; Bonanni, A.E.; Di Castelnuovo, A.; De Lucia, F.; Donati, M.B.; De Gaetano, G.; Iacoviello, L. Low income is associated with poor adherence to a Mediterranean diet and a higher prevalence of obesity: Cross-sectional results from the Moli-sani study. *BMJ Open* **2012**, *2*, e001685. [CrossRef]
63. Bonaccio, M.; Di Castelnuovo, A.; Bonanni, A.; Costanzo, S.; De Lucia, F.; Persichillo, M.; Zito, F.; Donati, M.B.; de Gaetano, G.; Iacoviello, L. Decline of the Mediterranean diet at a time of economic crisis. Results from the Moli-sani study. *Nutr. Metab. Cardiovasc. Dis.* **2014**, *24*, 853–860. [CrossRef]
64. Grosso, G.; Marventano, S.; Buscemi, S.; Scuderi, A.; Matalone, M.; Platania, A.; Giorgianni, G.; Rametta, S.; Nolfo, F.; Galvano, F.; et al. Factors Associated with Adherence to the Mediterranean Diet among Adolescents Living in Sicily, Southern Italy. *Nutrients* **2013**, *5*, 4908–4923. [CrossRef]
65. Grosso, G.; Marventano, S.; Giorgianni, G.; Raciti, T.; Galvano, F.; Mistretta, A. Mediterranean diet adherence rates in Sicily, southern Italy. *Public Health Nutr.* **2014**, *17*, 2001–2009. [CrossRef]
66. Grosso, G.; Pajak, A.; Mistretta, A.; Marventano, S.; Raciti, T.; Buscemi, S.; Drago, F.; Scalfi, L.; Galvano, F. Protective role of the Mediterranean diet on several cardiovascular risk factors: Evidence from Sicily, southern Italy. *Nutr. Metab. Cardiovasc. Dis.* **2014**, *24*, 370–377. [CrossRef]
67. Estruch, R.; Bach-Faig, A. Mediterranean diet as a lifestyle and dynamic food pattern. *Eur. J. Clin. Nutr.* **2018**. [CrossRef]
68. Sans, S. Mediterranean diet, active lifestyle and cardiovascular disease: A recipe for immortality? *Eur. J. Prev. Cardiol.* **2018**, *25*, 1182–1185. [CrossRef]
69. Yannakoulia, M.; Kontogianni, M.; Scarmeas, N. Cognitive health and Mediterranean Diet: Just diet or lifestyle pattern? *Ageing Res. Rev.* **2015**, *20*, 74–78. [CrossRef]

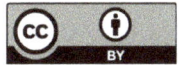

© 2019 by the authors. Licensee MDPI, Basel, Switzerland. This article is an open access article distributed under the terms and conditions of the Creative Commons Attribution (CC BY) license (http://creativecommons.org/licenses/by/4.0/).

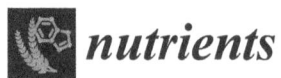

Review

Effect of Adherence to Mediterranean Diet during Pregnancy on Children's Health: A Systematic Review

Carlotta Biagi [1,*,†], **Mattia Di Nunzio** [2,†], **Alessandra Bordoni** [2,3], **Davide Gori** [4] **and Marcello Lanari** [1]

1. Pediatric Emergency Unit, Department of Medical and Surgical Sciences (DIMEC), St. Orsola Hospital, University of Bologna, Via Massarenti 11, 40138 Bologna (BO), Italy; marcello.lanari@unibo.it
2. Department of Agri-Food Sciences and Technologies (DISTAL), University of Bologna, Piazza Goidanich 60, 47521 Cesena, Italy; mattia.dinunzio@unibo.it (M.D.N.); alessandra.bordoni@unibo.it (A.B.)
3. Interdepartimental Center for Agro-Food Industrial Research (CIRI-AGRO), University of Bologna, via Quinto Bucci 336, 47521 Cesena (FC), Italy; alessandra.bordoni@unibo.it
4. Department of Biomedical and Neuromotor Sciences, University of Bologna, 40125 Bologna, Italy; davide.gori4@unibo.it
* Correspondence: carlottabiagi@yahoo.it; Tel.: +39-051-214-4540
† Both authors contributed equally to this work.

Received: 30 March 2019; Accepted: 27 April 2019; Published: 1 May 2019

Abstract: The traditional Mediterranean diet has been shown to be a healthy eating pattern that protects against the development of many diseases in adults and children. Pregnancy is a critical period of plasticity during which foetal development may be significantly influenced by different environmental factors, including maternal nutrition. In this context, several studies have examined the potential benefits of adherence to a Mediterranean diet during pregnancy on birth outcomes, considering the Mediterranean diet as a whole rather than focusing on the effect of its individual components. In this review, we systematically summarized and discussed results of studies investigating the protective role of Mediterranean diet against foetal growth, prematurity, neural tube defects and other congenital pathologies, asthma and allergy, body weight and metabolic markers. Although current data are insufficient and randomized control trials are needed, growing evidence suggests the beneficial effect of the Mediterranean diet during pregnancy on children's health. In this sense, strategies aiming to promote adherence to this dietary pattern might be of considerable importance to public health.

Keywords: Mediterranean diet; pregnancy; offspring; child health

1. Introduction

The Developmental Origins of Health and Disease (DOHaD) hypothesis posits that in utero exposure plays a critical role in the risk of disease in adulthood. Maternal diet during pregnancy contributes to the in-utero environment [1]; nutritional stress/stimulus applied during critical periods of early development permanently influences organism's physiology and metabolism, with the consequences of this metabolic programming often being observed much later in life [2,3]. Although the DOHaD hypothesis is well documented in animals [4], evidence connecting maternal diet quality during pregnancy and offspring risk factors is scarce and inconsistent in humans. Most studies have investigated the associations of specific nutrients, foods, or food groups intake during pregnancy with offspring health without considering the overall diet [5,6].

Foetal growth restriction (FGR) and risk of new-borns small for gestational age (SGA), prematurity, neural tube defects (NTDs), congenital heart defects (CHDs), gastroschisis, asthma and allergy, overweight and metabolic disorders represent leading causes of childhood diseases that are supposed to be connected to maternal nutrition.

FGR is defined as an estimated foetal weight or abdominal circumference below the 5th or the 10th centile according to gestational age (GA) and sex, and it affects about 5–10% of all pregnancies [7]. FGR is associated with an increased risk for childhood morbidity (mainly hypoglycaemia, developmental delay and infectious diseases) and with about half of all foetal deaths [8,9]. It is also associated with chronic diseases in adult life including coronary heart disease, stroke, type-2 diabetes mellitus, adiposity, metabolic syndrome and osteoporosis [10,11]. New-borns are considered SGA when their body weight is lower than the 10th centile according to neonatal growth curves adjusted for gestational age at delivery and sex [12]. Not all SGA new-borns are pathologically growth restricted, as a proportion of babies (18–22%) are constitutionally small but healthy [12]. However, FGR significantly overlaps SGA, and they are often considered as a single entity. FGR and SGA can arise from several maternal, foetal and placental problems [13]; however, maternal nutrition has been recognized as one of the most important environmental factors influencing foetal growth and development [14–17].

Preterm birth is defined as any birth before 37 weeks of GA [18]. Preterm birth, especially before 34 weeks of GA, is the leading cause of perinatal morbidity and mortality in developed country [19]. There are multiple risk factors for premature birth including having a previous premature birth, pregnancy with multiple babies, infection, drug or alcohol use, and age. A well-balanced diet during pregnancy has been reported to reduce the odds of a premature birth [20].

NTDs are a major health burden that affect 0.5–2/1000 pregnancies worldwide and represent a preventable cause of stillbirth, infant death and significant lifelong morbidity [21]. CHDs and gastroschisis are other common malformations representing major causes of mortality, morbidity and disability of perinatal origin [22,23]. The aetiology of these congenital malformations is multifactorial and both genetic predisposition and environmental influences contribute to them, with nutritional deficits serving as potential contributing factors [24,25].

The prevalence of asthma and allergic diseases (atopic dermatitis/eczema, allergic rhino-conjunctivitis) has increased worldwide over the past few decades with the highest incidence occurring in children [26]. Globalization and consequent deviation from traditional to Western diet might be one of the environmental changes involved in the recent increased of the atopic diseases. In fact, decreased antioxidant (fruit and vegetables), increased n-6 polyunsaturated fatty acids (PUFA) (margarine, vegetable oil), and decreased n-3 PUFA (fish oil) intakes might lead to oxidative stress and inflammation and might contribute to the higher incidence of asthma and allergies [27,28].

Due to the importance of maternal diet during pregnancy as influencer of child health, actions to improve its quality are urgently needed. In this light, a good adherence to the Mediterranean diet (MD) could represent a good strategy. MD is characterized by increased consumption of unprocessed and plant foods, olive oil, and fish, whereas consumption of red meat, animal fats, sugars and salt are minimal. The MD is rich in mono-unsaturated fatty acids (MUFA), omega-3 PUFA and antioxidant polyphenols, and it is been recommended for its overall health benefits and potential for disease prevention [29]. Several observational and intervention studies support the role of the MD in preventing obesity, type 2 diabetes mellitus and metabolic syndrome in adults [30,31], while some recent studies suggest a protective role against obesity development in children [32–34]. In pregnancy, a higher adherence to the MD has been associated with lower risk of preterm birth, and higher birth weight [20].

The aim of this systematic review is to verify the association between maternal adherence to the MD during pregnancy and children health outcomes, and to provide clinicians with levels and quality of evidence on the efficacy of MD in improving paediatric health outcomes.

2. Methods

2.1. Study Selection

This systematic review was performed according to the Preferred Reporting Items for Systematic Reviews and Meta-analyses guidelines (PRISMA) [35].

We searched electronic databases (September 17, 2018) Medline, EMBASE and Clinical Trials. The search process was conducted using the following keywords: (pregnancy OR gravidity OR pregnant OR pregnant women OR pregnan*) OR (child OR children OR childhood OR paediatric OR paediatric OR paediatric* OR paediatric OR offspring OR new-born OR new-borns OR neonate OR neonates Or neonatal OR toddler OR toddlers) AND ("Diet, Mediterranean" (Mesh) OR Mediterranean diet* OR Med Diet OR Mediterranean diet). Inclusion criteria were: (i) English language; (ii) systematic recording of diet during the gestational period (daily register or food frequency questionnaire—FFQ) in healthy women; (iii) assessment of "small for gestational age", prematurity, foetal growth, neural tube defects, asthma, wheeze, atopy, insulin resistance and metabolic syndrome, childhood overweight, metabolic markers, epigenetic and congenital pathologies in the offspring.

Exclusion criteria were: (i) irrelevant titles not indicating the research topic; (ii) evaluation of dietary patterns different from the MD; (iii) dietary intervention including single/few nutrients or single/few aspects of dietary intake; (iv) dietary intervention with inadequate description of the dietary treatment. There was no restriction regarding period or publication status.

Titles and abstracts of studies initially identified from databases (602 studies) were checked by two independent investigators (C.B. and M.D.N.) and disagreements among reviewers were resolved through a mediator (M.L.). After first screening, duplicates, reviews, letters, abstracts and articles without full-text in English language were also excluded. The detailed selection process is presented in Figure 1.

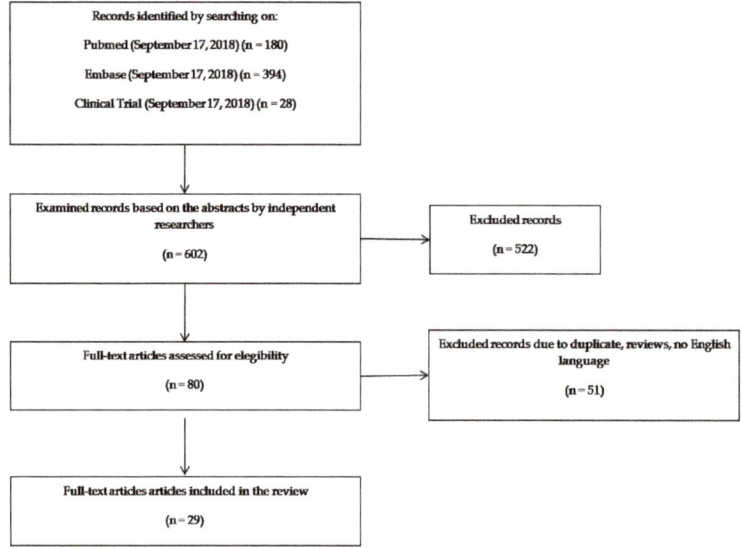

Figure 1. diagram of search strategy and study selection.

2.2. Study Quality Assessment

Two researchers (C.B. and M.D.N.) independently and blindly assessed the risk of bias of included studies using the parameters defined by the Cochrane Tool for Quality Assessment [36] and the Strengthening the Reporting of Observational Studies in Epidemiology (STROBE) [37]. Disagreement was resolved primarily through discussion and consensus between the researchers. If consensus was not reached, another blind reviewer (D.G) acted as third arbiter.

The Cochrane Tool analyses seven bias groups: sequence generation and allocation concealment (both within the domain of selection bias or allocation bias), blinding of participants and personnel (performance bias), blinding of outcome assessors (detection bias), incomplete outcome data (attrition bias), selective reporting (reporting bias) and an auxiliary domain: "other bias". For each bias group, it is possible to assign a value of "high," "low" or "unclear" risk of bias when it is not specified if a specific bias is present or not. Every bias judgment helps to assign a global assessment to every RCT according to the Agency for Healthcare Research and Quality (AHRQ) standards (good, fair and poor).

The STROBE statement is a 22 items tool specifically designed to evaluate observational studies quality. Items are associated with the different sections of an article, such as title and abstract (item 1), introduction (items 2 and 3), methods (items 4–12), results (items 13–17), discussion (items 18–21), and other information (item 22 on funding). Eighteen items are identical for the three different study designs, while four (specifically items 6, 12, 14, and 15) are differentially designed for each study type (i.e., cohort or case control). STROBE does not provide a scoring stratification. As a rule, the higher the score, the higher the quality of the study. We hence created three score thresholds corresponding to three levels of items scored: 0–14 as poor quality, 15–25 as intermediate quality and 26–33 as good quality of the study.

3. Results

3.1. Search Findings

The initial search identified 602 studies, with 522 records excluded following abstract review (Figure 1). Of the 80 articles retrieved, 51 were excluded because of duplicates, reviews, letters, abstracts and articles without full-text in English language. In the end, 29 studies were included in the analysis. Included studies were published between 2008 and 2018.

3.2. Studies Characteristics

A detailed description of the selected articles is reported in Table 1.

Table 1. Summary of the included studies.

Author	Geographic Area	Study Design	Included Participants	Assessment of Dietary Habits	Assessment of Adherence to MD	Outcomes	Results
Timmermans et al. (2012) [38]	Netherlands	Prospective population-based cohort study	3207 mothers with a spontaneously conceived live-born singleton pregnancy	Semi-quantitative FFQ (293 items) self-administered during early pregnancy (GA < 18 weeks)	Logistic regression analysis was used to identify a comparable dietary pattern, which was labeled MD as it was characterized by higher intakes of pasta, rice, vegetable oils, fish, vegetables and alcohol, and lower intakes of meat, potatoes and fatty sauces. All women were categorized into equal tertiles based on their probability score for the diet, namely: low MDA, medium MDA and high MDA.	Fetal growth	Low MDA resulted associated with lower birth weight (difference in grams at birth −72 [95% CI: −110.8 to 33.3])
Chatzi et al. (2012) [39]	Spain (INMA cohort) and Greece (RHEA cohort)	Prospective population-based cohort study	Spain: 2461 mother-newborn pairs. Greece: 889 mother-newborn pairs	Semi-quantitative FFQ (100 items in IMNA cohort and 250 items in RHEA cohort) administered by trained interviewers during first (IMNA cohort) or mid trimester (RHEA cohort) of pregnancy	Trichopoulou's score [40] modified for pregnancy	Fetal growth	High MDA was associated with lower risk of delivering a FGR infant (OR 0.5 [95% CI: 0.3–0.9]) in the INMA-Mediterranean cohort. In all cohort high MD adherence increased birth weight in smoking mothers
Sauders et al. (2014) [41]	Guadeloupe (French Caribbean Island)	Prospective mother-child cohort study	728 pregnant women with a live-born singleton pregnancy without major congenital malformations	Semi-quantitative FFQ (214 items) administered by trained interviewers in the days after delivery	Trichopoulou's score [40]	Fetal growth and prematurity	No overall associations with FGR. No overall association with prematurity. Decreased risk in overweight and obese woman (adjOR 0.7 [95% CI: 0.6–0.9])
Gomez-Roig et al. (2017) [42]	Spain	Cross-sectional study	46 mothers with SGA fetuses 81 mothers with appropriate for gestational age (AGA) fetuses	Semi-quantitative FFQ (127 items) administered by trained interviewers during the third trimester of pregnancy	Trichopoulou's score [40]	SGA infants	High MD score was associated with a lower risk of SGA (OR 0.18 [95% CI: 0.74–0.501]) for the third consumer quartile

Table 1. Cont.

Author	Geographic Area	Study Design	Included Participants	Assessment of Dietary Habits	Assessment of Adherence to MD	Outcomes	Results
Peraita-Costa et al. (2018) [43]	Spain	Cross-sectional population-based study	492 mothers	Semi-quantitative FFQ (16 items) self-administered after delivery	Modified KidMed score [44]	SGA infants	The newborns born to women with low MDA presented a higher risk of being SGA (adjOR 1.68 [95% CI: 1.02–5.46]) when adjusting for parental BMI and multiple gestation, but not when adjusting for all significant possible confounders.
Parlapani et al. (2017) [45]	Greece	Single-center, prospective, observational cohort study	82 women who delivered preterm singletons at post conceptional age < 34 weeks	Semi-quantitative FFQ (156 items) self-administered immediately before or after delivery	Panagiotakos dietary score [46]	Fetal growth and prematurity-associated complications	Low MD adherence increased the risk of IUGR, low birth weight, bronchopulmonary dysplasia and necrotizing enterolitis in preterm infants (<34 weeks)
Martinez-Galiano et al. (2018) [47]	Spain	Prospective multicenter matched case-control study (matching criterion: maternal age at delivery)	518 mothers of singleton SGA infants 518 mothers of singleton infants with normal weight for GA	Semi-quantitative FFQ (137 items) administered by trained interviewers within 2 days after delivery	PREDIMED score [48], Trichopoulou's score [40], Panagiotakos' score [46]	SGA infants	MDA and daily consumption of 5 gr of olive oil was associated to a reduced risk of SGA in newborns (adjOR 0.59 [95% CI: 0.38–0.98])
Assaf-Balut et al. (2017) [49]	Spain	Prospective randomized controlled intervention trial	500 mothers allocated to intervention (MD diet supplemented with extra virgin olive oil and pistachios) and 500 allocated to control (standard diet with limited fat intake)	Semi-quantitative FFQ (14 items) administered by trained interviewed during 4 study visits (at first ultrasound visit at 24–28 GA, at 36–38 GA, and at delivery) to evaluate the adherence to the intervention	MDA screener score [50]	SGA infants and prematurity	MD supplemented with extravergin olive oil and pistachios significantly reduced prematurity rate (p 0.023) and SGA (p 0.001) in the intervention group
Carmichael et al. (2013) [51]	United States	Cross-sectional study	5738 mothers with a singleton pregnancy who delivered non-malformed infants	Semi-quantitative FFQ (58 items) administered by telephone interview 6 weeks–24 months after delivery	Trichopoulou's score [40] and DQI incorporating pregnancy-specific nutritional recommendations [52]	Prematurity	No association
Mikkelse et al. (2008) [53]	Denmark	Prospective cohort study	35657 pregnant women with a live-born singleton pregnancy	Semi-quantitative FFQ (360 items) self-administered at mid-pregnancy (week 25) by mail	Khoury's score [54]	Prematurity	High MDA reduced the risk of early preterm birth (adjOR 0.28 [95% CI: 0.11–0.76]). No associations with late preterm delivery.

Table 1. Cont.

Author	Geographic Area	Study Design	Included Participants	Assessment of Dietary Habits	Assessment of Adherence to MD	Outcomes	Results
Haugen et al. (2008) [55]	Norway	Prospective cohort study	26563 pregnant women with a live-born singleton pregnancy	Semi-quantitative FFQ (255 items) self-administered at week 18–22 of pregnancy	Khoury's score [54]	Prematurity	No association
Smith et al. (2015) [56]	United Kingdom	Population-based cohort study	922 mothers with singleton late and moderate preterm (LMPT) births; 965 mothers with singleton term births	Maternal interview shortly after delivery	MDA on the basis of the presence of at least 1 of the following major criteria: five portions of fruit and vegetables every day; fish more than twice a week; meat no more than twice a week; max two cups of coffee/d.	Late and moderately preterm (LMPT) birth	Higher risk of delivering LMPT in not adherent women (RR 1.81 [95% CI: 1.04–3.14])
Vujkovic et al. (2009) [57]	Netherlands	Retrospective multicenter case-control study	50 mothers of children with spina bifida; 81 control mothers	Semi-quantitative FFQ (200 items) administered 14 months after delivery and individually checked for consistency at the hospital or by telephone by the researcher.	Principal component factor analysis (PCA) and reduce rank regression (RRR) were used to identify a comparable dietary pattern, which was labeled MD as it was characterized by high intake of vegetables, fruits, vegetable oils, legumes, fish, alcohol and cereal products and low intakes of potatoes and sweets.	NTDs	Low MDA according to both PCA and RRR, was associated with an increased risk of spina bifida (OR 2.7 [95% CI: 1.2–6.1] and OR 3.5 [95% CI: 1.5–7.9], respectively)
Carmichael et al. (2012) [58]	United States	Retrospective multicenter case-control study	936 mothers of children with NTDs; 2475 mothers of children with orofacial clefts; 6147 control mothers	Semi-quantitative FFQ (58 items) administered by telephone interviews 6 weeks–24 months after delivery	Trichopoulou's score [40] and DQI [52] incorporating pregnancy-specific nutritional recommendations	NTDs and orofacial clefts	High Trichopoulou score and DQI score were protective for NTDs, with a stronger association observed for anencephaly (adjOR 0.64 [95% CI: 0.45–0.92] and 0.49 [95% CI: 0.31–0.75], respectively)

Table 1. *Cont.*

Author	Geographic Area	Study Design	Included Participants	Assessment of Dietary Habits	Assessment of Adherence to MD	Outcomes	Results
Botto et al. (2016) [59]	USA	Population based, multicenter case-control study	9885 case mothers 9468 control mothers	Semi-quantitative FFQ (58 items) administered by telephone interviews 6 weeks–24 months after delivery	Trichopoulou's score [40] and the DQI [52] incorporating pregnancy-specific nutritional recommendations	Congenital Heart Defects	High Trichopoulou's score was protective only for perimembranous ventricular septal defects (14%, OR 0.86 [95% CI: 0.69–1.07]). High DQI was protective for tetralogy of Fallot (OR 0.63 [95% CI: 0.49–0.80]), conotruncal defects (OR 0.76 [95% CI: 0.64–0.91]), atrial septal defects (OR 0.77 [95% CI: 0.63–0.94]) and for all septal defects (OR 0.86 [95% CI: 0.75–1.00]).
Feldkamp et al. (2014) [60]	USA	Population based, multicenter case-control study	1125 gastroschisis cases 9483 controls	58-item FFQ (58 items) administered by a computerized-assisted telephone interview (CATI) to case and control mothers 6wk to 24 months after delivery	Trichopoulou's score [40] and the DQI [52] incorporating pregnancy-specific nutritional recommendations	Gastroschisis	High Trichopoulou's score (quartile 2, adjOR 0.62 [95% CI: 0.33–1.16]; quartile 3, adjOR 0.51 [95% CI: 0.28–0.94]; quartile 4, adjOR 0.50 [95% CI: 0.28, 0.90]) and DQI score (quartile 2, adjOR 0.58 [95% CI: 0.40–0.86]; quartile 3, adjOR 0.52 [95% CI: 0.36–0.79]; quartile 4, adjOR 0.48 [95% CI: 0.32–0.76]) were protective for gastroschisis.
Chatzi et al. (2008) [61]	Spain	Cohort study	460 children	Semi-quantitative FFQ (42 items) referred to the pregnancy and administered to mothers 3 months after delivery by a face-to-face interview. Semi-quantitative FFQ (96 items) administered to the parents of the children at 6.5 year of age by an interviewer	Trichopoulou's score [40]	Wheeze, atopic wheeze and atopy at 6.5 years	High MDS in mothers was protective for persistent wheeze (adjOR 0.22 [95% CI:0.08–0.58]), atopic wheeze (adjOR0.30 [95% CI:0.10–0.90]), and atopy (adjOR 0.55 [95% CI: 0.31–0.97]) in children at 6.5 years

Table 1. *Cont.*

Author	Geographic Area	Study Design	Included Participants	Assessment of Dietary Habits	Assessment of Adherence to MD	Outcomes	Results
De Batlle et al. (2008) [62]	Mexico	Cross-sectional study	1476 children	Semi-quantitative FFQ (70 items) referred to the pregnancy and self-administered at the children age of 6–7 years	Trichopoulou's score [40]	Asthma, Wheezing, rhinitis, sneezing, itchy-watery eyes at 6-7 years	High MDS was protective for current sneezing (OR 0.71 [95% CI: 0.53–0.97]).
Castro-Rodriguez et al. (2010) [63]	Spain	Cohort study	1409 infants	Semi-quantitative FFQ (11 items) referred to the pregnancy and self-administered at the children's aged of 15–18 months	MDS modified from Psaltopoulou [64]	Wheeze at 12 months	MD (p 0.036) and olive oil (p 0.002) were associated with less wheezing. Only olive oil intake remained inversely associated with wheezing (adjOR 0.57 [95% CI: 0.4–0.9])
Chatzi et al. (2013) [65]	Spain (INMA cohort) and Greece (RHEA cohort)	Cohort study	Spain: 1771 mother-newborn pairs. Greece: 745 mother-newborn pairs	Semi-quantitative FFQ (100 items in INMA cohort and 250 items in RHEA cohort) administered by trained interviewers at mean 13.8 weeks of GA (INMA cohort) or 14.6 weeks of GA (RHEA cohort)	Trichopoulou's score [40] modified for pregnancy considering dairy food protective and not including in the score alcohol consumption.	Wheeze and eczema at 12 months	No associations between MD score and wheeze and eczema
Alvarez-Zallo et al. (2018) [66]	Spain	Cohort study	1087 mother-infant pairs	Semi-quantitative FFQ (11-items) referred to the pregnancy and self-administered at the children aged 12–15 months	MDS modified from Psaltopoulou [64]	Wheeze and eczema at 12-15 months	No associations between MD score and wheezing, recurrent wheezing and eczema
Lange et al. (2010) [67]	United States	Cohort study	1376 mother-infant pairs	Semi-quantitative FFQ (166 items) self-administered at the first and second trimesters visits	MD score modified from Trichopoulou [40], Alternate Healthy Eating Index modified for pregnancy [68] and PCA to look at Western and Prudent diets	Wheeze, asthma and atopy at 3 years	No associations between dietary patterns and asthma, atopy or wheezing

Table 1. *Cont.*

Author	Geographic Area	Study Design	Included Participants	Assessment of Dietary Habits	Assessment of Adherence to MD	Outcomes	Results
Castro-Rodriguez et al. (2016) [69]	Spain	Cohort study	1000 mother-newborn pairs	Semi-quantitative FFQ (11 items) regarding the consumption of foods during pregnancy self-administered at the time point of 1.5 years of children's life. Semi-quantitative FFQ (11 items) regarding the consumption of food by the child self-administered at the time point of 4 years of life	MDS modified from Psaltopoulou [66]	Wheeze, dermatitis and allergic rhinitis at 4 years	No associations between MD score and wheezing, rhinitis and dermatitis
Gesteiro et al. (2012) [70]	Spain	Cross sectional study	35 women	169 items FFQ conducted by a trained dietician 3–5 after delivery	Healthy eating index (HEI) adapted for the Spanish population [71] and by a modified MDA scores used in the PREDIMED study [72]	Various insulin sensitivity/resistance biomarkers at birth	Low HEI- or low MDA-score diet delivered infants with high insulinaemia (p 0.048 or p 0.017, respectively). HOMA-IR (p 0.031 or p 0.049, respectively) and glycaemia (p 0.018 or p 0.048, respectively). The relative risk (RR) of high-neonatal glycaemia and insulinaemia were 7.6 (p 0.008) and 6.7 (p 0.017) for low vs. high HEI-score groups. High HOMA-IR and high glucose RR were, respectively, 3.4 (p 0.043) and 3.9 (p 0.016) in neonates from the <7 MDA- vs. >7 MDA-score group.

Table 1. Cont.

Author	Geographic Area	Study Design	Included Participants	Assessment of Dietary Habits	Assessment of Adherence to MD	Outcomes	Results
Chatzi et al. (2017) [73]	USA (Project Viva cohort) and Greece (RHEA cohort)	Prospective mother–child cohort study	997 mother–child pairs from Project Viva and 569 pairs from the RHEA study	In Project Viva, mothers reported their diet since the time of their last menstrual period at study enrolment (median 9.9 weeks gestation) using a validated semi-quantitative FFQ. RHEA participants completed a validated FFQ at mean 14.6 weeks gestation.	Trichopoulou's score [40]	BMI z-score, waist circumference, skin-fold thickness, systolic and diastolic blood pressure	In the pooled analysis, for each 3-point increment in the MDS, offspring BMI z-score was lower by 0.14 units (95% CI: −0.15 to −0.13), waist circumference by 0.39cm (95% CI: −0.64 to −0.14), the sum of skin-fold thicknesses by 0.63mm (95% CI: 0.98 to −0.28), systolic blood pressure by −1.03 mmHg (95% CI: −1.65 to −0.42) and diastolic blood pressure by −0.57 mmHg (95% CI: −0.98 to −0.16).
Fernández-Barrés et al. (2016) [74]	Spain	Population based cohort study	1827 pairs of mother and children	Validated 101 items FFQ conducted from first to third trimester	Relative Mediterranean diet score (rMED) [75]	BMI and waist circumference	A significant association between higher adherence to MD and lower waist circumference (−0.62 cm [95% CI: −1.1 to −0.14]).
Gesteiro et al. (2015) [76]	Spain	Cross sectional study	35 women	Complete 169 items FFQ guided by a trained dietician conducted at first trimester	Modified MDA scores used in the PREDIMED study [72]	Cord blood lipoprotein and homocysteine concentrations	Mothers at the low MDA-score delivered neonates with high cord blood LDL-c (p 0.049), Apo B (p 0.040), homocysteine (p 0.026) and Apo A1/Apo B ratio (p 0.024).
Mantzoros et al. (2010) [77]	USA	Prospective cohort study	780 women	Slightly modified semi-quantitative FFQ at both the first and second trimester	Trichopoulou's score [40]	Cord blood leptin and adiponectin concentrations	Closer adherence to a Mediterranean pattern diet during pregnancy was not associated with cord blood leptin (p 0.38) or adiponectin (p 0.93)
Gonzalez-Nahm et al. (2017) [78]	USA	Cohort study	390 women whose infants had DNA methylation data available from cord blood leukocytes	150 items FFQ at preconception or at first trimester	Modified Trichopoulou's score [40]	Methylation at the MEG3-IG region	Infants of mothers with a low adherence to a Mediterranean diet had a greater odd of hypo-methylation at the MEG3-IG differentially methylated region (OR 2.80 [95% CI: 1.35–5.82])

adjOR: adjusted odds ratio; BMI: body mass index; CI: confidence interval; GA: gestational age; FFQ: food frequency questionnaire; MEG3-IG: maternally expressed gene 3 - intergenic region; MD: Mediterranean Diet; MDA: Mediterranean Diet adherence; NTDs: neural tube defects; OR odds ratio; PTD: preterm delivery; RR: relative risk; SGA: small for gestational age; LMPT: Late and moderately preterm; HOMA-IR: homeostatic model assessment for insulin resistance.

Risk of FGR and of SGA new-borns were the outcomes addressed by the higher number of studies (8 out of 29 studies), followed by asthma and allergy in the offspring (7 out of 29), and prematurity risk (6 out of 29). Two studies [41,49] recurred in 2 different outcomes, FGR and prematurity, owing to multiple comparison groups between the articles. All studies except [49] were observational studies: 16 cohort studies, 5 case-control and 7 cross sectional studies.

3.3. Risk of bias and Quality of Reporting

We conducted the quality analysis based on the aforementioned methods and tools for analysis. Table 2 shows the main quality results scored by the papers included. Of the 29 articles included for quality analysis, 16 (55%) were cohort studies, 5 (17%) were case-control studies and 7 (24%) were cross sectional studies. One paper (3%) had an RCT study design. Six cohort studies (38%) were of good quality, 7 (44%) of intermediate quality and 3 (18%) of poor quality. All the 5 case control studies were of intermediate quality. Among cross sectional studies, five (71%) were of intermediate quality and 2 (29%) of poor quality.

Table 2. Risk of bias of the included studies.

Author	Study Type	Tool for Assessment	Quality
Timmermans et al. (2012) [38]	Cohort	STROBE	24/33—Intermediate
Chatzi et al. (2012) [39]	Cohort	STROBE	27/33—Good
Sauders et al. (2014) [41]	Cohort	STROBE	24/33—Intermediate
Gomez-Roig et al. (2017) [42]	Cross Sectional	STROBE	12/33—Poor
Peraita-Costa et al. (2018) [43]	Cross Sectional	STROBE	16/33—Intermediate
Parlapani et al. (2017) [45]	Cohort	STROBE	21/33—Intermediate
Martinez-Galiano et al. (2018) [47]	Case-Control	STROBE	22/33—Intermediate
Assaf-Balut et al. (2017) [49]	RCT	Cochrane ROB Tool	Poor quality due to blindness and allocation concealment
Carmichael et al. (2013) [51]	Cross Sectional	STROBE	11/33—Poor
Mikkelsen et al. (2008) [53]	Cohort	STROBE	19/33—Intermediate
Haugen et al. (2008) [55]	Cohort	STROBE	22/33—Intermediate
Smith et al. (2015) [56]	Cohort	STROBE	26/33—Good
Vujkovic et al. (2009) [57]	Case-Control	STROBE	21/33—Intermediate
Carmicheal et al. (2012) [58]	Case-Control	STROBE	17/33—Intermediate

Table 2. Cont.

Author	Study Type	Tool for Assessment	Quality
Botto et al. (2016) [59]	Case-Control	STROBE	18/33—Intermediate
Feldkamp et al. (2014) [60]	Case-Control	STROBE	23/33—Intermediate
Chatzi et al. (2008) [61]	Cohort	STROBE	25/33—Intermediate
De Batlle et al. (2008) [62]	Cross Sectional	STROBE	12/33—Poor
Castro-Rodriguez et al. (2010) [63]	Cohort	STROBE	26/33—Good
Chatzi et al. (2013) [65]	Cohort	STROBE	28/33—Good
Alvarez-Zallo et al. (2018) [66]	Cohort	STROBE	14/33—Poor
Lange et al. (2010) [67]	Cohort	STROBE	31/33—Good
Castro-Rodriguez et al. (2016) [69]	Cross Sectional	STROBE	18/33—Intermediate
Gesteiro et al. (2012) [70]	Cross Sectional	STROBE	16/33—Intermediate
Chatzi et al. (2017) [73]	Cohort	STROBE	26/33—Good
Fernández-Barrés et al. (2016) [74]	Cohort	STROBE	27/33—Good
Gesteiro et al. (2015) [76]	Cross Sectional	STROBE	22/33—Intermediate
Mantzoros et al. (2010) [77]	Cohort	STROBE	25/33—Intermediate
Gonzalez-Nahm et al. (2017) [78]	Cohort	STROBE	13/33—Poor

3.4. Evidence Synthesis

Results coming from the 29 selected articles are reported below according to the main outcome of the study.

3.4.1. Foetal Growth Restriction and Small for Gestational Age

Evidence for this outcome comes from 8 papers (Table 1, Table 2): an RCT of poor quality, 4 cohort studies (1 good, 3 intermediate quality), 2 cross sectional studies (1 intermediate and 1 poor quality) and 1 case-control study of intermediate quality. Cohort studies reached the best scores for quality.

In few studies, adherence to MD was assessed in early pregnancy since the trajectory of foetal growth is set at this stage [11]. The Generation R prospective observational study [38] evaluated the association between dietary patterns in the early phase of pregnancy (GA < 18 weeks) and foetal size/weight at birth in 3207 pregnant women living in Rotterdam. To test their adherence to MD over the preceding three months, a semiquantitative FFQ including 293 food items was self-administered at enrolment (median GA = 13.5 weeks). Women were categorised into tertiles of adherence to the MD (low, medium and high) based on their intake of vegetables, vegetable oil, fish, fruits, pasta and rice, meat, potatoes and fatty sauces. Low adherence to the MD in early pregnancy resulted associated with decreased intra-uterine size and lower birth weight compared to high adherence (difference in grams at birth −72 [95% CI: −110.8 to −33.3]).

Chatzi et al. [39] analysed the impact of MD adherence (MDA) during the first trimester of pregnancy on foetal growth in the Spanish multicentre INMA cohort (2461 mother-new-born pairs), divided into the Atlantic area and the Mediterranean area cohort, and during the mid-trimester in the Greek RHEA cohort (889 mother-new-born pairs). Semi-quantitative FFQ respectively were administered by trained interviewers. Maternal MDA was evaluated through a score including 100 or 250 food items modified from the MD score by Trichopoulou [40]. The modified score was specifically designed for pregnant women, and it considered dairy food protective and did not include alcohol consumption. Food intake and MD score differed significantly across cohorts, mean MD score being higher in the INMA-Mediterranean and RHEA cohorts compared to the INMA-Atlantic cohort. Women with high MD adherence had a significantly lower risk of delivering an FGR infant (OR 0.5 [95% CI: 0.3–0.9]) only in the INMA-Mediterranean cohort. Of note, in all cohorts, high MD adherence increased child weight at birth in smoking mothers, thus suggesting a counteraction of the detrimental effect of smoking. In most studies, adherence to the MD was evaluated in the last trimester of pregnancy or after delivery. Saunders and colleagues [41] found no association between maternal adherence to MD and the risk of FGR in 728 pregnant women enrolled in Guadeloupe. A semi-quantitative FFQ including 214 food items was administered by trained interviewers in the days following delivery, and adherence to the MD was evaluated using the Trichopoulou 9-level score [40].

In a Spanish cross-sectional prospective study [42], a semi-quantitative FFQ comprising 127 food items was administered by trained interviewers to 127 women (46 and 81 mothers with SGA and appropriate for gestational age foetuses, respectively) during the third trimester of pregnancy. Adherence to the MD was calculated according to Trichopoulou [40]. A good adherence appeared a protective factor for SGA, with an OR 0.18 (95% CI: 0.74–0.501) for the third consumer quartile.

An association between low maternal MDA and risk of SGA in new-borns was evidenced in another Spanish retrospective, cross-sectional population-based study involving 492 pregnant women [43]. A 16 items semi-quantitative FFQ was self-administered after delivery, and adherence to the MD was evaluated according to a modified version of the KidMed score [44] considering optimal (>7 score) and low (<7 score) adherence. Women with low MD adherence had a higher risk of delivery SGA babies (adjOR 1.68 [95% CI: 1.02–5.46]) when adjusting for parental body mass index (BMI) and multiple gestation, but not when adjusting for all significant possible confounders.

The single-centre, prospective, observational cohort study by Parlapani et al. [45] evaluated the relation between MD adherence and size at birth in 82 pregnant women who delivered preterm singletons (post-conceptional age <34 weeks). MD adherence was calculated according to the Dietary Score of Panagiotakos et al. [46] based on a self-administered semi-quantitative FFQ (156 food items). Neonates from mothers in the high-MD adherence group were less likely to be SGA (OR 3.3 [95% CI: 1.24–8.78]).

Interestingly, a recent multi-centre, matched case-control, Spanish study [47] evaluated the effect of MD adherence and olive oil intake during pregnancy on the risk of SGA infants using three different scores: PREDIMED score [48], Trichopoulou' s score [40] and Panagiotakos' score [46]. Five hundred eighteen mothers of SGA infants and 518 mothers of infants with normal weight for GA were enrolled, and a137-items semi-quantitative FFQ was administered by trained interviewers within two days after delivery. Independent of the score, adherence to the MD and daily consumption of 5 gr of olive oil was associated to a reduced risk of SGA in the new-born (adjOR 0.59 [95% CI: 0.38–0.98]).

To date, only one intervention study correlating adherence to the MD and SGA has been published [49]. The primary aim of this Spanish, randomized, controlled trial was the evaluation of the incidence of gestational diabetes mellitus (GDM) in pregnant women at 8–12 weeks GA. Five hundred women were randomly assigned to intervention group (MD supplemented with extra virgin olive oil and pistachios) or control group (standard diet with limited fat intake); secondary neonatal outcomes included SGA and prematurity (<37 GA). MD adherence was assessed according to the Mediterranean Diet Adherence Screener (MEDAS) score [50] based on a semi-quantitative 14-items FFQ administered by trained interviewers during the 4 study visits (first ultrasound visit, 24–28 GA, 36–38 GA, delivery). According to this score, women in the interventional group had a good adherence to the intervention. A significant reduction of SGA (p 0.001) was observed in the intervention arm.

3.4.2. Prematurity

Evidence for this outcome comes from 6 papers (Table 1, Table 2): an RCT of poor quality, 4 cohort studies (1 good, 3 intermediate quality) and 1 cross sectional study of poor quality. Cohort studies reached the best scores for quality.

MDA was not significantly associated with the risk of preterm delivery in 5738 American women who delivered non-malformed infants and participated as controls in the National Birth Defects Prevention Study, a multicentre, population-based, case-control study conducted in the United States [51]. MD adherence in the year before pregnancy was evaluated 6 weeks-24 months after delivery administering by telephone interview the computer-based semi-quantitative 58-item FFQ developed in the Nurses' Health Study [79]. The MD Trichopoulou's score [40] and the Diet Quality Index (DQI) incorporating pregnancy-specific nutritional recommendations [52] were calculated and they were not associated with preterm delivery. Notwithstanding, results should be interpreted with caution due to the poor quality of this study and the very low overall incidence of early preterm delivery (about 1%). Moreover, the study examined dietary habits during the year before pregnancy and subsequent substantial changes were not considered.

Saunders et al. [41] reported no overall associations between MD adherence during pregnancy and the risk of preterm delivery in a French Caribbean population having a dietary pattern similar to MD. However, a decreased risk was reported in overweight and obese woman (adjOR 0.7 [95%CI: 0.6–0.9]).

In 2008, adherence to the MD during pregnancy was reported to be associated with reduced risk of early preterm birth (<35 weeks of GA) in Denmark [53] but not in Norway [55]. In the Danish prospective cohort studies 35657 women [53] received a semi-quantitative FFQ (360-item) by mail in mid-pregnancy (gestation week 25). The questionnaire covered the diet during the previous four weeks. In the Norwegian cohort (26563 women) a semi-quantitative FFQ (255 items) investigating dietary habits before pregnancy was self-administered at week 18–22 of gestation [55]. For both studies, adherence to MD was assessed based on 5 major criteria defined by Khoury [54]: consumption of fish twice a week or more, 5 or more vegetable/fruit servings per day, use olive or rapeseed oil, meat at most twice a week, and no more than 2 cups of coffee per day. High MD adherence was associated with reduced the risk of early preterm birth (adjOR 0.28 [95% CI: 0.11–0.76]) in the Danish cohort. In both studies no association emerged regarding the risk of late preterm delivery (35–36 weeks of GA).

An association between MD and preterm delivery was also evidenced by Smith and colleagues [56], who analysed the associations between late and moderately preterm (LMPT) birth (32–37 weeks of GA) and maternal lifestyle factors (smoking, alcohol, drug use and diet) in a population-based case-cohort study involving the mothers of 922 LMPT and 965 term singletons born in UK. Lifestyle and dietary information during pregnancy were obtained via maternal interview shortly after delivery, and women were considered adherent to MD if their diet included at least 1 of the following: 5 portions of fruits and vegetables every day, fish more than twice a week, meat less than twice a week, maximum of 2 cup of coffee a day. Although not adherent women (2.6%) were almost twice as likely to deliver LMPT as adherent women (RR 1.81 [95% CI: 1.04–3.14]), it is worth considering that the "not adherent" diet was very poor, and the effect could be related to the highly unbalanced dietary pattern.

To date, the already mentioned randomized, controlled, trial by Assaf-Balut [49] is the only available intervention study on this topic. It demonstrated that an early nutritional intervention based on MD supplemented with extra virgin olive oil and pistachios significantly reduces the rate of prematurity (p 0.023).

3.4.3. Neural Tube Defects

Evidence for this outcome comes from 2 cross sectional studies of intermediate quality (Table 1, Table 2).

The case-control study by Vujkovic et al. involved 50 mothers of children with spina bifida and 81 control mothers [57]. Validated semi-quantitative FFQ (200 food items) were filled out 14 months after delivery covering the nutrient intake 3 months before the study moment. All FFQ were individually checked for consistency at the hospital or by telephone by the researchers. Principal component factor analysis (PCA) and reduce rank regression (RRR) were used to identify a comparable dietary pattern, which was labelled Mediterranean as it was characterised by high intake of vegetables, fruits, vegetable oils, legumes, fish, alcohol and cereal products and low intakes of potatoes and sweets. Low adherence to the MD, according to both PCA and RRR, was associated to a significantly increased risk of spina bifida compared with high adherence (OR 2.7 [95% CI: 1.2–6.1] and OR 3.5 [95% CI: 1.5–7.9]), respectively.

The multi-centre, population-based, case-control study by Carmicheal et al. [58] was conducted in the United States between 1997 and 2005 and it included 936 cases with NTDs, 2475 with orofacial clefts and 6147 controls. Telephone interviews were conducted between 6 weeks and 24 months after delivery to investigate the mother average intake of foods in the year before pregnancy using a semi-quantitative 58-item FFQ. The MD score of Trichopoulou [40], and the DQI incorporating pregnancy-specific nutritional recommendations [52] were calculated. Higher MD score and DQI appeared associated with reduced birth defect risks (adjOR 0.64 [95% CI: 0.45–0.92]), with a stronger association for anencephaly (adjOR 0.49 [95% CI: 0.31–0.75]). Association was still present after adjusting for maternal intake of mineral/vitamin supplements.

3.4.4. Congenital Heart Defects and Gastroschisis

We found two studies assessing the effects of maternal adherence to the MD on two congenital anomalies, CHDs and gastroschisis (Table 1). Both papers had a cross sectional design and scored intermediate quality (Table 2).

In the year 1997–2009, the National Birth Defects Prevention Study [59], a population-based, multicentre, case–control study enrolled 9885 mothers of babies with major CHDs and 9468 mothers of unaffected babies. Maternal interviews administrated 13 months for cases and 9 months for controls after delivery were standardised, computer-based and conducted primarily by telephone in English or Spanish. Interviews included a validated semiquantitative 58-items FFQ focused on consumption in the year before pregnancy. Maternal diet quality was assessed by the DQI for pregnancy [52] and the MD score of Trichopoulou [40]. Quartile 1 (Q1) and 4 (Q4) reflected the worst and best diet quality. An inverse association between better diet quality scores and risk for selected conotruncal and septal defects was present, where the inverse associations were typically weaker for MDS compared with DQI-P. For MDS, a significantly estimated risk reduction (Q4 vs. Q1) was associated only for perimembranous ventricular septal defects (14%, OR 0.86 [95% CI: 0.69–1.07]). For DQI-P, an estimated risks reductions were 37% for tetralogy of Fallot (OR 0.63 [95% CI: 0.49–0.80]), 24% for all conotruncal defects (OR 0.76 [95% CI: 0.64–0.91]), 23% for atrial septal defects (OR 0.77 [95% CI: 0.63–0.94]) and 14% for all septal defects (OR 0.86 [95% CI: 0.75–1.00]).

The National Birth Defects Prevention Study also investigated the relationship between maternal diet quality during the year before conception and gastroschisis in 1125 case mothers and 9483 control mothers (estimated delivery dates between 1997 and 2009) [60]. Diet quality was assessed by DQI [52] and Trichopoulou score [40] based on a validated semiquantitative 58-item FFQ administered as part of the computerized-assisted telephone interview (CATI). A statistically significant decrease of gastroschisis was associated to increasing diet quality for both the DQI and MDS. When stratified by maternal race/ethnicity, this finding was confined to Hispanic women. Among Hispanic women, the risk of gastroschisis decreased significantly with increasing DQI quartiles: quartile 2, aOR 0.58 (95% CI: 0.40–0.86); quartile 3, aOR 0.52 (95% CI: 0.36–0.79); and quartile 4, aOR0.48 (95% CI: 0.32–0.76). Increasing diet quality, as measured by the MDS, showed reduced risk of gastroschisis among women, mostly Hispanic, who were born outside the United States: quartile 2, aOR 0.62 (95% CI: 0.33–1.16); quartile 3, aOR 0.51 (95% CI: 0.28–0.94); and quartile 4, aOR 0.50 (95% CI: 0.28–0.90).

3.4.5. Asthma and Allergy

We retrieved 7 studies exploring the effect of maternal adherence to the MD and incidence of asthma and/or allergic diseases in the offspring (Table 1). Five studies were cohort studies (3 good, 1 intermediate quality and 1 of poor quality) and 2 were cross sectional studies (1 intermediate and 1 poor quality) (Table 2).

Two studies examined the incidence of allergic diseases in the offspring at 6.5 years of age. In the cross-sectional study by Chatzi et al. [61], involving 460 Spanish children, a semi-quantitative 42-item FFQ was administered to mothers three months after delivery by a face-to-face interview to investigate their dietary habits during pregnancy. Children dietary pattern at 6.5 years was evaluated using a semi-quantitative 96-item FFQ administered to parents by an interviewer. MD adherence was evaluated using the Trichopoulou score [40]. A high MDS during pregnancy resulted to be protective for persistent wheeze (adjOR 0.22 [95% CI: 0.08–0.58]), atopic wheeze (adjOR 0.30 [95% CI: 0.1–0.9]) and atopy (adjOR 0.55 [95% CI: 0.31–0.97]) in children. Results were confirmed even including children MDS in the multivariate models.

The cross-sectional study by De Batlle et al. [62] was conducted in Mexico on a random sample of 1476 children. Maternal adherence to the MD during pregnancy was assessed using a validated semi-quantitative 70-item FFQ self-administered at the children age of 6–7 years [80]. High adherence to MD, calculated according to the score of Trichopoulou [40], was associated to reduced risk of current sneezing (OR 0.71 [95% CI: 0.53–0.97]) in children but no associations were found for other endpoints. However, results of this study should be interpreted cautiously because of the reliability of maternal dietary recall after more than 6 years.

Other studies surveyed the offspring at earlier times: 3 studies at 12–18 months of life [63,65,66], one study at 3 years [67], and one study at 4 years [69]. In all of them the outcome was asthma/wheezing; 3 studies included also atopy/atopic eczema [65,67,69] and another study included also rhinitis [69]. Castro-Rodriguez et al. [63] performed an observational study on a Spanish cohort of 1409 infants aged 15–18 months. When children came to receive vaccination at 15–18 months of age, parents were asked to complete a questionnaire emphasizing on wheezing during the first year of life and also on epidemiological and risk/protective factors. At the same time a self-administered semi-quantitative 11-items FFQ were administered to mothers to collect data on their food intake during pregnancy. Maternal adherence to the MD, measured according to the score by Psaltopoulou [64], and consumption of olive oil were both significantly associated with less wheezing in children, but association was only confirmed for olive oil consumption after multivariate analysis. Similarly, other studies did not evidence any association between maternal adherence to the MD and development of wheeze or eczema in the first 15 months of life [65,66]; wheeze, asthma or allergy at 3 years of age [67]; wheezing, rhinitis and dermatitis in the children at 4 years of age [69]. Details of these studies are reported in Table 1.

3.4.6. Body Weight and Metabolic Markers

Evidence for these outcomes comes from 4 cohort studies (2 good, 1 intermediate quality and 1 of poor quality), 2 cross sectional studies of intermediate quality. Cohort studies reached the best scores for quality.

The quality of the diet during the first trimester of pregnancy and its relation to insulin sensitivity/resistance in the new-borns was evaluated in a cross-sectional study involving 35 women [70] who completed a 169-items FFQ 3–5 weeks after delivery. The FFQ was administered by trained dietician, and adherence to the MD was assessed by the healthy eating index (HEI) adapted for the Spanish population [71] and by a modified MDA scores used in the PREDIMED study [72]. Women with low HEI- or MDA scores delivered infants with high insulinaemia (p 0.048 and p 0.017, respectively), homeostatic model assessment for insulin resistance (HOMA-IR) (p 0.031 and p 0.049, respectively) and glycaemia (p 0.018 and p 0.048, respectively). The relative risk (RR) of high-neonatal glycaemia and insulinaemia was 7.6 (p 0.008) and 6.7 (p 0.017) for low vs. high HEI-score groups. High HOMA-IR and high glucose RR were, respectively, 3.4 (p 0.043) and 3.9 (p 0.016) in neonates from the <7 MDA- vs. >7 MDA-score group. These RRs were not affected by potential confounders.

Chatzi et al. [73] evaluated the association between maternal adherence to the MD in early pregnancy and offspring obesity and cardiometabolic risk in two cohorts with different socio-economic characteristics and different geographic locations. Project Viva, a prospective mother–child cohort began in Massachusetts, USA in 1999 (997 mother-child pairs), while the RHEA study, a population-based mother-child cohort study, started in Crete, Greece in 2007 (569 mother-child pairs). In Project Viva, at study enrolment (median 9.9 weeks' gestation) mothers reported their diet since the time of their last menstrual period using a validated semi-quantitative FFQ. RHEA participants completed a validated FFQ at mean 14.6 weeks gestation. Overall dietary pattern was examined using the Trichopoulou score [40]. Different parameters were evaluated in the children in mid-childhood (median 7.7 years, Viva project) and in early childhood (median 4.2 years, RHEA project). After pooling analysis calculated using mixed models, including cohort and child age at outcome assessment as random effects and all other covariates as fixed effects, for each 3-point increment in the MD score, ranged from 0 (minimal adherence to the MD) to 9 (maximal adherence), offspring BMI z-score was lower by 0.14 units (95% CI: −0.15 to −0.13), waist circumference by 0.39 cm (95% CI: −0.64 to −0.14), and the sum of skin-fold thicknesses by 0.63 mm (95% CI: −0.98 to −0.28). The Authors also observed a lower systolic (−1.03 mmHg [95% CI: −1.65 to −0.42]) and diastolic blood pressure (−0.57 mmHg [95% CI: −0.98 to −0.16]) in offspring.

Fernández-Barrés et al. [74] analysed 1827 mother–child pairs from the Spanish "Infancia y Medio Ambiente" cohort study, recruited between 2003 and 2008, to evaluate associations between adherence to the MD during pregnancy and childhood overweight and abdominal obesity risk. A validated 101-items FFQ was administered to evaluate dietary habits from first to third trimester of pregnancy, and the Mediterranean diet (rMD) score [75] was calculated. No association was evidenced between rMD score and body mass index z-score of children at 4 years of age, whereas there was a significant association between higher maternal adherence to the MD and lower waist circumference in children (−0.62 cm [95% CI: −1.1 to −0.14).

In a cross-sectional study, Gesteiro et al. [76] analysed the MD adherence in 35 Spanish women during the first trimester of pregnancy, who completed 169-items FFQ guided by a trained dietician. Adherence to the MD was calculated with a modified version of the score used in the PREDIMED study [72]. At birth, neonates from mothers with the lower MD score (<7) showed higher cord blood LDL-c (p 0.049), Apo B (p 0.040), Apo A1/Apo B ratio (p 0.024) and increased homocysteine levels (p 0.026).

In a cohort study, Mantzoros and colleagues [77] evaluated the relation between maternal adherence to the MD during pregnancy and cord blood adiponectin and/or leptin level, which have been associated with post-natal body size and adiposity in the first years of life, in 780 American women. Maternal diet assessment at both the first and second trimester was performed using a semi-quantitative FFQ slightly modified for use in pregnancy and MD score calculated accordingly to Trichopoulou [40]. Closer adherence to a MD during pregnancy was not associated with cord blood leptin or adiponectin (p 0.38 and p 0.93, respectively).

Gonzalez-Naqhm et al. [78] evaluated in 390 women enrolled in the Newborn Epigenetic Study the relation between MD adherence, assessed by a 150 items FFQ at preconception or at first trimester, and DNA methylation in cord blood leukocytes at birth. Infants of mothers with low adherence to the MD had greater odds of hypomethylation of the MEG3-IG region (OR 2.80 [95% CI: 1.35–5.82]). Sex-stratified models showed that this association was present in girls only. The MEG3-IG region may be an upstream regulator of the MEG3 DMR, which has been associated with type 2 diabetes [78]. Hypomethylation of MEG3- IG region could explain the association between MD and improvements of type 2 diabetes [81].

4. Discussion and Conclusions

In the present review, we systematically summarized studies carried out to verify the protective effect on the offspring of maternal adherence to the MD during pregnancy. All but one of the 29 studies included in the review were observational (cross-sectional, cohort, and case–control) studies.

Although maternal nutrition has been recognized as one of the most important environmental factors influencing foetal growth and development [14–17], we found intermediate evidence linking maternal adherence to the MD pattern to FGR and risk of SGA new-borns, with cohort studies that reached the best scores for quality (Table 2). A confirmation that adherence to the MD during pregnancy could represent a strategy for reducing the incidence of FGR and SGA new-borns could come from a randomized controlled trial that is recruiting patients in Spain [82]. This study is randomizing women at high risk for growth restricted foetuses into two different behavioural strategies program: a stress reduction program based on mindfulness techniques or a nutrition interventional program based on MD. The trial will last till February 2021.

We founded intermediate evidence supporting a protective effect of MD on preterm delivery, with cohort studies reaching the best scores for quality. The MD pattern, including low amount of sugars, could result in better blood glucose regulation during pregnancy. Although glucose intolerance is associated with a shorter duration of gestation independently of other known risk factors for prematurity [83], not all studies investigating the effect of MDA during pregnancy on preterm delivery found no significant correlation (Table 1). The heterogeneity of results could be in part explained by differences in the definition of preterm delivery (<37 weeks versus earlier periods). Of note, the only randomized controlled trial found in the literature [49] showed that an early nutritional intervention with MD supplemented with extra virgin olive oil and pistachios significantly reduces the rate of preterm delivery.

Since long ago, many studies demonstrated that appropriate intake of folate during pregnancy can prevent the recurrence of NTDs [84]. Although it is known that the MD provides appropriate amount of folate, to date only two cross sectional studies [57,58] have investigated the effects of maternal adherence to the MD on NTDs incidence in offspring. Maternal MD adherence and risk of NTDs appeared significantly related, but the low number of studies reduces the level of evidence. In addition, it is not clear whether the MD protective effect is simply due to the correct folic acid intake or other MD components contribute as well. Anyway, to improve adherence to the MD in the periconception period could be considered a good strategy to reduce the incidence of NTDs. Regarding CHDs and gastroschisis, the number of studies is too low to draw any conclusion.

At present, there is low evidence of a link between maternal adherence to the MD and incidence of asthma and/or allergic diseases in the offspring. This is also due to quality coming from these studies was much more mixed, particularly for cohort studies. Additional studies are needed to better clarify the role of maternal adherence to the MD on this outcome.

Obesity and metabolic syndrome (MetS) are two of the most common chronic diseases among children. Recent evidence suggests these conditions have their roots in utero as maternal obesity, dyslipidaemia, and hyperglycaemia are associated with child cardiometabolic health and developing insulin resistance and obesity later in life [85,86]. Although studies considered in this review indicate that higher adherence to the MD during pregnancy is a potential protective factor against abdominal obesity [73,74] and positively influences lipoprotein and homocysteine concentration [76], and insulin resistance in new-borns [70], the use of different endpoints to evaluate outcomes reduces the level of evidence.

Overall, most of the studies included in this review showed beneficial association between MD adherence during pregnancy and children's health. The strength of the association varied in the different health outcomes, and the level of evidence was affected by the high heterogeneity among the study design. Heterogeneity was mainly related to the methodology used for assessment of MD adherence. Epidemiological studies commonly use the FFQ to assess usual food consumption. Although an FFQ does not have the same accuracy as a dietary record or a 24 h dietary recall, it can reasonably report intake over a large period [87]. There are many kinds of FFQ, and not all have been validated. Anyway, they differ for the number of food items, the way of administration (self-administration or interviewer-administration), the quantification of consumed foods, etc. Furthermore, there are many ways to analyse results from FFQ, which are often used to extrapolate an index of overall diet quality based on an a priori scoring system [88]. The use of different scores for the assessment of adherence to the MD represents a possible confounding factor while comparing different studies.

In addition, the consumption rate of specific food groups was seldom considered. The so-called MD was inspired by the eating habits of people in the Mediterranean area (mainly Greece, Southern Italy and Spain). MD provides an optimal intake of "positive" nutrients (polyunsaturated fats, fibres, vitamins etc.) and a low intake of "negative" nutrients (e.g., saturated fats, sugars, sodium) through the proportionally high consumption of olive oil, legumes, unrefined cereals, fruits, and vegetables, moderate to high consumption of fish, moderate consumption of dairy products (mostly as cheese and yogurt), moderate wine consumption, and low consumption of non-fish meat products. The proportion of Mediterranean foods in the diet is different in different Mediterranean countries, even in people having the same level of adherence, and it largely depends on the characteristics of the study sample, i.e., ethnic origin of the enrolled population. Culture-driven dietary preferences vary among population and influence the intake of specific food subgroups. These differences are likely incompletely captured in the semiquantitative FFQ, particularly in their shorter version, because of the limited number of food items that are evaluated. Therefore, the sensitivity of MD adherence as predictor of children outcomes could be affected by regional variations of MD.

Another confounding factor is the stage of pregnancy considered for evaluation of adherence to the MD, as well as the time elapsed between the considered period and the administration of the FFQ. Not explored social and environmental factors could have a role.

How a good adherence to the MD during pregnancy could have positive effect in offspring not only during foetal life but also in later life is still unclear. The induction of epigenetics modification represents a possible explanation [78], but further studies are needed to confirm it. In addition to the epigenetics hypothesis, it is known that various nutrients may influence pregnancy outcomes by altering both maternal and foetal metabolism due to their roles in modulating oxidative stress, enzyme function, signal transduction and transcription pathways that occur early in pregnancy.

In conclusion, a good maternal diet quality in general, and the adherence to the MD in particular, are associated with a reduced occurrence of some negative outcomes in babies. Although it is still unclear whether an intervention to promote the MD could effectively reduce the prevalence of some childhood diseases, and randomized control trials are needed to better clarify it, current preconception care recommendations should carefully consider the benefit of MD, reinforcing advice on correct dietary habits. Strategies aiming to promote adherence to MD dietary pattern may be of considerable importance to public health. In addition, they have low cost and no side effects.

Author Contributions: C.B., M.D.N., A.B., and M.L. contributed to the design of the review and interpretation of findings. D.G., C.B. and M.D.N. performed the literature search and data extraction. D.G., C.B. and M.D.N performed the quality assessment process. C.B., M.D.N., A.B. and M.L. contributed to the writing of the manuscript. All authors read, revised, and approved the final manuscript.

Funding: This research received no external funding.

Conflicts of Interest: The authors declare no conflict of interest.

References

1. Hambidge, K.M.; Krebs, N.F. Strategies for optimizing maternal nutrition to promote infant development. *Reprod Health* **2018**, *15*, 87. [CrossRef]
2. Simeoni, U.; Armengaud, J.B.; Siddeek, B.; Tolsa, J.F. Perinatal origins of adult disease. *Neonatology* **2018**, *113*, 393–399. [CrossRef]

3. Rodriguez-Rodriguez, P.; Ramiro-Cortijo, D.; Reyes-Hernandez, C.G.; Lopez de Pablo, A.L.; Gonzalez, M.C.; Arribas, S.M. Implication of oxidative stress in fetal programming of cardiovascular disease. *Front. Physiol.* **2018**, *9*, 602. [CrossRef] [PubMed]
4. Reynolds, C.M.; Vickers, M.H. Utility of small animal models of developmental programming. *Methods Mol. Biol.* **2018**, *1735*, 145–163. [PubMed]
5. Trivedi, M.K.; Sharma, S.; Rifas-Shiman, S.L.; Camargo, C.A., Jr.; Weiss, S.T.; Oken, E.; Gillman, M.W.; Gold, D.R.; DeMeo, D.L.; Litonjua, A.A. Folic acid in pregnancy and childhood asthma: A US cohort. *Clin. Pediatr. (Phila)* **2018**, *57*, 421–427. [CrossRef] [PubMed]
6. Vinding, R.K.; Stokholm, J.; Sevelsted, A.; Chawes, B.L.; Bonnelykke, K.; Barman, M.; Jacobsson, B.; Bisgaard, H. Fish oil supplementation in pregnancy increases gestational age, size for gestational age, and birth weight in infants: A randomized controlled trial. *J. Nutr.* **2019**, *149*, 628–634. [CrossRef] [PubMed]
7. Nardozza, L.M.; Caetano, A.C.; Zamarian, A.C.; Mazzola, J.B.; Silva, C.P.; Marcal, V.M.; Lobo, T.F.; Peixoto, A.B.; Araujo Junior, E. Fetal growth restriction: Current knowledge. *Arch. Gynecol. Obstet.* **2017**, *295*, 1061–1077. [CrossRef] [PubMed]
8. Baschat, A.A. Neurodevelopment after fetal growth restriction. *Fetal. Diagn. Ther.* **2014**, *36*, 136–142. [CrossRef]
9. Pallotto, E.K.; Kilbride, H.W. Perinatal outcome and later implications of intrauterine growth restriction. *Clin. Obstet. Gynecol.* **2006**, *49*, 257–269. [CrossRef]
10. Calkins, K.; Devaskar, S.U. Fetal origins of adult disease. *Curr. Probl. Pediatr. Adolesc. Health Care* **2011**, *41*, 158–176. [CrossRef] [PubMed]
11. Gluckman, P.D.; Hanson, M.A.; Cooper, C.; Thornburg, K.L. Effect of in utero and early-life conditions on adult health and disease. *N. Engl. J. Med.* **2008**, *359*, 61–73. [CrossRef] [PubMed]
12. McCowan, L.M.; Harding, J.E.; Stewart, A.W. Customized birthweight centiles predict SGA pregnancies with perinatal morbidity. *BJOG* **2005**, *112*, 1026–1033. [CrossRef] [PubMed]
13. ACOG Practice bulletin no. 134: Fetal growth restriction. *Obstet. Gynecol.* **2013**, *121*, 1122–1133.
14. Brantsaeter, A.L.; Haugen, M.; Samuelsen, S.O.; Torjusen, H.; Trogstad, L.; Alexander, J.; Magnus, P.; Meltzer, H.M. A dietary pattern characterized by high intake of vegetables, fruits, and vegetable oils is associated with reduced risk of preeclampsia in nulliparous pregnant Norwegian women. *J. Nutr.* **2009**, *139*, 1162–1168. [CrossRef] [PubMed]
15. Brantsaeter, A.L.; Olafsdottir, A.S.; Forsum, E.; Olsen, S.F.; Thorsdottir, I. Does milk and dairy consumption during pregnancy influence fetal growth and infant birthweight? A systematic literature review. *Food Nutr. Res.* **2012**, *56*, 20050. [CrossRef] [PubMed]
16. Olsen, S.F. Consumption of marine n-3 fatty acids during pregnancy as a possible determinant of birth weight. A review of the current epidemiologic evidence. *Epidemiol. Rev.* **1993**, *15*, 399–413. [CrossRef] [PubMed]
17. Scholl, T.O.; Hediger, M.L.; Schall, J.I.; Khoo, C.S.; Fischer, R.L. Dietary and serum folate: Their influence on the outcome of pregnancy. *Am. J. Clin. Nutr.* **1996**, *63*, 520–525. [CrossRef] [PubMed]
18. Goldenberg, R.L.; Culhane, J.F.; Iams, J.D.; Romero, R. Epidemiology and causes of preterm birth. *Lancet* **2008**, *371*, 75–84. [CrossRef]
19. Saigal, S.; Doyle, L.W. An overview of mortality and sequelae of preterm birth from infancy to adulthood. *Lancet* **2008**, *371*, 261–269. [CrossRef]
20. Brantsaeter, A.L.; Haugen, M.; Myhre, R.; Sengpiel, V.; Englund-Ögge, L.; Nilsen, R.M.; Borgen, I.; Duarte-Salles, T.; Papadopoulou, E.; Vejrup, K.; et al. Diet matters, particularly in pregnancy—Results from MoBa studies of maternal diet and pregnancy outcomes. *Norsk. Epidemiologi.* **2014**, *24*, 63–77. [CrossRef]
21. Salih, M.A.; Murshid, W.R.; Seidahmed, M.Z. Classification, clinical features, and genetics of neural tube defects. *Saudi. Med. J.* **2014**, *35*, S5–S14.
22. Bhide, P.; Gund, P.; Kar, A. Prevalence of congenital anomalies in an Indian maternal cohort: Healthcare, prevention, and surveillance implications. *PLoS ONE* **2016**, *11*, e0166408. [CrossRef]
23. Carpenter, J.L.; Wiebe, T.L.; Cass, D.L.; Olutoye, O.O.; Lee, T.C. Assessing quality of life in pediatric gastroschisis patients using the Pediatric Quality of Life Inventory survey: An institutional study. *J. Pediatr. Surg.* **2016**, *51*, 726–729. [CrossRef]
24. Bibbins-Domingo, K.; Grossman, D.C.; Curry, S.J.; Davidson, K.W.; Epling, J.W., Jr.; Garcia, F.A.; Kemper, A.R.; Krist, A.H.; Kurth, A.E.; Landefeld, C.S.; et al. Folic acid supplementation for the prevention of neural tube defects: US preventive services task force recommendation statement. *JAMA* **2017**, *317*, 183–189. [PubMed]

25. Goodman, J.R.; Peck, J.D.; Landmann, A.; Williams, M.; Elimian, A. An evaluation of nutritional and vasoactive stimulants as risk factors for gastroschisis: A pilot study. *J. Matern. Fetal. Neonatal. Med.* **2019**, *32*, 2346–2353. [CrossRef] [PubMed]
26. Pearce, N.; Ait-Khaled, N.; Beasley, R.; Mallol, J.; Keil, U.; Mitchell, E.; Robertson, C. Worldwide trends in the prevalence of asthma symptoms: Phase III of the international study of asthma and allergies in childhood (ISAAC). *Thorax* **2007**, *62*, 758–766. [CrossRef]
27. Devereux, G.; Seaton, A. Diet as a risk factor for atopy and asthma. *J. Allergy Clin. Immunol.* **2005**, *115*, 1109–1117. [CrossRef] [PubMed]
28. Seaton, A.; Godden, D.J.; Brown, K. Increase in asthma: A more toxic environment or a more susceptible population? *Thorax* **1994**, *49*, 171–174. [CrossRef] [PubMed]
29. Corella, D.; Coltell, O.; Macian, F.; Ordovas, J.M. Advances in understanding the molecular basis of the mediterranean diet effect. *Annu. Rev. Food Sci. Technol.* **2018**, *9*, 227–249. [CrossRef] [PubMed]
30. Agnoli, C.; Sieri, S.; Ricceri, F.; Giraudo, M.T.; Masala, G.; Assedi, M.; Panico, S.; Mattiello, A.; Tumino, R.; Giurdanella, M.C.; et al. Adherence to a Mediterranean diet and long-term changes in weight and waist circumference in the EPIC-Italy cohort. *Nutr. Diabetes* **2018**, *8*, 22. [CrossRef] [PubMed]
31. Carlos, S.; De La Fuente-Arrillaga, C.; Bes-Rastrollo, M.; Razquin, C.; Rico-Campa, A.; Martinez-Gonzalez, M.A.; Ruiz-Canela, M. Mediterranean diet and health outcomes in the SUN cohort. *Nutrients* **2018**, *10*, 439. [CrossRef]
32. Bacopoulou, F.; Landis, G.; Rentoumis, A.; Tsitsika, A.; Efthymiou, V. Mediterranean diet decreases adolescent waist circumference. *Eur. J. Clin. Invest.* **2017**, *47*, 447–455. [CrossRef]
33. Mistretta, A.; Marventano, S.; Antoci, M.; Cagnetti, A.; Giogianni, G.; Nolfo, F.; Rametta, S.; Pecora, G.; Marranzano, M. Mediterranean diet adherence and body composition among Southern Italian adolescents. *Obes. Res. Clin. Pract.* **2017**, *11*, 215–226. [CrossRef] [PubMed]
34. Tognon, G.; Hebestreit, A.; Lanfer, A.; Moreno, L.A.; Pala, V.; Siani, A.; Tornaritis, M.; De Henauw, S.; Veidebaum, T.; Molnar, D.; et al. Mediterranean diet, overweight and body composition in children from eight European countries: Cross-sectional and prospective results from the IDEFICS study. *Nutr. Metab. Cardiovasc. Dis.* **2014**, *24*, 205–213. [CrossRef] [PubMed]
35. Moher, D.; Liberati, A.; Tetzlaff, J.; Altman, D.G. Preferred reporting items for systematic reviews and meta-analyses: The PRISMA statement. *Int. J. Surg.* **2010**, *8*, 336–341. [CrossRef]
36. Greenhalgh, T.; Peacock, R. Effectiveness and efficiency of search methods in systematic reviews of complex evidence: Audit of primary sources. *BMJ* **2005**, *331*, 1064–1065. [CrossRef] [PubMed]
37. von Elm, E.; Altman, D.G.; Egger, M.; Pocock, S.J.; Gotzsche, P.C.; Vandenbroucke, J.P. The Strengthening the Reporting of Observational Studies in Epidemiology (STROBE) statement: Guidelines for reporting observational studies. *Int. J. Surg.* **2014**, *12*, 1495–1499. [CrossRef] [PubMed]
38. Timmermans, S.; Steegers-Theunissen, R.P.; Vujkovic, M.; den Breeijen, H.; Russcher, H.; Lindemans, J.; Mackenbach, J.; Hofman, A.; Lesaffre, E.E.; Jaddoe, V.V.; et al. The Mediterranean diet and fetal size parameters: The Generation R Study. *Br. J. Nutr.* **2012**, *108*, 1399–1409. [CrossRef]
39. Chatzi, L.; Mendez, M.; Garcia, R.; Roumeliotaki, T.; Ibarluzea, J.; Tardon, A.; Amiano, P.; Lertxundi, A.; Iniguez, C.; Vioque, J.; et al. Mediterranean diet adherence during pregnancy and fetal growth: INMA (Spain) and RHEA (Greece) mother-child cohort studies. *Br. J. Nutr.* **2012**, *107*, 135–145. [CrossRef]
40. Trichopoulou, A.; Costacou, T.; Bamia, C.; Trichopoulos, D. Adherence to a Mediterranean diet and survival in a Greek population. *N. Engl. J. Med.* **2003**, *348*, 2599–2608. [CrossRef] [PubMed]
41. Saunders, L.; Guldner, L.; Costet, N.; Kadhel, P.; Rouget, F.; Monfort, C.; Thome, J.P.; Multigner, L.; Cordier, S. Effect of a Mediterranean diet during pregnancy on fetal growth and preterm delivery: Results from a French Caribbean Mother-Child Cohort Study (TIMOUN). *Paediatr. Perinat. Epidemiol.* **2014**, *28*, 235–244. [CrossRef] [PubMed]
42. Gomez Roig, M.D.; Mazarico, E.; Ferrero, S.; Montejo, R.; Ibanez, L.; Grima, F.; Vela, A. Differences in dietary and lifestyle habits between pregnant women with small fetuses and appropriate-for-gestational-age fetuses. *J. Obstet. Gynaecol. Res.* **2017**, *43*, 1145–1151. [CrossRef] [PubMed]
43. Peraita-Costa, I.; Llopis-Gonzalez, A.; Perales-Marin, A.; Sanz, F.; Llopis-Morales, A.; Morales-Suarez-Varela, M. A retrospective cross-sectional population-based study on prenatal levels of adherence to the Mediterranean diet: Maternal profile and effects on the newborn. *Int. J. Environ. Res. Public Health* **2018**, *15*, 1530. [CrossRef] [PubMed]

44. Serra-Majem, L.; Ribas, L.; Ngo, J.; Ortega, R.M.; Garcia, A.; Perez-Rodrigo, C.; Aranceta, J. Food, youth and the Mediterranean diet in Spain. Development of KIDMED, Mediterranean Diet Quality Index in children and adolescents. *Public Health Nutr.* **2004**, *7*, 931–935. [CrossRef] [PubMed]
45. Parlapani, E.; Agakidis, C.; Karagiozoglou-Lampoudi, T.; Sarafidis, K.; Agakidou, E.; Athanasiadis, A.; Diamanti, E. The Mediterranean diet adherence by pregnant women delivering prematurely: Association with size at birth and complications of prematurity. *J. Matern. Fetal. Neonatal Med.* **2017**, *13*, 1–8. [CrossRef] [PubMed]
46. Panagiotakos, D.B.; Pitsavos, C.; Stefanadis, C. Dietary patterns: A Mediterranean diet score and its relation to clinical and biological markers of cardiovascular disease risk. *Nutr. Metab. Cardiovasc. Dis.* **2006**, *16*, 559–568. [CrossRef] [PubMed]
47. Martinez-Galiano, J.M.; Olmedo-Requena, R.; Barrios-Rodriguez, R.; Amezcua-Prieto, C.; Bueno-Cavanillas, A.; Salcedo-Bellido, I.; Jimenez-Moleon, J.J.; Delgado-Rodriguez, M. Effect of adherence to a Mediterranean diet and olive oil intake during pregnancy on risk of small for gestational age infants. *Nutrients* **2018**, *10*, 1234. [CrossRef]
48. Martinez-Gonzalez, M.A.; Fernandez-Jarne, E.; Serrano-Martinez, M.; Wright, M.; Gomez-Gracia, E. Development of a short dietary intake questionnaire for the quantitative estimation of adherence to a cardioprotective Mediterranean diet. *Eur. J. Clin. Nutr.* **2004**, *58*, 1550–1552. [CrossRef] [PubMed]
49. Assaf-Balut, C.; Garcia de la Torre, N.; Duran, A.; Fuentes, M.; Bordiu, E.; Del Valle, L.; Familiar, C.; Ortola, A.; Jimenez, I.; Herraiz, M.A.; et al. A Mediterranean diet with additional extra virgin olive oil and pistachios reduces the incidence of gestational diabetes mellitus (GDM): A randomized controlled trial: The St. Carlos GDM prevention study. *PLoS ONE* **2017**, *12*, e0185873. [CrossRef]
50. Schroder, H.; Fito, M.; Estruch, R.; Martinez-Gonzalez, M.A.; Corella, D.; Salas-Salvado, J.; Lamuela-Raventos, R.; Ros, E.; Salaverria, I.; Fiol, M.; et al. A short screener is valid for assessing Mediterranean diet adherence among older Spanish men and women. *J. Nutr.* **2011**, *141*, 1140–1145. [CrossRef]
51. Carmichael, S.L.; Yang, W.; Shaw, G.M. Maternal dietary nutrient intake and risk of preterm delivery. *Am. J. Perinatol.* **2013**, *30*, 579–588. [PubMed]
52. Bodnar, L.M.; Siega-Riz, A.M. A Diet Quality Index for Pregnancy detects variation in diet and differences by sociodemographic factors. *Public Health Nutr.* **2002**, *5*, 801–809. [CrossRef] [PubMed]
53. Mikkelsen, T.B.; Osterdal, M.L.; Knudsen, V.K.; Haugen, M.; Meltzer, H.M.; Bakketeig, L.; Olsen, S.F. Association between a Mediterranean-type diet and risk of preterm birth among Danish women: A prospective cohort study. *Acta Obstet. Gynecol. Scand.* **2008**, *87*, 325–330. [CrossRef]
54. Khoury, J.; Henriksen, T.; Christophersen, B.; Tonstad, S. Effect of a cholesterol-lowering diet on maternal, cord, and neonatal lipids, and pregnancy outcome: A randomized clinical trial. *Am. J. Obstet. Gynecol.* **2005**, *193*, 1292–1301. [CrossRef]
55. Haugen, M.; Meltzer, H.M.; Brantsaeter, A.L.; Mikkelsen, T.; Osterdal, M.L.; Alexander, J.; Olsen, S.F.; Bakketeig, L. Mediterranean-type diet and risk of preterm birth among women in the Norwegian Mother and Child Cohort Study (MoBa): A prospective cohort study. *Acta Obstet. Gynecol. Scand.* **2008**, *87*, 319–324. [CrossRef]
56. Smith, L.K.; Draper, E.S.; Evans, T.A.; Field, D.J.; Johnson, S.J.; Manktelow, B.N.; Seaton, S.E.; Marlow, N.; Petrou, S.; Boyle, E.M. Associations between late and moderately preterm birth and smoking, alcohol, drug use and diet: A population-based case-cohort study. *Arch Dis. Child. Fetal. Neonatal Ed.* **2015**, *100*, F486–F491. [CrossRef] [PubMed]
57. Vujkovic, M.; Steegers, E.A.; Looman, C.W.; Ocke, M.C.; van der Spek, P.J.; Steegers-Theunissen, R.P. The maternal Mediterranean dietary pattern is associated with a reduced risk of spina bifida in the offspring. *BJOG* **2009**, *116*, 408–415. [CrossRef] [PubMed]
58. Carmichael, S.L.; Yang, W.; Feldkamp, M.L.; Munger, R.G.; Siega-Riz, A.M.; Botto, L.D.; Shaw, G. Reduced risks of neural tube defects and orofacial clefts with higher diet quality. *Arch. Pediatr. Adolesc. Med.* **2012**, *166*, 121–126. [CrossRef]
59. Botto, L.D.; Krikov, S.; Carmichael, S.L.; Munger, R.G.; Shaw, G.M.; Feldkamp, M.L. Lower rate of selected congenital heart defects with better maternal diet quality: A population-based study. *Arch. Dis. Child. Fetal. Neonatal Ed.* **2016**, *101*, F43–F49. [CrossRef]

60. Feldkamp, M.L.; Krikov, S.; Botto, L.D.; Shaw, G.M.; Carmichael, S.L. Better diet quality before pregnancy is associated with reduced risk of gastroschisis in Hispanic women. *J. Nutr.* **2014**, *144*, 1781–1786.
61. Chatzi, L.; Torrent, M.; Romieu, I.; Garcia-Esteban, R.; Ferrer, C.; Vioque, J.; Kogevinas, M.; Sunyer, J. Mediterranean diet in pregnancy is protective for wheeze and atopy in childhood. *Thorax* **2008**, *63*, 507–513. [CrossRef]
62. de Batlle, J.; Garcia-Aymerich, J.; Barraza-Villarreal, A.; Anto, J.M.; Romieu, I. Mediterranean diet is associated with reduced asthma and rhinitis in Mexican children. *Allergy* **2008**, *63*, 1310–1316. [CrossRef]
63. Castro-Rodriguez, J.A.; Garcia-Marcos, L.; Sanchez-Solis, M.; Perez-Fernandez, V.; Martinez-Torres, A.; Mallol, J. Olive oil during pregnancy is associated with reduced wheezing during the first year of life of the offspring. *Pediatr. Pulmonol.* **2010**, *45*, 395–402.
64. Psaltopoulou, T.; Naska, A.; Orfanos, P.; Trichopoulos, D.; Mountokalakis, T.; Trichopoulou, A. Olive oil, the Mediterranean diet, and arterial blood pressure: The Greek European Prospective Investigation into Cancer and Nutrition (EPIC) study. *Am. J. Clin. Nutr.* **2004**, *80*, 1012–1018. [CrossRef]
65. Chatzi, L.; Garcia, R.; Roumeliotaki, T.; Basterrechea, M.; Begiristain, H.; Iniguez, C.; Vioque, J.; Kogevinas, M.; Sunyer, J. Mediterranean diet adherence during pregnancy and risk of wheeze and eczema in the first year of life: INMA (Spain) and RHEA (Greece) mother-child cohort studies. *Br. J. Nutr.* **2013**, *110*, 2058–2068. [CrossRef]
66. Alvarez Zallo, N.; Aguinaga-Ontoso, I.; Alvarez-Alvarez, I.; Marin-Fernandez, B.; Guillen-Grima, F.; Azcona-San Julian, C. Influence of the Mediterranean diet during pregnancy in the development of wheezing and eczema in infants in Pamplona, Spain. *Allergol. Immunopathol. (Madr)* **2018**, *46*, 9–14. [CrossRef]
67. Lange, N.E.; Rifas-Shiman, S.L.; Camargo, C.A., Jr.; Gold, D.R.; Gillman, M.W.; Litonjua, A.A. Maternal dietary pattern during pregnancy is not associated with recurrent wheeze in children. *J. Allergy Clin. Immunol.* **2010**, *126*, 250–255. [CrossRef]
68. Rifas-Shiman, S.L.; Rich-Edwards, J.W.; Kleinman, K.P.; Oken, E.; Gillman, M.W. Dietary quality during pregnancy varies by maternal characteristics in Project Viva: A US cohort. *J. Am. Diet. Assoc.* **2009**, *109*, 1004–1011. [CrossRef] [PubMed]
69. Castro-Rodriguez, J.A.; Ramirez-Hernandez, M.; Padilla, O.; Pacheco-Gonzalez, R.M.; Perez-Fernandez, V.; Garcia-Marcos, L. Effect of foods and Mediterranean diet during pregnancy and first years of life on wheezing, rhinitis and dermatitis in preschoolers. *Allergol. Immunopathol. (Madr)* **2016**, *44*, 400–409. [CrossRef] [PubMed]
70. Gesteiro, E.; Rodriguez Bernal, B.; Bastida, S.; Sanchez-Muniz, F.J. Maternal diets with low healthy eating index or Mediterranean diet adherence scores are associated with high cord-blood insulin levels and insulin resistance markers at birth. *Eur. J. Clin. Nutr.* **2012**, *66*, 1008–1015. [CrossRef] [PubMed]
71. Kennedy, E.T.; Ohls, J.; Carlson, S.; Fleming, K. The Healthy Eating Index: Design and applications. *J. Am. Diet. Assoc.* **1995**, *95*, 1103–1108. [CrossRef]
72. Estruch, R.; Martinez-Gonzalez, M.A.; Corella, D.; Salas-Salvado, J.; Ruiz-Gutierrez, V.; Covas, M.I.; Fiol, M.; Gomez-Gracia, E.; Lopez-Sabater, M.C.; Vinyoles, E.; et al. Effects of a Mediterranean-style diet on cardiovascular risk factors: A randomized trial. *Ann. Intern. Med.* **2006**, *145*, 1–11. [CrossRef] [PubMed]
73. Chatzi, L.; Rifas-Shiman, S.L.; Georgiou, V.; Joung, K.E.; Koinaki, S.; Chalkiadaki, G.; Margioris, A.; Sarri, K.; Vassilaki, M.; Vafeiadi, M.; et al. Adherence to the Mediterranean diet during pregnancy and offspring adiposity and cardiometabolic traits in childhood. *Pediatr. Obes.* **2017**, *12*, 47–56. [CrossRef] [PubMed]
74. Fernandez-Barres, S.; Romaguera, D.; Valvi, D.; Martinez, D.; Vioque, J.; Navarrete-Munoz, E.M.; Amiano, P.; Gonzalez-Palacios, S.; Guxens, M.; Pereda, E.; et al. Mediterranean dietary pattern in pregnant women and offspring risk of overweight and abdominal obesity in early childhood: The INMA birth cohort study. *Pediatr. Obes.* **2016**, *11*, 491–499. [CrossRef] [PubMed]
75. Romaguera, D.; Norat, T.; Vergnaud, A.C.; Mouw, T.; May, A.M.; Agudo, A.; Buckland, G.; Slimani, N.; Rinaldi, S.; Couto, E.; et al. Mediterranean dietary patterns and prospective weight change in participants of the EPIC-PANACEA project. *Am. J. Clin. Nutr.* **2010**, *92*, 912–921. [CrossRef]
76. Gesteiro, E.; Bastida, S.; Rodriguez Bernal, B.; Sanchez-Muniz, F.J. Adherence to Mediterranean diet during pregnancy and serum lipid, lipoprotein and homocysteine concentrations at birth. *Eur. J. Nutr.* **2015**, *54*, 1191–1199. [CrossRef]
77. Mantzoros, C.S.; Sweeney, L.; Williams, C.J.; Oken, E.; Kelesidis, T.; Rifas-Shiman, S.L.; Gillman, M.W. Maternal diet and cord blood leptin and adiponectin concentrations at birth. *Clin. Nutr.* **2010**, *29*, 622–626. [CrossRef]

78. Gonzalez-Nahm, S.; Mendez, M.; Robinson, W.; Murphy, S.K.; Hoyo, C.; Hogan, V.; Rowley, D. Low maternal adherence to a Mediterranean diet is associated with increase in methylation at the MEG3-IG differentially methylated region in female infants. *Environ. Epigenet.* **2017**, *3*, dvx007. [CrossRef]
79. Willett, W.C.; Sampson, L.; Stampfer, M.J.; Rosner, B.; Bain, C.; Witschi, J.; Hennekens, C.H.; Speizer, F.E. Reproducibility and validity of a semiquantitative food frequency questionnaire. *Am. J. Epidemiol.* **1985**, *122*, 51–65. [CrossRef] [PubMed]
80. Hernandez-Avila, M.; Romieu, I.; Parra, S.; Hernandez-Avila, J.; Madrigal, H.; Willett, W. Validity and reproducibility of a food frequency questionnaire to assess dietary intake of women living in Mexico City. *Salud. Publica. Mex.* **1998**, *40*, 133–140. [CrossRef]
81. Forouhi, N.G.; Misra, A.; Mohan, V.; Taylor, R.; Yancy, W. Dietary and nutritional approaches for prevention and management of type 2 diabetes. *BMJ* **2018**, *361*, k2234. [CrossRef] [PubMed]
82. Clinical Trials.gov. Improving Mothers for a Better Prenatal Care Trial Barcelona (IMPACTBCN). Available online: https://clinicaltrials.gov/ct2/show/NCT03166332 (accessed on 17 September 2018).
83. Yang, X.; Hsu-Hage, B.; Zhang, H.; Zhang, C.; Zhang, Y. Women with impaired glucose tolerance during pregnancy have significantly poor pregnancy outcomes. *Diabetes Care* **2002**, *25*, 1619–1624. [CrossRef] [PubMed]
84. Czeizel, A.E.; Dudas, I.; Paput, L.; Banhidy, F. Prevention of neural-tube defects with periconceptional folic acid, methylfolate, or multivitamins? *Ann. Nutr. Metab.* **2011**, *58*, 263–271. [CrossRef] [PubMed]
85. Guillemette, L.; Hay, J.L.; Kehler, D.S.; Hamm, N.C.; Oldfield, C.; McGavock, J.M.; Duhamel, T.A. Exercise in pregnancy and children's cardiometabolic risk factors: A systematic review and meta-analysis. *Sports Med. Open* **2018**, *4*, 35. [CrossRef] [PubMed]
86. Plagemann, A. Perinatal programming and functional teratogenesis: Impact on body weight regulation and obesity. *Physiol. Behav.* **2005**, *86*, 661–668. [CrossRef] [PubMed]
87. Sampson, L. Food frequency questionnaires as a research instrument. *Clin. Nutr.* **1985**, *4*, 171–178.
88. Kazman, J.B.; Scott, J.M.; Deuster, P.A. Using item response theory to address vulnerabilities in FFQ. *Br. J. Nutr.* **2017**, *118*, 383–391. [CrossRef] [PubMed]

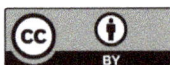

© 2019 by the authors. Licensee MDPI, Basel, Switzerland. This article is an open access article distributed under the terms and conditions of the Creative Commons Attribution (CC BY) license (http://creativecommons.org/licenses/by/4.0/).

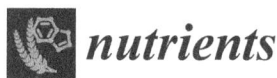

Review

Mediterranean Diet Pyramid: A Proposal for Italian People. A Systematic Review of Prospective Studies to Derive Serving Sizes

Annunziata D'Alessandro [1,*], Luisa Lampignano [2] and Giovanni De Pergola [3]

1. Medical Endocrinologist, General Internal Medicine A.S.L. Bari, v.le Iapigia 38/g, 70126 Bari, Italy
2. National Institute of Gastroenterology "S. de Bellis", Research Hospital, Castellana Grotte, 70013 Bari, Italy; luisalampignano@gmail.com
3. Department of Biomedical Sciences and Human Oncology, Section of Internal Medicine and Oncology, School of Medicine, Policlinico, University of Bari "Aldo Moro", p.zza Giulio Cesare 11, 70124 Bari, Italy; gdepergola@libero.it
* Correspondence: a.dalessandro2011@libero.it

Received: 4 May 2019; Accepted: 31 May 2019; Published: 7 June 2019

Abstract: In the last decade, a number of meta-analyses of mostly observational studies evaluated the relation between the intake of food groups and the risk of noncommunicable diseases (NCDs). In this study, we systematically reviewed dose-response meta-analyses of prospective studies with the aim to derive the quantities of food to consume to attain a protective (Mediterranean food) or a non-adverse (non-Mediterranean food) effect toward selected NCDs such as cardiovascular disease (CVD) including coronary heart disease (CHD) and stroke, type 2 diabetes (T2DM), colorectal (CRC) and breast cancer. These derived quantities, wherever possible, were suggested for a quantification of food servings of the Mediterranean Diet Pyramid proposed for Italian People (MDPPI). This pyramid came from the Modern Mediterranean Diet Pyramid developed in 2009 for Italian people. A weekly menu plan was built on the advice about frequency of intakes and serving sizes of such pyramid and the nutritional composition of this diet was compared with the Reference Italian Mediterranean Diet followed in 1960 in Nicotera. The diet built according the advice of MDPPI was very similar to that of Nicotera in the late 1950s that has been chosen as Italian Reference Mediterranean Diet with the exception of percentage of energy provided by cereals that was lower and of fruits and vegetables that was higher. Saturated fatty acids were only the 6% of daily energy intake. Also the Mediterranean Adequacy Index (MAI) was very similar to that of the aforementioned diet.

Keywords: Mediterranean diet; Mediterranean diet pyramid; noncommunicable diseases

1. Introduction

According to the 2018 Global Health Observatory Data of the World Health Organization (WHO), noncommunicable diseases (NCDs) such as cardiovascular disease (CVD), type 2 diabetes (T2DM), cancer and chronic respiratory diseases represent the leading cause of death in the world [1]. In Italy 91% of deaths are caused by NCDs and 10% of them are premature deaths because it affects people in a 30 to 70-year-old span [2].

Some lifestyle modifications and among them the adoption of healthy dietary choices as well as increasing the intake of fresh fruit and vegetable, whole grains and healthy fats, represent useful measures for the prevention of NCDs [3].

The Dietary Guidelines Advisory Committee included the Mediterranean Diet among highly beneficial dietary patterns for the prevention of overweight and obesity, CVD, T2DM, CRC and post-menopause breast cancer based upon prospective cohort studies, randomized clinical trials (RCTs) and high-quality systematic reviews [4].

The definition of dietary pattern takes into account several factors linked to habitually consumed food and beverages: quantities, proportions, combination or variety and frequency of intake [5].

The Mediterranean Diet is a dietary pattern that was identified in the early 1960s in South Italy, Crete and other areas of Greece [6]. At that time the food intake habits of three cohorts of the Seven Countries Study, Corfu and Crete in Greece and Nicotera in South Italy were almost identical [7]. The dietary habits characterized by higher consumption of vegetables and lower consumption of animal food were considered important determinants of the very low mortality for CHD observed in the Corfu and Crete cohorts at 25-year of follow-up [8].

During the last decade, a number of meta-analyses of mostly observational studies evaluated the association between the intake of food groups and the development of NCDs.

In the present study we performed a systematic review of dose-response meta-analyses of prospective studies, which evaluated the association between the intake of food groups belonging to a variant of the Modern Mediterranean Diet Pyramid (www.inran.it) and the risk of CVD, including CHD and stroke, T2DM, CRC and breast cancer. This variant was the MDPPI [9] (Figure 1).

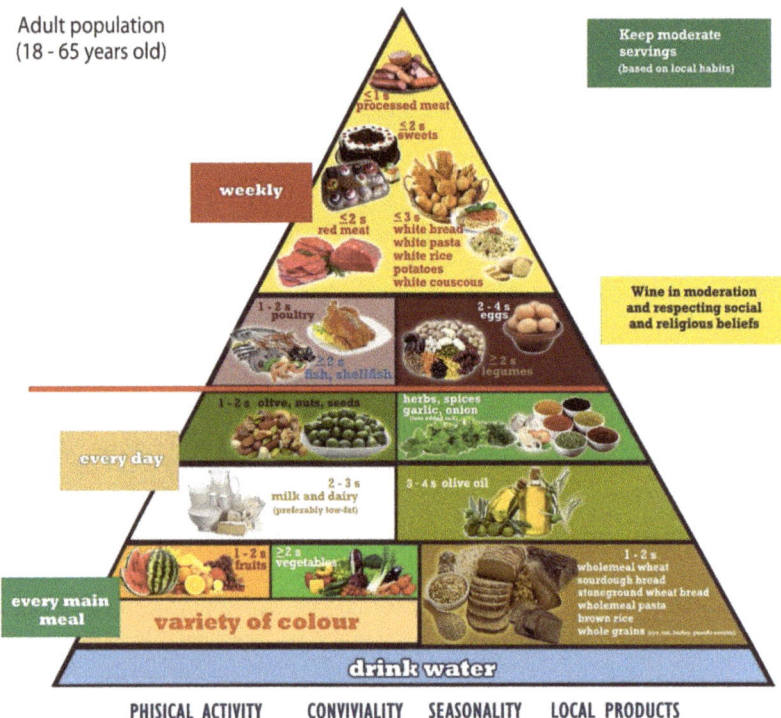

Figure 1. Proposal of Mediterranean Diet Pyramid for Italian People [9].

In particular, we derived from these meta-analyses the serving sizes of food to be consumed in order to obtain a protective (Mediterranean food) or a not detrimental (non-Mediterranean food) effect toward selected NCDs. A weekly menu plan was built on the advice about frequency of intakes and serving sizes of MDPPI and the nutritional composition of this diet was compared with the Reference Italian Mediterranean Diet followed in 1960 in Nicotera [10].

2. First Section

2.1. Methods

The criteria for systematic reviews (PRISMA statement) were followed [11].

We searched on Medline and Google Scholar for dose-response meta-analyses investigating the association between food groups of the MDPPI such as whole grains, vegetables, fruits, milk, cheese, yogurt, nuts, olive oil, herbs, spices, fish, legumes, eggs, refined grains, sweets/cakes/cookies, potatoes, red meat, processed meat, poultry, and red wine, on CVD, CHD, stroke, T2DM, CRC, and breast cancer risk, up to December 2018.

Inclusion criteria were as follows: (1) linear and/or nonlinear dose-response meta-analyses of prospective studies (cohort studies, follow-up of RCTs, case-cohort studies, nested case-control studies); (2) summary relative risks (RRs) or summary hazard ratios (HRs) with 95% confidence intervals (CIs); (3) I^2 statistic or *p*-value for heterogeneity; (4) exposure expressed in metric units (e.g., grams per day, milliliters per day; unit per day or per week, for eggs).

The publications were selected if the word meta-analysis appeared in the title and/or in the abstract. They were assessed for eligibility after reading the full text.

2.2. Results

Out of 95 dose-response meta-analyses that were identified, 36 were excluded while 59 met inclusion criteria and were withheld for this systematic review.

Twelve dose-response meta-analyses were evaluated for whole grain intake [12–23]; 11 for vegetable intake [17,18,20,21,24–30]; 12 for fruit intake [17,18,20,21,24–31]; 13 for milk intake [20,32–43]; 8 for cheese intake [20,33,35–39,44]; 6 for yogurt intake [33,35–38,41]; 8 for nut intake [17,18,21,41,45–48]; 2 for olive oil intake [49,50]; 9 for fish intake [17,18,20,21,41,51–54]; 4 for legume intake [17,18,20,21]; 3 for egg intake [55–57]; 2 for refined grain intake [17,18]; 1 for potato intake [58]; 13 for red meat intake [17,18,20,21,41,59–66]; 13 for processed meat intake [17,18,20,21,41,59–62,64–67]; 3 for poultry intake [41,61,68]; 2 for red wine intake [69,70].

No dose-response meta-analyses were identified for spice, herb and sweet/cake/cookie intakes.

2.2.1. Whole Grains

Table 1 reports the summary of linear dose-response meta-analyses of prospective studies on whole grain intake and CVD, CHD, stroke, type 2 diabetes (T2DM), and CRC.

A meta-analysis reported both a dose-response analysis for specific whole grains and for total whole grains [12]. Each increment intake of 90 g/day reduced CVD risk by 22% [16], CHD risk by 19% [16], and CRC risk by 17% [19,20]. Each increment intake of 90 g/day of specific whole grains reduced CVD mortality by 17% [12]. A meta-analysis reported that each increment intake of 30 g/day of whole grains reduced CHD risk by 5% [17]. In these meta-analyses, the heterogeneity was low or moderate (I^2 statistic < 50%).

Nonlinear dose-response analyses. The dose-response analysis of the association between whole grain intake and CVD mortality was nonlinear and above an intake of ~35 g/day [13] or of ~60 g/day [22] additional but more moderate benefits were evident. Two dose-response meta-analyses reported no evidence of nonlinearity between whole grain intake and reduction of CVD mortality [12,23].

There was evidence of a nonlinear association between whole grain intake and CVD, CHD and stroke with a reduction in risk up to 200 g/day for CVD, 210 g/day for CHD, and 120–150 g/day for stroke [16] and no reductions above these intakes. However, Bechthold et al., found evidence of a nonlinear dose-response association between whole grain intake and CHD with a decreased risk of 17% with increasing intake up to ~100 g/day and no benefits with further intakes [17]. In a meta-analysis, no association was evident for whole grain intake and stroke risk in the nonlinear dose-response analysis [17].

There was evidence of a nonlinear dose-response association between whole grain intake and T2DM risk with a 25% of risk reduction along with an increasing intake up to ~50 g/day and minimal benefits above this level of intake [18].

The intake of whole grains was associated with a linear decrease in the risk of CRC [19,21]; the risk decreased by ~20% along an increasing intake up to ~120 g/day and further benefits were evident for higher intakes up to ~200 g/day [21].

Table 1. Summary of linear dose-response meta-analyses of prospective studies on whole grain intake and CVD, CHD, stroke, T2DM and CRC.

Authors, Year, Reference	No. of Studies	Each Increment Intake Per Day	RR (95% CI)	I² Statistic	p-Value for Heterogeneity	Begg's or Egger's Test p-Value
Benisi-Kohansal 2016 [12]	3	90 g	CVD mortality 0.83 (0.76–0.91) *	0.00%	0.860	NR
Chen 2016 [13]	10	50 g	CVD mortality 0.70 (0.61–0.79)	64.80%	0.002	0.370/0.140
Li 2016 [14]	8	30 g	CVD mortality 0.95 (0.92–0.98)	68.60%	<0.001	0.276/0.202
Wei 2016 [15]	8	90 g	CVD mortality 0.74 (0.66–0.83)	76.30%	<0.001	0.107/0.834
Aune 2016 [16]	10	90 g	CVD 0.78 (0.73–0.85)	40.00%	0.090	0.310
Bechthold 2017 [17]	5	30 g	CHD 0.95 (0.92–0.98)	46.00%	0.110	NR
Aune 2016 [16]	7	90 g	CHD 0.81 (0.75–0.87)	9.00%	0.360	0.110
Bechthold 2017 [17]	4	30 g	Stroke 0.99 (0.95–1.03)	65.00%	0.040	NR
Aune 2016 [16]	6	90 g	Stroke 0.88 (0.75–1.03)	56.00%	0.040	0.010
Schwingshackl 2017 [18]	12	30 g	T2DM 0.87 (0.82–0.93)	91.00%	NR	NR
Aune 2011 [19]	6	90 g	CRC 0.83 (0.78–0.89)	18.00%	0.300	1.000/0.540
Vieira 2017 [20]	6	90 g	CRC 0.83 (0.79–0.89)	18.00%	0.300	NS
Schwingshackl 2018 [21]	9	30 g	CRC 0.95 (0.93–0.97)	58.00%	0.0200	NR

* specific whole grains; CVD, cardiovascular disease; CHD, coronary heart disease; T2DM, type 2 diabetes mellitus; CRC, colorectal cancer; RR, relative risk; NR, not reported; NS, not significant.

2.2.2. Vegetables

Table 2 reports the summary of linear dose-response meta-analyses of prospective studies on vegetable intake and CVD, CHD, stroke, T2DM, CRC, and breast cancer.

Each daily increment intake of 200 g of vegetables reduced the risk of CVD by 10% [24], whereas a daily increment intake of 400 g reduced the CHD risk by 18% [25] and a daily increment intake of 100 g by 3% [17]. In these meta-analyses, the heterogeneity was below 50%.

Nonlinear dose-response analyses. There was evidence of nonlinearity for vegetable intake and CVD (although the association was almost linear) with a 28% risk reduction at intakes of 600 g/day [24]. The nonlinear dose-response analysis was significant for the association between vegetable intake and CVD risk with a reduction of 11% and 28% for a daily intake of 200 g and 600 g, respectively [29].

A nonlinear association of CHD risk with vegetable intake was evident [24,25] with a reduction in risk at the lower levels of intake up to ~200–300 g/day and light further reductions in RRs of 30% up to 550–600 g/day [24]. One dose-response meta-analysis reported that the association between vegetable intake and CHD was linear; an increasing intake of vegetables up to 400 g/day reduced the RRs of CHD by ~12% and higher intakes lead to further reductions in RRs [17].

For stroke risk, there was no evidence of nonlinearity: risk reduction of stroke was evident along with the entire range of vegetable intake with the strongest reductions in RRs of 20% for a daily intake of 400 g [30]. However, in two dose-response meta-analyses there was evidence of nonlinearity between vegetable intake and stroke risk with a 28% reduction in RRs at 500 g/day [24] or with ~12% reduction in RRs up to intakes of ~200 g/day [17] without additional benefits above these amounts.

The association between vegetable intake and T2DM risk was nonlinear [18,26,27]. A maximal reduction in RRs of 9% was evident at ~300 g/day of intakes with no additional benefits for higher intakes [18]. Similarly, in another meta-analysis, the T2DM risk decreased by 6% at intakes of ~200–300 g/day of vegetables without further benefits at higher intakes [27].

There was evidence of nonlinear dose-response between vegetable intake and CRC risk: the risk decreased along the entire range of intakes and the RR reduction were 7% up to ~200 g/day; minimal further reductions were evident for higher intakes [21].

There was no evidence of nonlinear dose-response association between vegetable intakes and breast cancer risk [28].

Table 2. Summary of linear dose-response meta-analyses of prospective studies on vegetable intake and CVD, CHD, stroke, T2DM, CRC, breast cancer.

Authors, Year, Reference	No. of Studies	Each Increment Intake Per Day	RR (95% CI)	I^2 Statistic	p-Value for Heterogeneity	Begg's or Egger's Test p-Value
Aune 2017 [24]	14	200 g	CVD 0.90 (0.87–0.93)	11.50%	0.330	0.530
Gan 2015 [25]	13	400 g	CHD 0.82 (0.73–0.92)	35.60%	0.068	0.880/0.381
Aune 2017 [24]	20	200 g	CHD 0.84 (0.79–0.90)	60.60%	<0.0001	0.001
Bechthold 2017 [17]	14	100 g	CHD 0.97 (0.96–0.99)	12.00%	0.320	NR
Aune 2017 [24]	13	200 g	Stroke 0.87 (0.79–0.96)	63.40%	0.001	0.150
Bechthold 2017 [17]	10	100 g	Stroke 0.92 (0.86–0.98)	79.00%	<0.001	NR
Li 2014 [26]	5	106 g	T2DM 0.98 (0.89–1.08)	45.80%	0.117	0.117
Wu 2015 [27]	7	106 g	T2DM 0.98 (0.95–1.01)	78.30%	0.000	0.130/0.150
Schwingshackl 2017 [18]	11	100 g	T2DM 0.98 (0.96–1.00)	62.00%	NR	NS
Vieira 2017 [20]	11	100 g	CRC 0.98 (0.96–0.99)	0.00%	0.480	NS
Schwingshackl 2018 [21]	15	100 g	CRC 0.97 (0.96–0.98)	0.00%	0.640	0.530
Aune 2012 [28]	9	200 g	Breast cancer 1.00 (0.95–1.06)	17.00%	0.290	NR

CVD, cardiovascular disease; CHD, coronary heart disease; T2DM, type 2 diabetes mellitus; CRC, colorectal cancer; RR, relative risk; NR, not reported; NS, not significant.

2.2.3. Fruits

Table 3 reports the summary of linear dose-response meta-analyses of prospective studies on fruit intake and CVD, CHD, stroke, T2DM, CRC, and breast cancer.

Table 3. Summary of linear dose-response meta-analyses of prospective studies on fruit intake and CVD, CHD, stroke, T2DM, CRC, breast cancer.

Authors, Year, Reference	No. of Studies	Each Increment Intake Per Day	RR (95% CI)	I^2 Statistic	p-Value for Heterogeneity	Begg's or Egger's Test p-Value
Aune 2017 [24]	17	200 g	CVD 0.87 (0.82–0.92)	79.10%	<0.0001	0.410
Gan 2015 [25]	15	300 g	CHD 0.84 (0.75–0.93)	31.70%	0.0780	0.367/0.591
Aune 2017 [24]	24	200 g	CHD 0.90 (0.86–0.94)	43.70%	0.0100	0.040
Bechthold 2017 [17]	13	100 g	CHD 0.94 (0.90–0.97)	71.00%	<0.0010	NR
Aune 2017 [24]	16	200 g	Stroke 0.82 (0.74–0.90)	72.90%	<0.0001	0.620
Bechthold 2017 [17]	10	100 g	Stroke 0.90 (0.84–0.97)	86.00%	0.0010	NR
Li 2014 [26]	7	106 g	T2DM 0. 94 (0.89–1.00)	0.00%	0.059	NR
Wu 2015 [27]	9	106 g	T2DM 0.99 (0.97–1.00)	18.60%	0.278	0.470/0.680
Schwingshackl 2017 [18]	13	100 g	T2DM 0.98 (0.97–1.00)	21.00%	NR	NS
Vieira 2017 [20]	13	100 g	CRC 0.96 (0.93–1.00)	68.00%	<0.0001	NS
Schwingshackl et al. 2018 [21]	16	100 g	CRC 0.97 (0.95–0.99)	61.00%	<0.0010	0.120
Aune 2012 [28]	10	200 g	Breast cancer 0.94 (0.89–1.00)	39.00%	0.1000	NR

CVD, cardiovascular disease; CHD, coronary heart disease; T2DM, type 2 diabetes mellitus; CRC, colorectal cancer; RR, relative risk; NR, not reported; NS, not significant.

Each daily increment intake of 300 g or 200 g of fruits reduced the RRs of CHD by 16% [25] and 10% [24], respectively. The RRs of T2DM were reduced by 6%, 1% and 2% for a daily increment intake of 106 g [26], 106 g [27] and 100 g [18], respectively. The breast cancer risk was reduced by 6% for each daily increment intake of 200 g [28]. In these linear dose-response meta-analyses, the heterogeneity was below 50%.

Nonlinear dose-response analyses. There was evidence of nonlinearity between fruit intake and CVD risk with the strongest inverse association at lower intakes (up to ~200–300 g/day) and light further reductions at greater intakes: at 800 g/day of intake the reduction in RRs was 27% [24]. Similarly, in another meta-analysis, the reduction in CVD risk was 14% at 200 g/day of intake and 16% at 500 g/day of intake [29].

Nonlinear association between fruit intake and CHD was found: most of the reduction in risk was up to ~200 g/day of intake [17,24,25] without benefit for greater intake [17] or with a light reduction for greater intakes [24,25].

In two dose-response meta-analyses, the association between fruit intake and stroke was nonlinear with a 20% of reduction in RRs for daily intakes of ~200–350 g [24] or ~200 g [17] and not benefits for greater intakes. One dose-response meta-analysis reported no evidence of nonlinearity between fruit intake and stroke with a reduction in RRs of 46% for a daily intake of 300 g [30].

Four dose-response meta-analyses reported evidence of nonlinear association between fruit intake and T2DM risk with most reduction in RRs for lower intakes [18,26,27,31]. For ~200 g of fruit intake the reduction in RRs was 13% [31] 10% [18] or 12% [27] and no benefits were evident for higher intakes.

A nonlinear dose-response association was detected between fruit intake and CRC with the greatest reduction in RRs by ~8% increasing the intake up to ~200 g/day and little further benefits above these intakes [21]

The inverse association between fruit intake and breast cancer was linear [28].

2.2.4. Milk

Table 4 reports the summary of linear dose-response meta-analyses of prospective studies on milk intake and CVD, CHD, stroke, T2DM, CRC, and breast cancer.

Table 4. Summary of linear dose-response meta-analyses of prospective studies on milk intake and CVD, CHD, stroke, T2DM, CRC, and breast cancer.

Authors, Year, Reference	No. of Studies	Each Increment Intake Per Day	RR (95% CI)	I^2 Statistic	p-Value for Heterogeneity	Begg's or Egger's Test p-Value
Soedamah-Muthu 2011 [32]	4	200 mL	CVD 0.94 (0.89–0.99)	0.00%	0.5020	NR
Guo 2017 [33]	12	244 g	CVD 1.01 (0.93–1.10)	92.40%	<0.0010	0.449
Soedamah-Muthu 2011 [32]	6	200 mL	CHD 1.00 (0.96–1.04)	26.90%	0.2330	NR
Mullie 2016 [34]	9	200 mL	CHD 1.01 (0.98–1.05)	16.00%	0.3000	0.680/0.050
Guo 2017 [33]	12	244 g	CHD 1.01 (0.96–1.06)	45.50%	0.0430	0.397
Soedamah-Muthu 2011 [32]	6	200 mL	Stroke 0.87 (0.72–1.07)	94.60%	0.0000	NR
de Goede 2016 [35]	14	200 g	Stroke 0.93 (0.88–0.98)	86.00%	<0.0010	0.060
Mullie 2016 [34]	10	200 mL	Stroke 0.91 (0.82–1.02)	92.00%	<0.0100	0.530/0.050
Aune 2013 [36]	7	200 g	T2DM 0.87 (0.72–1.04)	93.60%	<0.0001	0.410
Gao 2013 [37]	8	200 g	T2DM incidence 0.89 (0.79–1.01)	66.30%	0.0050	NR
Gijsbers 2016 [38]	12	200 g	T2DM incidence 0.97 (0.93–1.02)	57.40%	0.0070	0.071
Aune 2012 [39]	9	200 g	CRC 0.90 (0.85–0.94)	0.00%	0.6200	0.840/0.860
Vieira 2017 [20]	9	200 g	CRC 0.94 (0.92–0.96)	0.00%	0.9700	NS
Dong 2011 [40]	9	200 g	Breast cancer 0.98 (0.95–1.01)	NR	>0.3000	>0.050
Wu 2016 [41]	11	200 g	Breast cancer incidence 0.97 (0.93–1.01)	36.40%	NR	0.436/0.355

CVD, cardiovascular disease; CHD, coronary heart disease; T2DM, type 2 diabetes mellitus; CRC, colorectal cancer; RR, relative risk; NR, not reported; NS, not significant.

A daily increment intake of 200 mL of milk reduced the RRs of CVD by 6% [32]. A daily increment intake of 200 mL [32,34] or 244 g of milk [33] had a neutral effect on CHD risk. The RRs of CRC was reduced by 10% [39] or 6% [20] for each daily increment intake of 200 g of milk. The RRs of breast cancer and breast cancer incidence were reduced by 2% [40] and 3% [41] for each daily increment intake of 200 g of milk. In these meta-analyses, the heterogeneity was low below 50%.

Nonlinear dose-response analyses. An inverse and nonlinear association between milk intake and stroke was found with a maximal effect up to ~200 mL/day (reduction in RRs of 18%) [42] or up to 125 g/day (reduction in RRs of 14%) [35]; the reduction in RRs remained but was attenuated up to ~700 mL/day [42] or ~750 g/day [35].

There was evidence of an inverse linear association between low fat or skim milk intake and T2DM and of a nonlinear positive association between whole milk intake and T2DM [36].

The association between milk intake and reduced CRC risk was nonlinear with the strongest reduction in RRs (20–30%) from 500 to 800 g/day of intake and week association below 200 g/day of intake [39]. In a meta-analysis of 22 prospective cohort studies, no association between milk intake and breast cancer risk was found [43]. In another meta-analysis, a linear inverse association between skim milk intake and breast cancer incidence was found [41].

2.2.5. Cheese

Table 5 reports the summary of linear dose-response meta-analyses of prospective studies on cheese intake and CVD, CHD, stroke, T2DM, and CRC.

Table 5. Summary of linear dose-response meta-analyses of prospective studies on cheese intake and CVD, CHD, stroke, T2DM, and CRC.

Authors, Year, Reference	No. of Studies	Each Increment Intake Per Day	RR (95% CI)	I^2 Statistic	p-Value for Heterogeneity	Begg's or Egger's Test p-Value
Chen 2017 [44]	7	50 g	CVD 0.92 (0.83–1.02)	16.90%	0.301	>0.100
Guo 2017 [33]	11	10 g	CVD 0.98 (0.95–1.00)	82.60%	<0.001	NR
Chen 2017 [44]	8	50 g	CHD 0.90 (0.84–0.95)	0.00%	0.444	0.170/0.040
Guo 2017 [33]	10	10 g	CHD 0.99 (0.97–1.02)	40.30%	0.089	0.273
Chen 2017 [44]	5	50 g	Stroke 0.94 (0.84–1.04)	63.70%	0.026	>0.10
de Goede 2016 [35]	7	40 g	Stroke 0.97 (0.94–1.01)	31.20%	0.179	NR
Aune 2013 [36]	8	50 g	T2DM 0.92 (0.86–0.99)	0.00%	0.790	0.740
Gao 2013 [37]	7	30 g	T2DM incidence 0.80 (0.69–0.93)	59.00%	0.020	NR
Gijsbers 2016 [38]	13	10 g	T2DM incidence 1.00 (0.99–1.02)	61.70%	0.002	0.880
Aune 2012 [39]	7	50 g	CRC 0.96 (0.83–1.12)	28.00%	0.220	NR
Vieira 2017 [20]	7	50 g	CRC 0.94 (0.87–1.02)	10.00%	0.360	NS

CVD, cardiovascular disease; CHD, coronary heart disease; T2DM, type 2 diabetes mellitus; CRC, colorectal cancer; RR, relative risk; NR, not reported; NS, not significant.

A daily increment intake of 50 g reduced CVD and CHD risk by 8% and 10%, respectively [44]. The stroke risk was reduced by 3% with a daily increment intake of 40 g [35]. An increment intake of 50 g reduced the T2DM risk by 8% [36].

The risk of CRC was reduced by 4% [39] and 6% [20] with a daily increment intake of 50 g, respectively. In these dose-response meta-analyses, the heterogeneity was below 50%.

Nonlinear dose-response analyses. The association between cheese intake and CVD was nonlinear and almost U-shaped with a maximal risk reduction at ~40 g/day [44]. The association between cheese intake and CHD was linear with progressive risk reduction up to an intake of 120 g/day [44]. The association between cheese intake and stroke was inverse and nonlinear with a maximal risk reduction at 40 g/day [44] or at 25 g/day [35] without benefits for greater intakes.

Nonlinearity was found between cheese intake and T2DM with a maximal reduction in RRs up to 50 g/day and not further benefits for higher intakes [36].

2.2.6. Yogurt

Table 6 reports the summary of linear dose-response meta-analyses of prospective studies on yogurt intake and CVD, CHD, stroke, T2DM, and breast cancer.

Table 6. Summary of linear dose-response meta-analyses of prospective studies on yogurt intake and CVD, CHD, stroke, T2DM, and breast cancer.

Authors, Year, Reference	No. of Studies	Each Increment Intake Per Day	RR (95% CI)	I^2 Statistic	p-Value for Heterogeneity	Begg's or Egger's Test p-Value
Guo 2017 [33]	3	50 g	CVD 1.03 (0.97–1.09)	0.00%	0.499	NR
Guo 2017 [33]	3	50 g	CHD 1.03 (0.97–1.09)	0.00%	0.685	NR
de Goede 2016 [35]	3	100 g	Stroke 1.02 (0.90–1.17)	47.80%	0.147	NR
Aune 2013 [36]	7	200 g	T2DM 0.78 (0.60–1.02)	69.90%	0.003	0.370
Gao 2013 [37]	7	50 g	T2DM incidence 0.91 (0.82–1.00)	74.00%	0.001	NR
Gijsbers 2016 [38]	12	50 g	T2DM incidence 0.94 (0.90–0.97)	73.30%	0.000	0.180
Wu 2016 [41]	3	200 g	Breast cancer incidence 0.87 (0.72–1.06)	0.00%	NR	1.000/0.488

CVD, cardiovascular disease; CHD, coronary heart disease; T2DM, type 2 diabetes mellitus; RR, relative risk; NR, not reported.

A daily increment intake of 50 g [33] or 100 g [35] was not associated with CVD, CHD [33] and stroke risk [35]. A daily increment intake of 200 g reduced breast cancer incidence by 13% [41]. In these dose-response meta-analyses, the heterogeneity was below 50%.

Nonlinear dose-response analyses. The association between yogurt intake and T2DM risk was inverse and nonlinear with a maximal reduction at intakes of 120–140 g/day [36] or 80 g/day [38] and not further reductions at higher intakes. The association between yogurt intake and breast cancer risk was nonlinear [41].

2.2.7. Nuts

Table 7 reports the summary of linear dose-response meta-analyses of prospective studies on nut intake and CVD, CHD, stroke, T2DM, CRC and breast cancer.

Table 7. Summary of linear dose-response meta-analyses of prospective studies on nut intake and CVD, CHD, stroke, T2DM, CRC, breast cancer.

Authors, Year, Reference	No. of Studies	Each Increment Intake Per Day	RR (95% CI)	I^2 Statistic	p-Value for Heterogeneity	Begg's or Egger's Test p-Value
Luo 2014 [45]	4	28 g	CVD incidence 0.71 (0.59–0.85)	48.80%	0.119	0.090
Aune 2016 [46]	11	28 g	CVD 0.80 (0.72–0.89)	56.00%	0.001	NR
Grosso 2015 [47]	5	28 g	CVD mortality 0.61 (0.42–0.91)	75.00%	NR	NR
Aune 2016 [46]	11	28 g	CHD 0.71 (0.63–0.80)	47.00%	0.040	0.280
Bechthold 2017 [17]	4	28 g	CHD 0.67 (0.43–1.05)	85.00%	0.001	NR
Aune 2016 [46]	11	28 g	Stroke 0.93 (0.83–1.05)	14.00%	0.310	0.300
Bechthold 2017 [17]	6	28 g	Stroke 0.99 (0.84–1.17)	45.00%	0.110	NR
Luo 2014 [45]	4	28 g	T2DM incidence 1.03 (0.91–1.16)	63.90%	0.040	0.810
Schwingshackl 2017 [18]	7	28 g	T2DM 0.89 (0.71–1.12)	77.00%	NR	NR
Schwingshackl 2018 [21]	4	28 g	CRC 0.96 (0.76–1.21)	25.00%	0.260	NR
Wu 2016 [41]	3	28 g	Breast cancer incidence 0.96 (0.84–1.09)	0.00%	NR	0.100/0.955

CVD, cardiovascular disease; CHD, coronary heart disease; T2DM, type 2 diabetes mellitus; CRC, colorectal cancer; RR, relative risk; NR, not reported.

A daily increment of 28 g reduced the RRs of CVD incidence [45] and CHD [46] by 29%; the risk of stroke by 7% [46] or 1% [17]; the risk of CRC [18] and breast cancer incidence [41] by 4%. In these dose-response meta-analyses, the heterogeneity was below 50%.

Nonlinear dose-response analyses. The association between nut intake and CVD was nonlinear with a maximal reduction in risk up to intakes of ~15 g/day and no benefits above these values [46]. There was evidence of nonlinearity between nut intake and CHD risk with an inverse association that reached the maximal values at ~15–20 g of daily intakes without further reductions for greater intakes [46]. A nonlinear inverse association was reported between nut intake and CHD risk with maximal benefits in reduction of RRs (21%) up to ~10–15 g/day and no benefits above these intakes [17].

There was evidence of an inverse nonlinear association between nut intake and risk of stroke with a maximal reduction in RRs up to ~10–15 g of daily intake but a positive association at ~30 g of daily intake [46]. An inverse nonlinear association was found between nut intake and stroke risk with a 14% risk reduction at daily intake of 12 g without any further benefits for greater intakes [48]. However, in another meta-analysis no association was found between daily nut intake and risk of stroke in the nonlinear dose-response analysis [17]. There was no evidence of a nonlinear dose-response association between daily nut intake and T2DM [18] or CRC risk [21]. The association between nut intake and breast cancer was nonlinear [41].

2.2.8. Olive Oil

Table 8 reports the summary of linear dose-response meta-analyses of prospective studies on olive oil intake and CHD, stroke, and T2DM.

Table 8. Summary of linear dose-response meta-analyses of prospective studies on olive oil intake and CHD, stroke, T2DM.

Authors, Year, Reference	No. of Studies	Each Increment Intake Per Day	RR (95% CI)	I^2 Statistic	p-Value for Heterogeneity	Begg's or Egger's Test p-Value
Martínez-Gonzáles 2014 [49]	5	25 g	CHD 0.94 (0.78–1.14)	66.20%	0.020	NR
Martínez-Gonzáles 2014 [49]	3	25 g	Stroke 0.76 (0.67–0.86)	0.00%	0.440	0.110
Schwingshackl 2017 [50]	4	10 g	T2DM 0.91 (0.87–0.95)	0.00%	NR	NR

CHD, coronary heart disease; T2DM, type 2 diabetes mellitus; RR, relative risk; NR, not reported.

Each 25 g increment intake per day of olive oil reduced the RRs of stroke by 24% [49]. An increment intake of 10 g of olive oil reduced the RRs of T2DM by 9% [50]. In these dose-response meta-analyses, the heterogeneity was below 50%.

Nonlinear dose-response analyses. There was evidence of an inverse nonlinear association between olive oil intake and T2DM risk. A daily intake of ~15–20 g reduced the RRs of T2DM by 13%. Greater intakes did not bring further benefits. Excluding one study the association became linear [50].

2.2.9. Fish and Shellfish

Table 9 reports the summary of linear dose-response meta-analyses of fish intake and CVD, CHD, stroke, T2DM, CRC, breast cancer.

Table 9. Summary of linear dose-response meta-analyses of prospective studies on fish intake and CVD, CHD, stroke, T2DM, CRC, breast cancer.

Authors, Year, Reference	No. of Studies	Each Increment Intake Per Day	RR (95% CI)	I^2 Statistic	p-Value for Heterogeneity	Begg's or Egger's Test p-Value
Jayedi 2018 [51]	8	20 g	CVD mortality 0.96 (0.94–0.98)	0.00%	0.620	NR
Bechthold 2017 [17]	15	100 g	CHD 0.88 (0.79–0.99)	40.00%	0.060	NS
Zheng 2012 [52]	17	15 g	CHD mortality 0.94 (0.90–0.98)	63.10%	0.000	NR
Bechthold 2017 [17]	15	100 g	Stroke 0.86 (0.75–0.99)	25.00%	0.180	NR
Schwingshackl 2017 [18]	15	100 g	T2DM 1.09 (0.93–1.28)	84.00%	NR	NS
Vieira 2017 [20]	11	100 g	CRC 0.89 (0.80–0.99)	0.00%	0.520	NS
Schwingshackl 2018 [21]	16	100 g	CRC 0.93 (0.85–1.01)	12.00%	0.320	0.910
Zheng 2013 [53]	11	15 g	Breast cancer 1.00 (0.97–1.03)	64.00%	0.001	NS
Wu 2016 [41]	13	120 g	Breast cancer incidence 1.07 (0.94–1.21)	33.30%	NR	0.100/0.089

CVD, cardiovascular disease; CHD, coronary heart disease; T2DM, type 2 diabetes mellitus; CRC, colorectal cancer; RR, relative risk; NR, not reported; NS, not significant.

Each increment of 20 g/day decreased CVD mortality by 4% [51]. Each daily intake of 100 g reduced the RRs of CHD and stroke of 12% and 14%, respectively [17] and the CRC risk by 11% [20] or 7% [21]. A daily increment intake of 120 g increased the breast cancer incidence of 7% [41]. In these dose-response meta-analyses, the heterogeneity was below 50%.

Nonlinear dose-response analyses. The association between fish intake and CVD mortality was linear [51]. There was evidence of linearity of the association between fish intake and CHD mortality: for each 20g/day the reduction of RRs was 7% [54]. However, in another meta-analysis there was evidence of nonlinearity between fish intake and risk of CHD mortality that had greater risk reduction at ~30–60 g/day than for lower and higher intakes [52]. The nonlinear dose-response association between fish intake and CHD or stroke was significant and the risk of CHD decreased with greater daily intake up to ~15% at ~250 g/day; the risk of stroke decreased with greater daily intake up to ~10% at ~80–100 g/day [17].

No association between fish intake and T2DM [18], CRC [21], and breast cancer risk [53] was evident. A nonlinear association with fish intake and breast cancer incidence was found [41].

2.2.10. Legumes

Table 10 reports the summary of linear dose-response meta-analyses of prospective studies on legume intake and CHD, stroke, T2DM, and CRC.

A daily increment of 50 g reduced the risk of CHD by 4% [17]. No association was evident for a daily increment of 50 g of legumes on the risk of CRC [20]. In these dose-response meta-analyses, the heterogeneity was below 50%.

Nonlinear dose-response analyses. An inverse nonlinear dose-response association between legume intake and CHD was evident; the risk decreased by ~10% with increasing intakes up to ~100 g/day without no benefits for higher intakes. No association was evident between legume intake and stroke [17], T2DM [18], and CRC risk [21].

Table 10. Summary of linear dose-response meta-analyses of prospective studies on legume intake and CHD, stroke, T2DM, CRC.

Authors, Year, Reference	No. of Studies	Each Increment Intake Per Day	RR (95% CI)	I² Statistic	p-Value for Heterogeneity	Begg's or Egger's Test p-Value
Bechthold 2017 [17]	8	50 g	CHD 0.96 (0.92–1.01)	39.00%	0.120	NR
Bechthold 2017 [17]	6	50 g	Stroke 1.00 (0.88–1.13)	62.00%	0.020	NR
Schwingshackl 2017 [18]	12	50 g	T2DM 1.00 (0.92–1.09)	87.00%	NR	NR
Schwingshackl 2018 [21]	10	50 g	CRC 1.00 (0.92–1.08)	50.00%	0.040	0.590
Vieira 2017 [20]	4	50 g	CRC 1.00 (0.95–1.06)	33.00%	0.200	NS

CHD, coronary heart disease; T2DM, type 2 diabetes mellitus; CRC, colorectal cancer; RR, relative risk; NR, not reported; NS, not significant.

2.2.11. Eggs

Table 11 reports the summary of linear dose-response meta-analyses of prospective studies on egg intake and CHD, stroke, T2DM, and breast cancer.

Table 11. Summary of linear dose-response meta-analyses of prospective studies on egg intake and CHD, stroke, T2DM, breast cancer.

Authors, Year, Reference	No. of Studies	Each Increment Intake Per Day or Week	RR (95% CI)	I² Statistic	p-Value for Heterogeneity	Begg's or Egger's Test p-Value
Rong 2013 [55]	9	1egg/day	CHD 0.99 (0.85–1.15)	0.00%	0.970	>0.050/>0.050
Rong 2013 [55]	8	1egg/day	Stroke 0.91 (0.81–1.02)	0.00%	0.460	>0.050/>0.050
Tamez 2016 [56]	13	1egg/day	T2DM 1.13 (1.04–1.22)	85.00%	<0.001	0.460
Keum 2015 [57]	6	5eggs/week	Breast cancer 1.05 (0.99–1.11)	0.00%	0.927	0.620

CHD, coronary heart disease; T2DM, type 2 diabetes mellitus; RR, relative risk.

An increased intake of 1 egg/day was not associated with increased risk of CHD or stroke [55]. An increased intake of 5 eggs/week increased the risk of breast cancer of 5% [57]. No heterogeneity was detected between the studies.

Nonlinear dose-response analyses. No evidence of nonlinear dose-response was found between egg intake and risk of CHD and stroke [55]. The association between egg intake and breast cancer risk was linear with an increased risk for intakes ≥5 eggs/week [57].

2.2.12. Refined Grains

Table 12 reports the summary of linear dose-response meta-analyses of prospective studies on refined grain intake and CHD, stroke, T2DM.

Table 12. Summary of linear dose-response meta-analyses of prospective studies on refined grain intake and CHD, stroke, T2DM.

Authors, Year, Reference	No. of Studies	Each Increment Intake Per Day	RR (95% CI)	I² Statistic	p-Value for Heterogeneity	Begg's or Egger's Test p-Value
Bechthold 2017 [17]	4	30 g	CHD 1.01 (0.99–1.04)	0.00%	0.510	NR
Bechthold 2017 [17]	4	30 g	Stroke 1.00 (0.98–1.01)	0.00%	0.510	NR
Schwingshackl 2017 [18]	14	30 g	T2DM 1.01 (0.99–1.03)	59.00%	NR	NR

CHD, coronary heart disease; T2DM, type 2 diabetes mellitus; RR, relative risk; NR, not reported.

Each additional daily intake of 30 g of refined grains was not associated with the risk of CHD or stroke without heterogeneity between the studies [17].

Nonlinear dose-response analyses. The association between refined grain intake and CHD was linear and the RRs were greater than 1.00 for intakes higher than ~100–120 g/day [17].

There was no association between refined grain intake and risk of stroke [17]. The association between refined grain intake and T2DM was linear and direct. An intake of ~200–400 g/day was associated with an increased risk of 6–14% [18].

2.2.13. Potatoes

Table 13 reports the summary of linear dose-response meta-analyses of prospective studies on potato intake and CHD, stroke, T2DM, and CRC.

Table 13. Summary of linear dose-response meta-analyses on potato intake and CHD, stroke, T2DM, CRC.

Authors, Year, Reference	No. of Studies	Total Intake Per Day	RR (95% CI)	I² Statistic	p-Value for Heterogeneity	Begg's or Egger's Test p-Value
Schwingshackl 2018 [58]	7	150 g	CHD 1.03 (0.96–1.09)	0.00%	0.990	NR
Schwingshackl 2018 [58]	6	150 g	Stroke 0.98 (0.93–1.03)	3.00%	0.400	NR
Schwingshackl 2018 [58]	7	150 g	T2DM 1.18 (1.10–1.27)	30.00%	0.200	NR
Schwingshackl 2018 [58]	6	150 g	CRC 1.05 (0.92–1.20)	20.00%	0.280	NR

CHD, coronary heart disease; T2DM, type 2 diabetes mellitus; CRC, colorectal cancer; RR, relative risk; NR, not reported.

An increment in daily total potato intake of 150 g was not associated with the risk of CHD, stroke or CRC but was positively associated with T2DM risk (18% increase). No heterogeneity between the studies was found [58].

Nonlinear dose-response analyses. There was no association between total potato intake and CHD and stroke. There was no evidence of nonlinearity between total potato intake and T2DM or CRC risk. The risk of T2DM was positively associated with potato intake: at value up to ~260 g/day it reached ~51% mostly due to French fries intake [58].

The risk of CRC was positively associated with potato intake: for an intake higher than ~134 g/day, the risk the CRC increased up to 25% for a daily intake of ~190 g [58].

2.2.14. Red Meat

Table 14 reports the summary of linear dose-response meta-analyses of prospective studies on red meat intake and CVD, CHD, stroke, T2DM, CRC, and breast cancer.

Table 14. Summary of linear dose-response meta-analyses of prospective studies on red meat intake and CVD, CHD, stroke, T2DM, CRC, breast cancer.

Authors, Year, Reference	No. of Studies	Each Increment Intake Per Day	RR (95% CI)	I² Statistic	p-Value for Heterogeneity	Begg's or Egger's Test, p-Value
Abete 2014 [59]	6	100 g	CVD mortality 1.15 (1.05–1.26)	76.60%	<0.001	>0.100/>0.100
Bechthold 2017 [17]	3	100 g	CHD 1.15 (1.08–1.23)	0.00%	0.680	NR
Bechthold 2017 [17]	7	100 g	Stroke 1.12 (1.06–1.17)	0.00%	0.500	NR
Aune 2009 [60]	9	120 g	T2DM 1.20 (1.04–1.38)	68.30%	0.001	NR
Feskens 2013 [61]	14	100 g	T2DM 1.13 (1.03–1.23)	36.00%	NR	NR
Schwingshackl 2017 [18]	14	100 g	T2DM 1.17 (1.08–1.26)	83.00%	NR	NS
Larsson 2006 [62]	14	120 g	CRC 1.28 (1.18–1.39)	0.00%	0.790	NR
Alexander 2011 [63]	13	70 g	CRC 1.05 (0.97–1.13)	NR	<0.001	0.97
Chan 2011 [64]	8	100 g	CRC incidence 1.17 (1.05–1.13)	0.00%	0.483	NS
Vieira 2017 [20]	8	100 g	CRC 1.12 (1.00–1.25)	24.00%	0.240	NS
Zhao 2017 [65]	9	100 g	CRC 1.16 (1.05–1.29)	0.00%	0.600	NR
Schwingshackl 2018 [21]	21	100 g	CRC 1.12 (1.06–1.19)	27.00%	0.130	0.620
Guo 2015 [66]	11	120 g	Breast cancer 1.11 (1.05–1.16)	NR	>0.100	NR
Wu 2016 [41]	8	120 g	Breast cancer incidence 1.13 (1.01–1.26)	56.40%	NR	0.266/0.110

CVD, cardiovascular disease; CHD, coronary heart disease; T2DM, type 2 diabetes mellitus; CRC, colorectal cancer; RR, relative risk; NR, not reported; NS, not significant.

Each 100 g daily increment of red meat was associated with a 15% and a 12% increased risk of CHD and stroke, respectively [17]. The risk of T2DM was increased for the same daily intake by 13% [61]. The risk of CRC was increased by 28% for an increase in red meat intake of 120 g/day [62], and from 12% to 17% for an increase in red meat intake of 100 g/day [20,21,64,65]. A daily increment of 120 g of red meat intake increased the risk of breast cancer by 11% [66]. The heterogeneity between the studies was below 50%.

Nonlinear dose-response analyses. There was evidence of a nonlinear dose-response association between red meat intake and CHD risk: it increased by ~20% up to ~100 g of daily intake [17].

The association between red meat intake and stroke was linear with an increased risk of ~10% for increasing intakes up to ~100 g/day [17].

The association between read meat intake and T2DM risk was linear and direct with an increasing risk of ~20% for a daily intake up to ~100 g/day of intake [18]. The association between red meat intake and CRC risk was linear and positive and an intake of 150 g/day was associated with an increased risk of ~20% [21]. A linear association was observed between red meat intake and increased breast cancer incidence risk [41].

2.2.15. Processed Meat

Table 15 reports the summary of linear dose-response meta-analyses of prospective studies on processed meat intake and CVD, CHD, stroke, T2DM, CRC, and breast cancer.

Table 15. Summary of linear dose-response meta-analyses of prospective studies on processed meat intake and CVD, CHD, stroke, T2DM, CRC, breast cancer.

Authors, Year, Reference	No. of Studies	Each Increment Intake Per Day	RR (95% CI)	I^2 Statistic	p-Value for Heterogeneity	Begg's or Egger's Test p-Value
Abete 2014 [59]	6	50 g	CVD mortality 1.24 (1.09–1.40)	76.40%	0.0010	>0.100/>0.100
Wang 2016 [67]	10	50 g	CVD mortality 1.15 (1.07–1.24)	75.40%	<0.0100	≥0.370/≥0.540
Bechthold 2017 [17]	3	50 g	CHD 1.27 (1.09–1.49)	0.00%	0.5100	NR
Bechthold 2017 [17]	6	50 g	Stroke 1.17 (1.02–1.34)	56.00%	0.0500	NR
Aune 2009 [60]	8	50 g	T2DM 1.57 (1.28–1.93)	74.00%	<0.0001	NR
Feskens 2013 [61]	21	50 g	T2DM 1.32 (1.19–1.48)	89.00%	NR	NR
Schwingshackl 2017 [18]	14	50 g	T2DM 1.37 (1.22–1.55)	88.00%	NR	NR
Larsson 2006 [62]	11	30 g	CRC 1.09 (1.05–1.13)	0.00%	0.7800	NR
Chan 2011 [64]	9	50 g	CRC incidence 1.18 (1.10–1.28)	12.20%	0.3330	NS
Vieira 2017 [20]	10	50 g	CRC 1.18 (1.10–1.28)	11.00%	0.3400	NS
Zhao 2017 [65]	8	50 g	CRC 1.22 (1.12–1.33)	19.00%	0.2800	NR
Schwingshackl 2018 [21]	16	50 g	CRC 1.17 (1.10–1.23)	6.00%	0.3900	0.660
Guo 2015 [66]	7	50 g	Breast cancer 1.09 (1.03–1.16)	NR	>0.100	NR
Wu 2016 [41]	20	50 g	Breast cancer incidence 1.09 (1.02–1.17)	11.80%	0.3290	0.945/0.566

CVD, cardiovascular disease; CHD, coronary heart disease; T2DM, type 2 diabetes mellitus; CRC, colorectal cancer; RR, relative risk; NR, not reported; NS, not significant.

Each daily increment of 50 g of processed meat intake increased CHD risk by 27% [17]. Each daily increment intake of 30 g increased CRC risk by 9% [62]. Each daily increment intake of 50 g increased CRC risk from 17% to 22% [20,21,64,65]. In two dose-response meta-analyses, the risk of breast cancer was increased by 9% with each increment of 50 g/day of processed meat [41,66]. The heterogeneity between the studies was below 50%.

Nonlinear dose-response analyses. There was no evidence of nonlinear dose-response association between processed meat and CHD or stroke risk. No association was found between processed meat intake and CHD risk while the risk of stroke increased by ~15% with a processed meat intake up to 70 g/day [17]. A nonlinear positive dose-response association was evident between processed meat intake and T2DM with a risk increase of ~30% up to 50 g/day and moderate further increase in risk for additional intakes [18]. The dose response association between processed meat intake and increased CRC risk was linear and an intake up to ~60 g/day increased the risk of ~20% [21]. The relation between processed meat intake and increased risk of breast cancer incidence was linear [41].

2.2.16. Poultry

Table 16 reports the summary of linear dose-response meta-analyses of prospective studies on poultry intake and T2DM, CRC, and breast cancer.

Each daily 50 g increment of poultry intake reduced by 11% and 3% the risk of CRC incidence and mortality, respectively [68]. Each 120 g daily increment intake of poultry reduced the risk of breast cancer incidence by 3% [41]. The heterogeneity between the studies was below 50%.

Nonlinear dose-response analyses. No evidence of a nonlinear association between poultry intake and CRC incidence was found: along with the increment in poultry intake up to ~90 g/day the RRs decreased up to ~15% [68]. No association was found between poultry intake and risk of breast cancer incidence [41].

Table 16. Summary of linear dose-response meta-analyses of prospective studies on poultry intake and CVD, CHD, stroke, T2DM, CRC, breast cancer.

Authors, Year, Reference	No. of Studies	Each Increment Intake Per Day	RR (95% CI)	I² Statistic	p-Value for Heterogeneity	Begg's or Egger's Test p-Value
Feskens 2013 [61]	10	100 g	T2DM 1.04 (0.82–1.32)	51.00%	NR	NR
Shi 2015 [68]	16	50 g	CRC incidence 0.89 (0.81–0.97)	41.20%	0.043	0.140
Shi 2015 [68]	4	50 g	CRC mortality 0.97 (0.79–1.20)	0.00%	0.695	NR
Wu 2016 [41]	10	120 g	Breast cancer incidence 0.97 (0.85–1.11)	33.20%	NR	0.107/0.090

T2DM, type 2 diabetes mellitus; CRC, colorectal cancer; RR, relative risk; NR, not reported.

2.2.17. Wine

A dose-response meta-analysis of seven prospective studies evaluating the associations between alcohol intake and CVD mortality (fatal CVD, fatal CHD, fatal ischemic heart disease) showed a J-shaped curve with a maximal reduction in RRs of 34% at 24 g/day of alcohol intake from wine [69]. However, the reduction in risk of ~34% was similar for intakes from ~10 to 30 g of alcohol from wine.

A dose-response meta-analysis between wine intake and T2DM risk, carried out on 13 prospective studies, showed a U-shaped association: all levels of daily wine intakes < 80 g were associated with a risk reduction and the lowest risk (20% of reduction) was evident at 20–30 g of daily intake of wine [70].

3. Discussion

3.1. Whole Grains

The intake of whole grains had a protective effect toward CVD [16], CHD [16,17], stroke [16], T2DM [18], and CRC risk [19,21]. Overall, a whole grain intake above 210 g/day is not necessary to obtain benefits on CVD, CHD, stroke, T2DM, and CRC risk.

Biological plausibility of such protective actions should be found in a beneficial effect of whole grain toward cardio-metabolic risk factors. RCTs and its meta-analyses showed a beneficial effect of whole grains compared with refined grains against CVD risk factors such as systolic and pulse blood pressure in healthy persons [71], diastolic blood pressure in overweight and obese adults [72], total and LDL cholesterol in healthy individuals [73], post-prandial blood glucose and insulin and the maximal glucose and insulin response in healthy subjects [74], post-prandial blood glucose and peripheral insulin resistance in obese adults [75], low-grade inflammation in overweight and obese subjects [76]. Fiber and many bioactive components in bran and in the germ are involved in this protective activity [77].

The MDPPI suggests 1 or 2 servings, three times a day. We propose that each serving of whole grain is 30 g with a total amount of 90–180 g/day. Wholemeal wheat sourdough bread, stoneground heat bread, wholemeal pasta, brown rice, whole grain cereals should be eaten every day. The intake of whole grains should be made by substituting food based on refined flours in order to avoid the increase of daily energy intake [78]. The intake of whole grain sourdough bread typical of the Mediterranean Diet of the early 1960s in Nicotera and maybe in Crete and Corfu is particularly recommended for its low glycemic index (GI) (revised in [9]). Italian law allows defining, as whole grain food, the products obtained by whole grain flour as well as the ones derived from refined flour added with bran or middling but it establishes that in this last case the single components (flour, bran and middling) should be clearly indicated [79]. Therefore, consumers' choice should be made through a careful exam of the labels on foodstuffs. In the case of whole grain bread bought in bakeries, Italian law does not enforce the declaration of the quantities of the ingredients so it is impossible to establish the quantity of whole grain flour in the final product or whether it is a compound product of refined flour added with bran or middling [80].

3.2. Vegetables and Fruits

3.2.1. Vegetables

In the nonlinear dose-response analyses, the highest reduction in RRs for CVD was reported at intakes of 600 g/day [24,29]. The maximal reductions in RRs of CHD were evident at 550–600 g/day [17,24] and of stroke at 500 g/day [24], respectively. The benefits on T2DM risk were minimal and obtained at intakes up to ~200–300 g/day [18,27]. The benefits on CRC risk were found up to ~200 g/day of intakes and not above [21].

The MDPPI suggests at least 2 servings of vegetables during the three main meals or, as an alternative, in the breaks between the main meals as snack. We propose that each serving of vegetables in the MDPPI is 100 g.

3.2.2. Fruits

In dose-response analysis the associations between daily fruit intakes and CVD [24,29], CHD [17,24,25], stroke [17,24,30], T2DM [18,26,27,31], and CRC [21] had the highest reductions in RRs at intakes of ~200–300 g/day but for CVD risk further benefits were evident up to ~500–800 g/day of intakes [24,29].

The MDPPI recommends 1–2 servings, three times a day. We propose that each serving of fruits is 100 g.

The protective mechanisms of increasing vegetable and fruit intake toward CVD risk include decreasing blood pressure, regulation of lipids metabolism, reducing oxidative stress and low-grade inflammation [81–83]. The high content of antioxidants (flavonoids, vitamin C, Vitamin E, ß-carotene) reduces DNA damaging [84]. The protective effects of fruit intake toward T2DM depend on their richness in fiber that improves insulin sensitivity and reduces the risk of weight gain [31].

An increased intake of fruits and vegetables should be encouraged in their quantities as well as in their variety since different colors ensure the provision of different micronutrients in a well balanced diet [85]. The protective effect of the intake of fruits and vegetables over the risk of CVD depends on the richness in fiber, vitamins, minerals, phytochemicals which ensures antioxidant and anti-inflammatory effects as well as low glycemic load (GL) and energetic density [85].

3.3. Dairy (Milk, Cheese, Yogurt)

3.3.1. Milk

According to a nonlinear dose-response meta-analysis, a daily intake of ~100 mL of milk reduces the risk of stroke by ~12% [42]. The protective effect of skim milk intake toward T2DM or breast cancer incidence was more evident at greater intakes of ~600 g/day [36,41]. Also, the protective effect of milk intake toward CRC was more evident at greater intakes of ~500–800 g [39].

3.3.2. Cheese

In dose-response analysis the protective effect of cheese intake toward CVD, stroke and T2DM was evident for little intakes up to ~40 g/day [44], ~25 g/day [35], ~50 g/day [36], respectively without benefits for greater intakes.

3.3.3. Yogurt

The protective effect of little daily quantities of yogurt intake was evident toward T2DM. The highest reductions in RRs were found up to 120–140 g/day [36] or 80 g/day [38] without benefits for higher intakes.

Overall these data indicated that small daily quantities of dairy products could have a protective effect toward CVD, stroke, and T2DM risk. The protective effect of milk and low-fat dairy on stroke risk could be in relation to a reduced incidence of hypertension [86]. It is worth noting that in a number of cheeses many angiotensin I-converting enzyme inhibitory peptides were identified [87,88].

The MDPPI suggests 2–3 servings, a day. We propose that 1 serving of milk is 50 g, 1 serving of yogurt is 50 g, 1 serving of cheese is 30 g.

Low-fat dairy should be preferably chosen. There is evidence that low-fat dairy has a better beneficial effect than high-fat dairy in the prevention of T2DM [89] and of CVD mortality [90]. A review of a number of RCTs concluded that there was not enough evidence of an unfavorable effect of dairy products on the cardio-metabolic risk factors (lipids, blood pressure, inflammation, insulin resistance, vascular function) independently from their fat content, and that the possible unfavorable effect of saturated fatty acids could be nullified if they are consumed in the frame of the dairy food matrix [91].

Moreover, it should be considered that, in the evaluation of the cardio-metabolic effects of dairy food in the RCTs, the quality of diet of the control group is of fundamental importance. For instance, a recent RCT evaluated the cardio-metabolic effects of 5 iso-energetic diets (cheese, butter, carbohydrate, monounsaturated fatty acids and polyunsaturated fatty acids diets), and found that LDL cholesterol was significantly lower after the cheese diet compared to the butter diet, but significantly higher than the carbohydrate, the monounsaturated fatty acids and the polyunsaturated fatty acids diets. No meaningful difference was noted among the 5 diets on risk factors such as inflammation markers, blood pressure and glucose-insulin homeostasis [92]. The matrix effect in this study is limited to the metabolism of cholesterol for the lack of increase of LDL cholesterol after cheese intake compared to butter. Indeed, the calcium contained in cheese can link the saturated fatty acids in the intestine and increase their fecal excretion [92].

3.4. Nuts

In dose-response analyses the maximal reduction in risk were observed at ~15 g/day for CVD [46], at ~15–20 g/day [46] or at ~10–15 g/day [17] for CHD. Similarly, the maximal risk reduction was observed at ~10–15 g/day [46] or at 12 g/day [48] for stroke risk.

A favorable effect of nuts on CVD health is biologically plausible considering the unique composition of these monounsaturated fatty acids and polyunsaturated fatty acids, fiber, magnesium, arginine and polyphenols rich food [93]. Possible effects include a reduction of low-grade inflammation, oxidative stress, endothelial dysfunction and an improvement of the lipid profile and of insulin resistance [94].

The MDPPI recommends 1 or 2 servings, of nuts a day. We propose that 1 serving of nut is 15 g.

3.5. Olive Oil

The dose-response analysis showed a protective effect of olive oil intake toward T2DM risk. It decreased to 13% with increasing intake up to ~15–20 g/day and no benefits were evident above these intakes [18].

Olive oil has been defined as the hallmark of Mediterranean Diet [49]. In Nicotera, in the late 1950s, the intake of olive oil provided 13–17% of total daily energy [95].

A meta-analysis of RCTs supported a cardiovascular protective role of olive oil for its beneficial effects on low-grade inflammation and endothelial function [96]. The biological plausibility of a protective effect on T2DM risk depends on some extra virgin olive oil components. Indeed, the monounsaturated fatty acids (compared to the saturated fatty acids) [97] and the polyphenols improve insulin sensitivity in many ways and therefore the T2DM risk [98].

The MDPPI suggests an intake of 3–4 servings of extra virgin olive oil, per day. We propose that 1 serving of extra virgin olive oil is 10 g.

3.6. Spices and Herbs

No dose-response meta-analyses were identified for spice and herb intake and CVD, CHD, stroke, T2DM, CRC and breast cancer.

Because of their high phenolic component content, spices and herbs have antioxidant power, anti-inflammatory and anti-mutagen properties, and therefore they can have a role in the prevention of CVD, T2DM, cancer and other degenerative diseases that have the oxidative stress as an important cause [99]. Not only does their use add flavor to food but also contributes to the decrease of salt intake. The WHO recommends a reduction of < 5 g/day salt (<2 g/day sodium) in order to reduce blood pressure and CVD, CHD and stroke risks [100].

The MDPPI recommends a daily intake of herbs and spices.

3.7. Fish and Shellfish

The dose-response association between fish intake and CHD mortality had the maximal reduction in RRs at ~30–60 g of daily fish intake without any further benefits for lower and higher intakes [52]. In another meta-analysis, a daily intake of fish as little as 20 g reduced the CHD mortality of 7% [54].

In a broad review that evaluated the relationship between fish or fish oil intake and CHD mortality in prospective cohort studies and RCTs, the intake of 250 mg/day of eicosapentaenoic acid and docosahexaenoic acid reduced CHD mortality by 36% without further reductions for higher intakes [101]. These intakes are easily obtained with two-100 g servings a week of which at least one is blue fish (www.ieo.it/bda).

The n-3 polyunsaturated fatty acids of fish reduce the CVD risk with an anti-inflammatory, antiarrhythmic and antiplatelet aggregation effect [102]. An RCT meta-analysis reported that the intake of oily fish was associated with a significant reduction of plasma triglycerides and to a significant increase of HDL cholesterol [103]. Moreover, an RCT meta-analysis did not highlight any n-3 polyunsaturated fatty acids effect on insulin sensitivity [104].

The MDPPI suggests a fish intake ≥2 servings a week (preferably fatty fish). We propose that 1 serving of fish or shellfish is 100 g.

3.8. Legumes

A protective effect of legume intake on CHD risk was evident up to ~100 g/day without benefits for higher intakes [17].

Legumes include lentils, beans, chickpeas, peas, peanuts, soya and other podded plants [105]. Beans, lentils, chickpeas and peas are high in fiber, protein and low in fat and are also called pulses [106]. The above studies do not allow a differentiation between fresh and dry legumes.

The MDPPI recommends an intake of ≥2 servings a week of legumes. We propose that 1 serving of fresh legumes is 100 g and 1 serving of pulses is 50 g.

Coherently to the Mediterranean tradition, legumes should partially replace protein food of animal origin.

3.9. Eggs

No association between egg intake and CHD or stroke risk was found (up to 1 egg/day) whereas the association between egg intake and breast cancer showed an increment of the risk above an intake of 5 eggs/week (Table 11). The biological plausibility of a lack of an unfavorable effect of a higher intake of eggs over the risk of CHD and stroke is provided by RCTs that did not find a worsening in CVD risk markers (lipid profile, body weight) in greater consumers of eggs (up to 1 egg/day) [107]. An increase of the intake of cholesterol with the diet does not have a negative impact on the lipid profile because in about 75% of the population leads to a reduction of the absorption of the same and/or of its synthesis and therefore a moderate or absent difference in serum cholesterol (normal or hypo-responders subjects) [108]. In hyper-responding subjects, the dietary increase of cholesterol leads to an increase of LDL cholesterol but also of HDL cholesterol with minimal effects on the LDL/HDL ratio [109]. The saturated fatty acids and the trans-fatty acids represent the major determiners of the total and LDL cholesterol [110]. The increased risk of breast cancer at egg intake >5/week could happen in subjects whose serum cholesterol levels are influenced by dietary intake and an excess of cholesterol may increase the risk of breast cancer through an increase of sexual hormones that promote cellular proliferation [57].

The MDPPI advised an intake of 2–4 eggs/week.

3.10. Refined Grains

The nonlinear dose-response analyses indicated that the RRs of CHD [17] and T2DM [18] were greater than 1.00 for intakes higher than ~100–120 g/day. The risk of T2DM increased by 6–14% with an intake of 200–400 g/day of refined grains [18].

The biological plausibility of an absence of a protective effect of refined grains respect to the whole ones against CHD, stroke and T2DM depends on the removal of fiber, micronutrients and minerals following the elimination of the bran and germ with cardio-metabolic protective effects [111]. Just like white potatoes and added sugar, refined cereals have a high GI and can increase the GL of the diet. They produce rapid glycemic and insulinemic peaks after the intake making way to adverse events such as stimulating reward/craving in cerebral areas, activation of the hepatic de novo lipogenesis and enabling visceral adiposity (reviewed in [111]). A recent international consensus established that low GI/GL diets reduce the risk of T2DM development in both sexes and they also reduce CHD risk mostly in women. These protective effects have greater relevance in sedentary, overweight or insulin resistant subjects. Low GI diets could have a protective effect against some cancer types such as CRC and breast cancer (reviewed in [112]).

The MDPPI recommends the limit of intake of refined grains of 3 servings a week. We propose that 1 serving of refined cereals is 60 g.

3.11. Potatoes

In nonlinear dose-response meta-analyses no association was found between daily potato intake and CHD or stroke, instead, the association between potato intake and T2DM or CRC showed increased risk above ~134 g/day. The increased risk of T2DM was mainly due to French fries intakes [58].

The MDPPI recommends the limit of intake of potatoes of 3 servings a week. We propose that one serving of potatoes is 100 g.

3.12. Red Meat and Processed Meat

3.12.1. Red Meat

In nonlinear dose-response meta-analyses, a red meat intake up to 100 g/day increased the CHD risk by 20% and of stroke by 10% [17]. The association between red meat intake and increased risk of T2DM [18], CRC [21] and breast cancer [41] was linear.

The MDPPI recommends the intake of ≤2 servings of red meat a week. We propose that 1 serving of red meat is 100 g.

3.12.2. Processed Meat

In nonlinear dose-response meta-analyses, the association between processed meat intake and CHD was null [17]. Otherwise the risk of stroke [17], T2DM [18], CRC [21] increased by 15%, 30%, and 20% with increased intakes above 70 g/day, 50 g/day and 60 g/day, respectively.

The MDPPI recommends an intake of processed meat of ≤1 serving per week. We propose that 1 serving is 50 g.

The mechanisms that link the intake of meat to NCDs risk involve a number of substances.

Haem iron has a pro-oxidant action that increases oxidative stress. The saturated fatty acids (processed meat is particularly rich) increase LDL cholesterol. Advanced glycation end products (which are found in animal products rich in fats and proteins especially if processed) have a pro-inflammatory action. Nitrates and nitrites (used in meat preservation) facilitate endothelial dysfunction, atherosclerosis and insulin resistance. Salt (used in meat preservation) has a hypertensive effect and it is a possible risk factor for gastric cancer. Polycyclic aromatic hydrocarbons and heterocyclic aromatic amines (which are formed during meat cooking at high temperatures) are carcinogenic especially for CRC (reviewed in [113–115]). A greater intake of red meat was in relation to a higher risk of CRC cancer. In 2015 the International Agency for Research on Cancer classified the intake of red meat as "probably carcinogenic for humans" and processed meat as "carcinogenic for humans" [116].

3.13. Poultry

In nonlinear dose-response meta-analyses, an intake of ~90 g/day of poultry reduced CRC incidence by ~15% [68].

The MDPPI suggests that poultry intake should be ≤2 servings a week. We propose that one serving is 100 g.

3.14. Sweets and Cakes and Cookies

No dose-response meta-analyses were identified for sweet/cake/cookie intakes.

The vast majority of sweets contain carbohydrates, which are rapidly digested such as refined flours and high GI sugar, which can increase the GL diet. They are often rich in industrial trans fatty acids [117] that increase CHD and sudden death risk because of the unfavorable effects on the lipid profile, insulin resistance, visceral adiposity, endothelial inflammation and dysfunction [111]. An occasional intake of sweets probably does not have a negative impact on health as opposed to a regular intake.

The MDPPI recommends an intake of ≤2 servings of sweets a week. We propose that 1 serving is 25 g. This quantity was arbitrarily decided.

3.15. Wine

Based on 2 dose-response meta-analyses the greater protection against CVD mortality was evident at 15–30 g of daily intake of alcohol from wine [69], and against T2DM risk at 20–30 g/day of wine [70].

The cardio-metabolic protective effects of light to moderate alcohol intake depend on an increase of HDL cholesterol and of adiponectin, a reduction of the low-grade inflammation, an improvement of insulin sensitivity, and endothelial function (reviewed in [118]).

The MDPPI suggests a moderate intake of red wine during meals. We propose that 1 serving is 10 g of ethanol and up to 3 serving and up to 1 serving and half were indicated for men and women, respectively.

Although these quantities are obtained from a little number of meta-analyses, several reviews indicated similar intakes of alcohol as optimal [118–120]. A regular and moderate wine intake during meals is a "Mediterranean way of drinking" [121].

4. Second Section

Methods and Results

Based on frequencies and serving sizes indicated in Table 17 we built a weekly menu plan (Supplementary Table S1).

For some food groups, we calculated equivalents portions: 30 g-whole grain servings were 30 g of wholemeal pasta or whole rice or whole barley or whole spelled, 40 g of wholemeal sourdough bread, 20 g of breakfast cereals; 60 g-refined grain servings were 60 g of white pasta, 80 g of white bread; 100 g-fruit servings were 70 g of figs or grapes or prickly pears and 130 g of apricots or peaches or medlars. Nutritional diet composition is in Table 18.

Table 17. Mediterranean Diet Pyramid proposed for Italian people (MDPPI).

Food Groups	Frequency of Intake	Serving Size (g, mL, on Average)
Whole grains	1–2 servings every main meal (three meals)	30 g
Fruits	1–2 servings every main meal (three meals)	100 g
Vegetables	≥2 servings every main meal (three meals)	100 g
Milk and dairy (preferably low-fat)	2–3 servings/day	Milk 50 mL; Yogurt 50 g; Cheese 30 g
Nuts	1–2 servings/day	15 g
Extra Virgin Olive oil	3–4 servings/day	10 g
Herbs and spices	use them every day	
Fish and shellfish	≥2 servings/week	100 g
Poultry	1–2 servings/week	100 g
Legumes	≥2 servings/week	100 g fresh, 50 g dry
Eggs	2–4 servings/week	1 egg
Refined grains	≤3 servings/week	60 g
Potatoes	≤3 servings/week	100 g
Red meat	≤2 servings/week	100 g
Processed meat	≤1 serving/week	50 g
Sweets	≤2 servings/week	25 g
Red wine	≤2 glasses/day for men; ≤1 glass/day for women	15 g of alcohol

Table 18. Nutritional composition (mean of 7 days) and number of servings of weekly menu plan built on advice of Mediterranean Diet Pyramid for Italian People.

Energy intake: 1998.85 kcal/day	
Carbohydrates: 246.67 g (46.3%)	
Protein: 82.31 g (16.5%) vegetal protein 49.27 g and animal protein 30.64 g	
Fats: 71.08 g (32%): SFAs 13.26 g (6.1% of total kcal), MUFAs 36.13 g, PUFAs,11.82 g	
Fiber: 47.48 g	
Ethanol: 15 g	
Red Wine: 5.2% of total kcal	1 drink/day
Olive oil: 13.5% of total kcal	3 servings/day
Potatoes: 1.9% of total kcal	3 servings/week
Legumes: 6.7% of total kcal	1 serving/day
Refined grains: 3.9% of total kcal	3 servings/week
Whole grains: 27.4% of total kcal	2 servings at every main meal (6 servings/day)
Vegetables: 5.7% of total kcal	2 servings at every main meal (6 servings/day)
Fresh fruits: 11% of total kcal	2 servings at every main meal (6 servings/day)
Nuts: 9.1% of total kcal	2 servings/day
Processed meat: 0.9% of total kcal	1 serving/week
Red Meat: 1.4% of total kcal	2 servings/week
Poultry: 1.4% of total kcal	2 servings/week
Milk and dairy: 4.1% of total kcal	2 servings/day
Fish and shellfish: 3.5% of total kcal	3 servings/week
Eggs: 1.4% of total kcal	2 eggs/week
Sweets: 1.8% of total kcal	2 servings/week
MAI [77]: 8	
Average weekly GI: 46%	
Average weekly GL: 115.89	
Total calories provided from vegetable food: 77%	
Total calories provided from animal food: 23%	

SFAs, saturated fatty acids; MUFAs, monounsaturated fatty acids; PUFA, polyunsaturated fatty acids; MAI, Mediterranean Adequacy index; GI, glycemic index; GL, glycemic load.

5. Discussion

The diet built according the advice of MDPPI (Table 17) was very similar to that of Nicotera in the late 1950s that has been chosen as Italian Reference Mediterranean Diet [95] with the exception of percentage of energy provided by cereals that was lower and of fruits and vegetables that was higher. Indeed, Fidanza reported the following percentages of total energy of food groups: cereal (50–59%), virgin olive oil (13–17%), vegetables (2.2–3.6%), potatoes (2.3–4.4%), legumes (3–6%), fruits (2.6–3.6% including nuts that were about 3% of the weight of all fruits), fish (1.6–2.0%), red wine (1–6%), meat (2.6–5.0%), dairy (2–4%). The intake of eggs and animal fats was rare [95]. Saturated fatty acids were only the 6% of daily energy intake. Also the MAI was very close to the MAI of the diet in 1960 that was 9.4 for males and 11.4 for females living in Nicotera [122].

6. Conclusions

The MDPPI represents a modification proposal of the Modern Mediterranean Diet Pyramid presented during the third conference of CIISCAM (Centro Interuniversitario Internazionale di Studi sulle Culture Alimentari Mediterranee) in Parma, Italy, on November 3, 2009 (www.inran.it). In the MDPPI the modification interested cereal food, which were divided into two groups. The whole grain cereal derived foods, which are at the base of the pyramid and the foods derived from refined flour, which are at the top of the pyramid along with other food to be consumed with moderation. The presence at the bottom of the pyramid of wholemeal wheat sourdough bread and stoneground wheat bread is remarkable because they were typically used in Nicotera in the beginning of the 1960s and probably also in Crete and Corfu. They are rich in fiber and have a low GI (reviewed in [9]). Refined cereal foods are placed at the top of the pyramid for their possible unfavorable cardio-metabolic effects [111]. According to a recent survey the consumption of whole grain foods in Italy is quite low [123].

The present study is a systematic review of dose-response meta-analyses of prospective studies, which evaluated the relationship among food groups and selected nutrition-related NCDs such as CVD including CHD and stroke, T2DM, CRC and breast cancer. Our purpose has been to derive from these meta-analyses serving sizes of food group belonging to MDPPI with a protective (Mediterranean food) or a non-adverse (non-Mediterranean food) effect toward the above mentioned NCDs. Subsequently we have evaluated the compatibility of a weekly menu plan built according the MDPPI advice, with the Nicotera diet in the late 1950s. Only for sweets/cakes/cookies the lack of dose-response meta-analyses led us to define an arbitrarily serving size. In our opinion, the advice of the MDPPI as dietary pattern well defined into its characteristics as quantity and frequency of intake is compatible with the Reference Italian Mediterranean Diet. It is a plant-based dietary pattern [124] rich in high quality plant food that lowers the risk of T2DM [125] and CHD [126].

However, our study has some limitations. A first limit is given by the fact that the distinction between some food groups is not precise and there are overlaps. For example, the vegetable group includes beans, peas, potatoes, herbs as onions and garlic and so on; the legumes group includes peanuts that are often included in the nuts group. Another limit is that the single items of food groups could be not identical to those typical of Mediterranean area. The level of evidence that is variable in several meta-analyses depending on the quality of the studies considered, the strength of the associations and the presence of heterogeneity represent another limit.

All in all, we think that the MDPPI can represent a valid instrument for the definition of Mediterranean Diet that must also consider the types of food, the amounts, and their intake frequency. The indicated amounts are compatible both with the studies which evaluated the effect of the intake of food groups on different diet-correlated NCDs outcomes and the ones of the Italian Reference Mediterranean Diet of the late 1950s.

Supplementary Materials: The following are available online at http://www.mdpi.com/2072-6643/11/6/1296/s1, Table S1: Weekly menu plan based on advice of Mediterranean Diet Pyramid for Italian People.

Author Contributions: A.D. conceived the study, developed the selection criteria, performed the literature search and drafted the manuscript. L.L. planned the weekly menu and evaluated its nutritional composition. G.D.P. contributed to literature search and reviewed the manuscript. All the authors read and approved the final version of the manuscript.

Funding: This research received no external funding.

Acknowledgments: We acknowledge Giovanni Misciagna for his critical review.

Conflicts of Interest: The authors declare no conflict of interest.

References

1. WHO. Global Health Observatory Data. Available online: http://www.who.int (accessed on 13 December 2018).
2. WHO. Noncommunicable Diseases (NCD) Country Profiles, Italy. 2018. Available online: http://www.who.int (accessed on 13 December 2018).
3. Ezzati, M.; Riboli, E. Can noncommunicable diseases be prevented? Lessons from studies of populations and individuals. *Science* **2012**, *337*, 1482–1487. [CrossRef] [PubMed]
4. Kimokoti, R.W.; Millen, B.E. Nutrition for the Prevention of Chronic Diseases. *Med. Clin. N. Am.* **2016**, *100*, 1185–1198. [CrossRef] [PubMed]
5. Scientific Report of the 2015 Dietary Guidelines Advisory Committee. Available online: http://health.gov/dietaryguidelines/2015-scientific-report/ (accessed on 13 February 2018).
6. Fidanza, F. Who remembers the true Italian Mediterranean diet? *Diabetes Nutr. Metab.* **2001**, *14*, 119–120. [PubMed]
7. Alberti-Fidanza, A.; Fidanza, F.; Chiuchiù, M.P.; Verducci, G.; Fruttini, D. Dietary studies on two rural Italian population groups of the Seven Countries Study. 3. Trend of food and nutrient intake from 1960 to 1991. *Eur. J. Clin. Nutr.* **1999**, *53*, 854–860. [CrossRef] [PubMed]
8. Menotti, A.; Kromhout, D.; Blackburn, H.; Fidanza, F.; Buzina, R.; Nissinen, A. Food intake patterns and 25-year mortality from coronary heart disease: Cross-cultural correlations in the Seven Countries Study. The Seven Countries Study Research Group. *Eur. J. Epidemiol.* **1999**, *15*, 507–515. [CrossRef] [PubMed]
9. D'Alessandro, A.; De Pergola, G. Mediterranean diet pyramid: A proposal for Italian people. *Nutrients* **2014**, *6*, 4302–4316. [CrossRef]
10. Fidanza, F.; Alberti, A. The Healthy Italian Mediterranean Diet Temple Food Guide. *Nutr. Today* **2005**, 71–78. [CrossRef]
11. Moher, D.; Liberati, A.; Tetzlaff, J.; Altman, D.G. Preferred reporting items for systematic reviews and meta-analyses: The PRISMA statement. *Ann. Intern. Med.* **2009**, *151*, 264–269. [CrossRef]
12. Benisi-Kohansal, S.; Saneei, P.; Salehi-Marzijarani, M.; Larijani, B.; Esmaillzadeh, A. Whole-Grain Intake and Mortality from All Causes, Cardiovascular Disease, and Cancer: A Systematic Review and Dose-Response Meta-Analysis of Prospective Cohort Studies. *Adv. Nutr.* **2016**, *7*, 1052–1065. [CrossRef]
13. Chen, G.C.; Tong, X.; Xu, J.Y.; Han, S.F.; Wan, Z.X.; Qin, J.B.; Qin, L.Q. Whole-grain intake and total, cardiovascular, and cancer mortality: A systematic review and meta-analysis of prospective studies. *Am. J. Clin. Nutr.* **2016**, *104*, 164–172. [CrossRef]
14. Li, B.; Zhang, G.; Tan, M.; Zhao, L.; Jin, L.; Tang, X.; Jiang, G.; Zhong, K. Consumption of whole grains in relation to mortality from all causes, cardiovascular disease, and diabetes: Dose-response meta-analysis of prospective cohort studies. *Medicine* **2016**, *95*, e4229. [CrossRef]
15. Wei, H.; Gao, Z.; Liang, R.; Li, Z.; Hao, H.; Liu, X. Whole-grain consumption and the risk of all-cause, CVD and cancer mortality: A meta-analysis of prospective cohort studies. *Br. J. Nutr.* **2016**, *116*, 514–525. [CrossRef]
16. Aune, D.; Keum, N.; Giovannucci, E.; Fadnes, L.T.; Boffetta, P.; Greenwood, D.C.; Tonstad, S.; Vatten, L.J.; Riboli, E.; Norat, T. Whole grain consumption and risk of cardiovascular disease, cancer, and all cause and cause specific mortality: Systematic review and dose-response meta-analysis of prospective studies. *Br. Med. J.* **2016**, *353*, i2716. [CrossRef]

17. Bechthold, A.; Boeing, H.; Schwedhelm, C.; Hoffmann, G.; Knüppel, S.; Iqbal, K.; De Henauw, S.; Michels, N.; Devleesschauwer, B.; Schlesinger, S.; et al. Food groups and risk of coronary heart disease, stroke and heart failure: A systematic review and dose-response meta-analysis of prospective studies. *Crit. Rev. Food Sci. Nutr.* **2019**, *59*, 1071–1090. [CrossRef]
18. Schwingshackl, L.; Hoffmann, G.; Lampousi, A.M.; Knüppel, S.; Iqbal, K.; Schwedhelm, C.; Bechthold, A.; Schlesinger, S.; Boeing, H. Food groups and risk of type 2 diabetes mellitus: A systematic review and meta-analysis of prospective studies. *Eur. J. Epidemiol.* **2017**, *32*, 363–375. [CrossRef]
19. Aune, D.; Chan, D.S.; Lau, R.; Vieira, R.; Greenwood, D.C.; Kampman, E.; Norat, T. Dietary fibre, whole grains, and risk of colorectal cancer: Systematic review and dose-response meta-analysis of prospective studies. *Br. Med. J.* **2011**, *343*, d6617. [CrossRef]
20. Vieira, A.R.; Abar, L.; Chan, D.S.M.; Vingeliene, S.; Polemiti, E.; Stevens, C.; Greenwood, D.; Norat, T. Foods and beverages and colorectal cancer risk: A systematic review and meta-analysis of cohort studies, an update of the evidence of the WCRF-AICR Continuous Update Project. *Ann. Oncol.* **2017**, *28*, 1788–1802. [CrossRef]
21. Schwingshackl, L.; Schwedhelm, C.; Hoffmann, G.; Knüppel, S.; Laure Preterre, A.; Iqbal, K.; Bechthold, A.; De Henauw, S.; Michels, N.; Devleesschauwer, B.; et al. Food groups and risk of colorectal cancer. *Int. J. Cancer* **2018**, *142*, 1748–1758. [CrossRef]
22. Zhang, B.; Zhao, Q.; Guo, W.; Bao, W.; Wang, X. Association of whole grain intake with all-cause, cardiovascular, and cancer mortality: A systematic review and dose-response meta-analysis from prospective cohort studies. *Eur. J. Clin. Nutr.* **2018**, *72*, 57–65. [CrossRef]
23. Zong, G.; Gao, A.; Hu, F.B.; Sun, Q. Whole Grain Intake and Mortality from all causes, Cardiovascular Disease, and Cancer: A Meta-Analysis of Prospective Cohort Studies. *Circulation* **2016**, *133*, 2370–2380. [CrossRef]
24. Aune, D.; Giovannucci, E.; Boffetta, P.; Fadnes, L.T.; Keum, N.; Norat, T.; Greenwood, D.C.; Riboli, E.; Vatten, L.J.; Tonstad, S. Fruit and vegetable intake and the risk of cardiovascular disease, total cancer and all-cause mortality-a systematic review and dose-response meta-analysis of prospective studies. *Int. J. Epidemiol.* **2017**, *46*, 1029–1056. [CrossRef]
25. Gan, Y.; Tong, X.; Li, L.; Cao, S.; Yin, X.; Gao, C.; Herath, C.; Li, W.; Jin, Z.; Chen, Y.; et al. Consumption of fruit and vegetable and risk of coronary heart disease: A meta-analysis of prospective cohort studies. *Int. J. Cardiol.* **2015**, *183*, 129–137. [CrossRef]
26. Li, M.; Fan, Y.; Zhang, X.; Hou, W.; Tang, Z. Fruit and vegetable intake and risk of type 2 diabetes mellitus: Meta-analysis of prospective cohort studies. *Br. Med. J.* **2014**, *4*, e005497. [CrossRef]
27. Wu, Y.; Zhang, D.; Jiang, X.; Jiang, W. Fruit and vegetable consumption and risk of type 2 diabetes mellitus: A dose-response meta-analysis of prospective cohort studies. *Nutr. Metab. Cardiovasc. Dis.* **2015**, *25*, 140–147. [CrossRef]
28. Aune, D.; Chan, D.S.; Vieira, A.R.; Rosenblatt, D.A.; Vieira, R.; Greenwood, D.C.; Norat, T. Fruits, vegetables and breast cancer risk: A systematic review and meta-analysis of prospective studies. *Breast Cancer Res. Treat.* **2012**, *134*, 479–493. [CrossRef]
29. Zhan, J.; Liu, Y.J.; Cai, L.B.; Xu, F.R.; Xie, T.; He, Q.Q. Fruit and vegetable consumption and risk of cardiovascular disease: A meta-analysis of prospective cohort studies. *Crit. Rev. Food Sci. Nutr.* **2017**, *57*, 1650–1663. [CrossRef]
30. Hu, D.; Huang, J.; Wang, Y.; Zhang, D.; Qu, Y. Fruits and vegetables consumption and risk of stroke: A meta-analysis of prospective cohort studies. *Stroke* **2014**, *45*, 1613–1619. [CrossRef]
31. Li, S.; Miao, S.; Huang, Y.; Liu, Z.; Tian, H.; Yin, X.; Tang, W.; Steffen, L.M.; Xi, B. Fruit intake decreases risk of incident type 2 diabetes: An updated meta-analysis. *Endocrine* **2015**, *48*, 454–460. [CrossRef]
32. Soedamah-Muthu, S.S.; Ding, E.L.; Al-Delaimy, W.K.; Hu, F.B.; Engberink, M.F.; Willett, W.C.; Geleijnse, J.M. Milk and dairy consumption and incidence of cardiovascular diseases and all-cause mortality: Dose-response meta-analysis of prospective cohort studies. *Am. J. Clin. Nutr.* **2011**, *93*, 158–171. [CrossRef]
33. Guo, J.; Astrup, A.; Lovegrove, J.A.; Gijsbers, L.; Givens, D.I.; Soedamah-Muthu, S.S. Milk and dairy consumption and risk of cardiovascular diseases and all cause mortality: Dose-response meta-analysis of prospective cohort studies. *Eur. J. Epidemiol.* **2017**, *32*, 269–287. [CrossRef]

34. Mullie, P.; Pizot, C.; Autier, P. Daily milk consumption and all-cause mortality, coronary heart disease and stroke: A systematic review and meta-analysis of observational cohort studies. *BMC Public Health.* **2016**, *16*, 1236. [CrossRef]
35. de Goede, J.; Soedamah-Muthu, S.S.; Pan, A.; Gijsbers, L.; Geleijnse, J.M. Dairy Consumption and Risk of Stroke: A Systematic Review and Updated Dose Response Meta-Analysis of Prospective Cohort Studies. *J. Am. Heart Assoc.* **2016**, *5*, e002787. [CrossRef]
36. Aune, D.; Norat, T.; Romundstad, P.; Vatten, L.J. Dairy products and the risk of type 2 diabetes: A systematic review and dose-response meta-analysis of cohort studies. *Am. J. Clin. Nutr.* **2013**, *98*, 1066–1083. [CrossRef]
37. Gao, D.; Ning, N.; Wang, C.; Wang, Y.; Li, Q.; Meng, Z.; Liu, Y.; Li, Q. Dairy products consumption and risk of type 2 diabetes: Systematic review and dose response meta-analysis. *PLoS ONE.* **2013**, *8*, e73965. [CrossRef]
38. Gijsbers, L.; Ding, E.L.; Malik, V.S.; de Goede, J.; Geleijnse, J.M.; Soedamah-Muthu, S.S. Consumption of dairy foods and diabetes incidence: A dose-response meta-analysis of observational studies. *Am. J. Clin. Nutr.* **2016**, *103*, 1111–1124. [CrossRef]
39. Aune, D.; Lau, R.; Chan, D.S.M.; Vieira, R.; Greenwood, D.C.; Kampman, E.; Norat, T. Dairy products and colorectal cancer risk: A systematic review and meta-analysis of cohort studies. *Ann. Oncol.* **2012**, *23*, 37–45. [CrossRef]
40. Dong, J.Y.; Zhang, L.; He, K.; Qin, L.Q. Dairy consumption and risk of breast cancer: A meta-analysis of prospective cohort studies. *Breast Cancer Res. Treat.* **2011**, *127*, 23–31. [CrossRef]
41. Wu, J.; Zeng, R.; Huang, J.; Li, X.; Zhang, J.; Ho, J.C.; Zheng, Y. Dietary Protein Sources and Incidence of Breast Cancer: A Dose-Response Meta-Analysis of Prospective Studies. *Nutrients* **2016**, *8*, 730. [CrossRef]
42. Hu, D.; Huang, J.; Wang, Y.; Zhang, D.; Qu, Y. Dairy foods and risk of stroke: A meta-analysis of prospective cohort studies. *Nutr. Metab. Cardiovasc. Dis.* **2014**, *24*, 460–469. [CrossRef]
43. Zang, J.; Shen, M.; Du, S.; Chen, T.; Zou, S. The Association between Dairy Intake and Breast Cancer in Western and Asian Populations: A Systematic Review and Meta-Analysis. *J. Breast Cancer* **2015**, *18*, 313–322. [CrossRef]
44. Chen, G.C.; Wang, Y.; Tong, X.; Szeto, I.M.Y.; Smit, G.; Li, Z.N.; Qin, L.Q. Cheese consumption and risk of cardiovascular disease: A meta-analysis of prospective studies. *Eur. J. Nutr.* **2017**, *56*, 2565–2575. [CrossRef]
45. Luo, C.; Zhang, Y.; Ding, Y.; Shan, Z.; Chen, S.; Yu, M.; Hu, F.B.; Liu, L. Nut consumption and risk of type 2 diabetes, cardiovascular disease, and all-cause mortality: A systematic review and meta-analysis. *Am. J. Clin. Nutr.* **2014**, *100*, 256–269. [CrossRef]
46. Aune, D.; Keum, N.; Giovannucci, E.; Fadnes, L.T.; Boffetta, P.; Greenwood, D.C.; Tonstad, S.; Vatten, L.J.; Riboli, E.; Norat, T. Nut consumption and risk of cardiovascular disease, total cancer, all-cause and cause-specific mortality: A systematic review and dose-response meta-analysis of prospective studies. *BMC Med.* **2016**, *14*, 207. [CrossRef]
47. Grosso, G.; Yang, J.; Marventano, S.; Micek, A.; Galvano, F.; Kales, S.N. Nut consumption on all-cause, cardiovascular, and cancer mortality risk: A systematic review and meta-analysis of epidemiologic studies. *Am. J. Clin. Nutr.* **2015**, *101*, 783–793. [CrossRef]
48. Shao, C.; Tang, H.; Zhao, W.; He, J. Nut intake and stroke risk: A dose-response meta-analysis of prospective cohort studies. *Sci. Rep.* **2016**, *6*, 30394. [CrossRef]
49. Martínez-González, M.A.; Dominguez, L.J.; Delgado-Rodríguez, M. Olive oil consumption and risk of CHD and/or stroke: A meta-analysis of case-control, cohort and intervention studies. *Br. J. Nutr.* **2014**, *112*, 248–259. [CrossRef]
50. Schwingshackl, L.; Lampousi, A.M.; Portillo, M.P.; Romaguera, D.; Hoffmann, G.; Boeing, H. Olive oil in the prevention and management of type 2 diabetes mellitus: A systematic review and meta-analysis of cohort studies and intervention trials. *Nutr. Diabetes* **2017**, *7*, e262. [CrossRef]
51. Jayedi, A.; Shab-Bidar, S.; Eimeri, S.; Djafarian, K. Fish consumption and risk of all-cause and cardiovascular mortality: A dose-response meta-analysis of prospective observational studies. *Public Health Nutr.* **2018**, *21*, 1297–1306. [CrossRef]
52. Zheng, J.; Huang, T.; Yu, Y.; Hu, X.; Yang, B.; Li, D. Fish consumption and CHD mortality: An updated meta-analysis of seventeen cohort studies. *Public Health Nutr.* **2012**, *15*, 725–737. [CrossRef]
53. Zheng, J.S.; Hu, X.J.; Zhao, Y.M.; Yang, J.; Li, D. Intake of fish and marine n-3 polyunsaturated fatty acids and risk of breast cancer: Meta-analysis of data from 21 independent prospective cohort studies. *Br. Med. J.* **2013**, *346*, f3706. [CrossRef]

54. He, K.; Song, Y.; Daviglus, M.L.; Liu, K.; Van Horn, L.; Dyer, A.R.; Greenland, P. Accumulated evidence on fish consumption and coronary heart disease mortality: A meta-analysis of cohort studies. *Circulation* **2004**, *109*, 2705–2711. [CrossRef]
55. Rong, Y.; Chen, L.; Zhu, T.; Song, Y.; Yu, M.; Shan, Z.; Sands, A.; Hu, F.B.; Liu, L. Egg consumption and risk of coronary heart disease and stroke: Dose-response meta-analysis of prospective cohort studies. *Br. Med. J.* **2013**, *346*, e8539. [CrossRef]
56. Tamez, M.; Virtanen, J.K.; Lajous, M. Egg consumption and risk of incident type 2 diabetes: A dose-response meta-analysis of prospective cohort studies. *Br. J. Nutr.* **2016**, *115*, 2212–2218. [CrossRef]
57. Keum, N.; Lee, D.H.; Marchand, N.; Oh, H.; Liu, H.; Aune, D.; Greenwood, D.C.; Giovannucci, E.L. Egg intake and cancers of the breast, ovary and prostate: A dose response meta-analysis of prospective observational studies. *Br. J. Nutr.* **2015**, *114*, 1099–1107. [CrossRef]
58. Schwingshackl, L.; Schwedhelm, C.; Hoffmann, G.; Boeing, H. Potatoes and risk of chronic disease: A systematic review and dose-response meta-analysis. *Eur. J. Nutr.* **2018**. [CrossRef]
59. Abete, I.; Romaguera, D.; Vieira, A.R.; Lopez de Munain, A.; Norat, T. Association between total, processed, red and white meat consumption and all cause, CVD and IHD mortality: A meta-analysis of cohort studies. *Br. J. Nutr.* **2014**, *112*, 762–775. [CrossRef]
60. Aune, D.; Ursin, G.; Veierød, M.B. Meat consumption and the risk of type 2 diabetes: A systematic review and meta-analysis of cohort studies. *Diabetologia* **2009**, *52*, 2277–2287. [CrossRef]
61. Feskens, E.J.; Sluik, D.; van Woudenbergh, G.J. Meat consumption, diabetes, and its complications. *Curr. Diab. Rep.* **2013**, *13*, 298–306. [CrossRef]
62. Larsson, S.C.; Wolk, A. Meat consumption and risk of colorectal cancer: A meta-analysis of prospective studies. *Int. J. Cancer* **2006**, *119*, 2657–2664. [CrossRef]
63. Alexander, D.D.; Weed, D.L.; Cushing, C.A.; Lowe, K.A. Meta-analysis of prospective studies of red meat consumption and colorectal cancer. *Eur. J. Cancer Prev.* **2011**, *20*, 293–307. [CrossRef]
64. Chan, D.S.; Lau, R.; Aune, D.; Vieira, R.; Greenwood, D.C.; Kampman, E.; Norat, T. Red and processed meat and colorectal cancer incidence: Meta-analysis of prospective studies. *PLoS ONE* **2011**, *6*, e20456. [CrossRef]
65. Zhao, Z.; Feng, Q.; Yin, Z.; Shuang, J.; Bai, B.; Yu, P.; Guo, M.; Zhao, Q. Red and processed meat consumption and colorectal cancer risk: A systematic review and meta-analysis. *Oncotarget* **2017**, *8*, 83306–83314. [CrossRef]
66. Guo, J.; Wei, W.; Zhan, L. Red and processed meat intake and risk of breast cancer: A meta-analysis of prospective studies. *Breast Cancer Res. Treat.* **2015**, *151*, 191–198. [CrossRef]
67. Wang, X.; Lin, X.; Ouyang, Y.Y.; Liu, J.; Zhao, G.; Pan, A.; Hu, F.B. Red and processed meat consumption and mortality: Dose-response meta-analysis of prospective cohort studies. *Public Health Nutr.* **2016**, *19*, 893–905. [CrossRef]
68. Shi, Y.; Yu, P.W.; Zeng, D.Z. Dose-response meta-analysis of poultry intake and colorectal cancer incidence and mortality. *Eur. J. Nutr.* **2015**, *54*, 243–250. [CrossRef]
69. Costanzo, S.; Di Castelnuovo, A.; Donati, M.B.; Iacoviello, L.; de Gaetano, G. Wine, beer or spirit drinking in relation to fatal and nonfatal cardiovascular events: A meta-analysis. *Eur. J. Epidemiol.* **2011**, *26*, 833–850. [CrossRef]
70. Huang, J.; Wang, X.; Zhang, Y. Specific types of alcoholic beverage consumption and risk of type 2 diabetes: A systematic review and meta-analysis. *J. Diabetes Investig.* **2017**, *8*, 56–68. [CrossRef]
71. Tighe, P.; Duthie, G.; Vaughan, N.; Brittenden, J.; Simpson, W.G.; Duthie, S.; Mutch, W.; Wahle, K.; Horgan, G.; Thies, F. Effect of increased consumption of whole-grain foods on blood pressure and other cardiovascular risk markers in healthy middle-aged persons: A randomized controlled trial. *Am. J. Clin. Nutr.* **2010**, *92*, 733–740. [CrossRef]
72. Kirwan, J.P.; Malin, S.K.; Scelsi, A.R.; Kullman, E.L.; Navaneethan, S.D.; Pagadala, M.R.; Haus, J.M.; Filion, J.; Godin, J.P.; Kochhar, S.; et al. A Whole-Grain Diet Reduces Cardiovascular Risk Factors in Overweight and Obese Adults: A Randomized Controlled Trial. *J. Nutr.* **2016**, *146*, 2244–2251. [CrossRef]
73. Hollænder, P.L.; Ross, A.B.; Kristensen, M. Whole-grain and blood lipid changes in apparently healthy adults: A systematic review and meta-analysis of randomized controlled studies. *Am. J. Clin. Nutr.* **2015**, *102*, 556–572. [CrossRef]
74. Marventano, S.; Vetrani, C.; Vitale, M.; Godos, J.; Riccardi, G.; Grosso, G. Whole grain intake and glycaemic control in healthy subjects: A systematic review and meta-analysis of randomized controlled trials. *Nutrients* **2017**, *9*, 769. [CrossRef]

75. Malin, S.K.; Kullman, E.L.; Scelsi, A.R.; Haus, J.M.; Filion, J.; Pagadala, M.R.; Godin, J.P.; Kochhar, S.; Ross, A.B.; Kirwan, J.P. A whole–grain diet reduces peripheral insulin resistance and improves glucose kinetics in obese adults: A randomized-controlled trial. *Metabolism* **2018**, *82*, 111–117. [CrossRef]
76. Vitaglione, P.; Mennella, I.; Ferracane, R.; Rivellese, A.A.; Giacco, R.; Ercolini, D.; Gibbons, S.M.; La Storia, A.; Gilbert, J.A.; Jonnalagadda, S.; et al. Whole-grain wheat consumption reduces inflammation in a randomized controlled trial on overweight and obese subjects with unhealthy dietary and lifestyle behaviors: Role of polyphenols bound to cereal dietary fiber. *Am. J. Clin. Nutr.* **2015**, *101*, 251–261. [CrossRef]
77. Fardet, A. New hypotheses for the health-protective mechanisms of whole-grain cereals: What is beyond fibre? *Nutr. Res. Rev.* **2010**, *23*, 65–134. [CrossRef]
78. Mann, K.D.; Pearce, M.S.; Seal, C.J. Providing evidence to support the development of whole grain dietary recommendations in the United Kingdom. *Proc. Nutr. Soc.* **2017**, *76*, 369–377. [CrossRef]
79. Gazzetta Ufficiale, N. 4 of 7th January 2004. Available online: http://www.gazzettaufficiale.it/eli/id/2004/01/07/03A14210/sg (accessed on 15 February 2018).
80. Sette, S.; D'Addezio, L.; Piccinelli, R.; Hopkins, S.; Le Donne, C.; Ferrari, M.; Mistura, L.; Turrini, A. Intakes of whole grain in an Italian sample of children, adolescents and adults. *Eur. J. Nutr.* **2017**, *56*, 521–533. [CrossRef]
81. Li, B.; Li, F.; Wang, L.; Zhang, D. Fruit and Vegetables Consumption and Risk of Hypertension: A Meta-Analysis. *J. Clin. Hypertens.* **2016**, *18*, 468–476. [CrossRef]
82. Tang, G.Y.; Meng, X.; Li, Y.; Zhao, C.N.; Liu, Q.; Li, H.B. Effects of Vegetables on Cardiovascular Diseases and Related Mechanisms. *Nutrients* **2017**, *9*, 857. [CrossRef]
83. Zhao, C.N.; Meng, X.; Li, Y.; Li, S.; Liu, Q.; Tang, G.Y.; Li, H.B. Fruits for Prevention and Treatment of Cardiovascular Diseases. *Nutrients* **2017**, *9*, 598. [CrossRef]
84. Lampe, J.W. Health effects of vegetables and fruit: Assessing mechanisms of action in human experimental studies. *Am. J. Clin. Nutr.* **1999**, *70* (Suppl. 3), S475–S490. [CrossRef]
85. Alissa, E.M.; Ferns, G.A. Dietary fruits and vegetables and cardiovascular diseases risk. *Crit. Rev. Food Sci. Nutr.* **2017**, *57*, 1950–1962. [CrossRef] [PubMed]
86. Soedamah-Muthu, S.S.; Verberne, L.D.; Ding, E.L.; Engberink, M.F.; Geleijnse, J.M. Dairy consumption and incidence of hypertension: A dose-response meta-analysis of prospective cohort studies. *Hypertension* **2012**, *60*, 1131–1137. [CrossRef] [PubMed]
87. Smacchi, E.; Gobbetti, M. Peptides from several Italian cheeses inhibitory to proteolytic enzymes of lactic acid bacteria, pseudomonas fluorescens ATCC 948 and to the angiotensin I-converting enzyme. *Enzym. Microb. Technol.* **1998**, *22*, 687–694. [CrossRef]
88. Sieber, R.; Bütikofer, U.; Egger, C.; Portmann, R.; Walther, B.; Wechsler, D. ACE-inhibitory activity and ACE-inhibiting peptides in different cheese varieties. *Dairy Sci. Technol.* **2010**, *90*, 47–73. [CrossRef]
89. Tong, X.; Dong, J.Y.; Wu, Z.W.; Li, W.; Qin, L.Q. Dairy consumption and risk of type 2 diabetes mellitus: A meta-analysis of cohort studies. *Eur. J. Clin. Nutr.* **2011**, *65*, 1027–1031. [CrossRef] [PubMed]
90. Huo Yung Kai, S.; Bongard, V.; Simon, C.; Ruidavets, J.B.; Arveiler, D.; Dallongeville, J.; Wagner, A.; Amouyel, P.; Ferrières, J. Low-fat and high-fat dairy products are differently related to blood lipids and cardiovascular risk score. *Eur. J. Prev. Cardiol.* **2014**, *21*, 1557–1567. [PubMed]
91. Drouin-Chartier, J.P.; Côté, J.A.; Labonté, M.È.; Brassard, D.; Tessier-Grenier, M.; Desroches, S.; Couture, P.; Lamarche, B. Comprehensive Review of the Impact of Dairy Foods and Dairy Fat on Cardiometabolic Risk. *Adv. Nutr.* **2016**, *7*, 1041–1051. [CrossRef]
92. Brassard, D.; Tessier-Grenier, M.; Allaire, J.; Rajendiran, E.; She, Y.; Ramprasath, V.; Gigleux, I.; Talbot, D.; Levy, E.; Tremblay, A.; et al. Comparison of the impact of SFAs from cheese and butter on cardiometabolic risk factors: A randomized controlled trial. *Am. J. Clin. Nutr.* **2017**, *105*, 800–809. [CrossRef]
93. Kim, Y.; Keogh, J.B.; Clifton, P.M. Benefits of Nut Consumption on Insulin Resistance and Cardiovascular Risk Factors: Multiple Potential Mechanisms of Actions. *Nutrients* **2017**, *9*, 1271. [CrossRef]
94. de Souza, R.G.M.; Schincaglia, R.M.; Pimentel, G.D.; Mota, J.F. Nuts and Human Health Outcomes: A Systematic Review. *Nutrients* **2017**, *9*, 1311. [CrossRef]
95. Fidanza, F.; Alberti, A.; Lanti, M.; Menotti, A. Mediterranean Adequacy Index: Correlation with 25-year mortality from coronary heart disease in the Seven Countries Study. *Nutr. Metab. Cardiovasc. Dis.* **2004**, *14*, 254–258. [CrossRef]

96. Schwingshackl, L.; Christoph, M.; Hoffmann, G. Effects of Olive Oil on Markers of Inflammation and Endothelial Function-A Systematic Review and Meta-Analysis. *Nutrients* **2015**, *7*, 7651–7675. [CrossRef]
97. Risérus, U.; Willett, W.C.; Hu, F.B. Dietary fats and prevention of type 2 diabetes. *Prog. Lipid Res.* **2009**, *48*, 44–51. [CrossRef] [PubMed]
98. Guasch-Ferré, M.; Merino, J.; Sun, Q.; Fitó, M.; Salas-Salvadó, J. Dietary Polyphenols, Mediterranean Diet, Prediabetes, and Type 2 Diabetes: A Narrative Review of the Evidence. *Oxid. Med. Cell. Longev.* **2017**, *2017*, 6723931. [CrossRef] [PubMed]
99. Srinivasan, K. Antioxidant potential of spices and their active constituents. *Crit. Rev. Food Sci. Nutr.* **2014**, *54*, 352–372. [CrossRef] [PubMed]
100. WHO. Sodium Intake for Adults and Children. Available online: http://www.who.int/nutrition/publications/guidelines (accessed on 20 March 2018).
101. Mozaffarian, D.; Rimm, E.B. Fish intake, contaminants, and human health: Evaluating the risks and the benefits. *J. Am. Med. Assoc.* **2006**, *296*, 1885–1899. [CrossRef] [PubMed]
102. Kris-Etherton, P.M.; Harris, W.S.; Appel, L.J. Fish consumption, fish oil, omega-3 fatty acids, and cardiovascular disease. *Circulation.* **2002**, *106*, 2747–2757. [CrossRef] [PubMed]
103. Alhassan, A.; Young, J.; Lean, M.E.J.; Lara, J. Consumption of fish and vascular risk factors: A systematic review and meta-analysis of intervention studies. *Atherosclerosis* **2017**, *266*, 87–94. [CrossRef] [PubMed]
104. Akinkuolie, A.O.; Ngwa, J.S.; Meigs, J.B.; Djoussé, L. Omega-3 polyunsaturated fatty acid and insulin sensitivity: A meta-analysis of randomized controlled trials. *Clin. Nutr.* **2011**, *30*, 702–707. [CrossRef]
105. Zhu, B.; Sun, Y.; Qi, L.; Zhong, R.; Miao, X. Dietary legume consumption reduces risk of colorectal cancer: Evidence from a meta-analysis of cohort studies. *Sci. Rep.* **2015**, *5*, 8797. [CrossRef]
106. Viguiliouk, E.; Blanco Mejia, S.; Kendall, C.W.; Sievenpiper, J.L. Can pulses play a role in improving cardiometabolic health? Evidence from systematic reviews and meta-analyses. *Ann. N. Y. Acad. Sci.* **2017**, *1392*, 43–57. [CrossRef] [PubMed]
107. Geiker, N.R.W.; Larsen, M.L.; Dyerberg, J.; Stender, S.; Astrup, A. Egg consumption, cardiovascular diseases and type 2 diabetes. *Eur. J. Clin. Nutr.* **2018**, *72*, 44–56. [CrossRef] [PubMed]
108. Clayton, Z.S.; Fusco, E.; Kern, M. Egg consumption and heart health: A review. *Nutrition* **2017**, *37*, 79–85. [CrossRef] [PubMed]
109. Herron, K.L.; Vega-Lopez, S.; Conde, K.; Ramjiganesh, T.; Shachter, N.S.; Fernandez, M.L. Men classified as hypo-or hyperresponders to dietary cholesterol feeding exhibit differences in lipoprotein metabolism. *J. Nutr.* **2003**, *133*, 1036–1042. [CrossRef] [PubMed]
110. Fuller, N.R.; Sainsbury, A.; Caterson, I.D.; Markovic, T.P. Egg Consumption and Human Cardio-Metabolic Health in People with and without Diabetes. *Nutrients* **2015**, *7*, 7399–7420. [CrossRef] [PubMed]
111. Mozaffarian, D. Dietary and Policy Priorities for Cardiovascular Disease, Diabetes, and Obesity: A Comprehensive Review. *Circulation* **2016**, *133*, 187–225. [CrossRef]
112. Augustin, L.S.; Kendall, C.W.; Jenkins, D.J.; Willett, W.C.; Astrup, A.; Barclay, A.W.; Björck, I.; Brand-Miller, J.C.; Brighenti, F.; Buyken, A.E.; et al. Glycemic index, glycemic load and glycemic response: An International Scientific Consensus Summit from the International Carbohydrate Quality Consortium (ICQC). *Nutr. Metab. Cardiovasc. Dis.* **2015**, *25*, 795–815. [CrossRef]
113. Kim, Y.; Keogh, J.; Clifton, P. A review of potential metabolic etiologies of the observed association between red meat consumption and development of type 2 diabetes mellitus. *Metabolism* **2015**, *64*, 768–779. [CrossRef]
114. Battaglia Richi, E.; Baumer, B.; Conrad, B.; Darioli, R.; Schmid, A.; Keller, U. Health Risks Associated with Meat Consumption: A Review of Epidemiological Studies. *Int. J. Vitam. Nutr. Res.* **2015**, *85*, 70–78. [CrossRef]
115. Rohrmann, S.; Linseisen, J. Processed meat: The real villain? *Proc. Nutr. Soc.* **2016**, *75*, 233–241. [CrossRef]
116. Bouvard, V.; Loomis, D.; Guyton, K.Z.; Grosse, Y.; Ghissassi, F.E.; Benbrahim-Tallaa, L.; Guha, N.; Mattock, H.; Straif, K. International Agency for Research on Cancer Monograph Working Group. Carcinogenicity of consumption of red and processed meat. *Lancet Oncol.* **2015**, *16*, 1599–1600. [CrossRef]
117. Report from the Commission to the European Parliament and the Council 2015. Available online: https://ec.europa.eu/.../fs_labelling-nutrition_trans-fats-report_en (accessed on 23 February 2019).
118. O'Keefe, J.H.; Bhatti, S.K.; Bajwa, A.; Di Nicolantonio, J.J.; Lavie, C.J. Alcohol and cardiovascular health: The dose makes the poison . . . or the remedy. *Mayo Clin. Proc.* **2014**, *89*, 382–393. [CrossRef] [PubMed]

119. Lippi, G.; Franchini, M.; Favaloro, E.J.; Targher, G. Moderate red wine consumption and cardiovascular disease risk: Beyond the "French paradox". *Semin. Thromb. Hemost.* **2010**, *36*, 59–70. [CrossRef] [PubMed]
120. Poli, A.; Marangoni, F.; Avogaro, A.; Barba, G.; Bellentani, S.; Bucci, M.; Cambieri, R.; Catapano, A.L.; Costanzo, S.; Cricelli, C.; et al. Moderate alcohol use and health: A consensus document. *Nutr. Metab. Cardiovasc. Dis.* **2013**, *23*, 487–504. [CrossRef] [PubMed]
121. Giacosa, A.; Barale, R.; Bavaresco, L.; Faliva, M.A.; Gerbi, V.; La Vecchia, C.; Negri, E.; Opizzi, A.; Perna, S.; Pezzotti, M.; et al. Mediterranean way of drinking and longevity. *Crit. Rev. Food Sci. Nutr.* **2016**, *56*, 635–640. [CrossRef] [PubMed]
122. De Lorenzo, A.; Alberti, A.; Andreoli, A.; Iacopino, L.; Serranò, P.; Perriello, G. Food habits in a southern Italian town (Nicotera) in 1960 and 1996: Still a reference Italian Mediterranean diet? *Diabetes Nutr. Metab.* **2001**, *14*, 121–125.
123. Ruggiero, E.; Bonaccio, M.L.; Di Castelnuovo, A.; Bonanni, A.; Costanzo, S.; Persichillo, M.; Bracone, F.; Cerletti, C.; Donati, M.B.; de Gaetano, G.; et al. Consumption of whole grain food and its determinants in a general Italian population: Results from the INHES Study. *Nutr. Metab. Cardiovasc. Dis.* **2019**. [CrossRef]
124. Harvard, T.H. Chan School of Public Health. Diet Review: Mediterranean Diet. Available online: https://www.hsph.harvard.edu/nutritionsource/healthy-weight/diet-reviews/mediterranean-diet/ (accessed on 16 March 2019).
125. Satija, A.; Bhupathiraju, S.N.; Rimm, E.B.; Spiegelman, D.; Chiuve, S.E.; Borgi, L.; Willett, W.C.; Manson, J.E.; Sun, Q.; Hu, F.B. Plant-Based Dietary Patterns and Incidence of Type 2 Diabetes in US Men and Women: Results from Three Prospective Cohort Studies. *PLoS Med.* **2016**, *13*, e1002039. [CrossRef]
126. Satija, A.; Bhupathiraju, S.N.; Spiegelman, D.; Chiuve, S.E.; Manson, J.E.; Willett, W.C.; Rexrode, K.M.; Rimm, E.B.; Hu, F.B. Healthful and Unhealthful Plant-Based Diets and the Risk of Coronary Heart Disease in U.S. Adults. *J. Am. Coll. Cardiol.* **2017**, *70*, 411–422. [CrossRef]

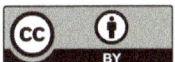

© 2019 by the authors. Licensee MDPI, Basel, Switzerland. This article is an open access article distributed under the terms and conditions of the Creative Commons Attribution (CC BY) license (http://creativecommons.org/licenses/by/4.0/).

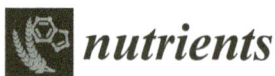

Review

Obesity and the Mediterranean Diet: A Review of Evidence of the Role and Sustainability of the Mediterranean Diet

Santa D'Innocenzo [1],*, Carlotta Biagi [2] and Marcello Lanari [2]

1. Prochild Project, Department of Medical and Surgical Sciences (DIMEC), St. Orsola-Malpighi Hospital, University of Bologna, 40138 Bologna, Italy
2. Pediatric Emergency Unit, Department of Medical and Surgical Sciences (DIMEC), St. Orsola-Malpighi Hospital, University of Bologna, 40138 Bologna, Italy; carlottabiagi@yahoo.it (C.B.); marcello.lanari@unibo.it (M.L.)
* Correspondence: santa@santadinno.com; Tel.: +39-0335-5444472

Received: 30 March 2019; Accepted: 30 May 2019; Published: 9 June 2019

Abstract: Several different socio-economic factors have caused a large portion of the population to adopt unhealthy eating habits that can undermine healthcare systems, unless current trends are inverted towards more sustainable lifestyle models. Even though a dietary plan inspired by the principles of the Mediterranean Diet is associated with numerous health benefits and has been demonstrated to exert a preventive effect towards numerous pathologies, including obesity, its use is decreasing and it is now being supplanted by different nutritional models that are often generated by cultural and social changes. Directing governments' political actions towards spreading adherence to the Mediterranean Diet's principles as much as possible among the population could help to tackle the obesity epidemic, especially in childhood. This document intends to reiterate the importance of acting in certain age groups to stop the spread of obesity and proceeds with a critical review of the regulatory instruments used so far, bearing in mind the importance of the scientific evidence that led to the consideration of the Mediterranean Diet as not just a food model, but also as the most appropriate regime for disease prevention, a sort of complete lifestyle plan for the pursuit of healthcare sustainability.

Keywords: Mediterranean Diet; public health policy; childhood obesity; healthy lifestyle; health communication

1. Introduction: Mediterranean Diet, When Evidence Speaks

The Mediterranean Diet (MD) has been identified as having proved to be the most effective amongst many others in terms of prevention of obesity-related diseases [1]. In view of this scientific evidence in a prevention activity, the purpose of this review is to critically evaluate the methods that can inform and gently persuade consumers to adopt the MD principles in order to tackle childhood obesity, for the pursuit of healthcare sustainability.

MD is characterized by a high intake of vegetables, fruits, nuts, cereals, whole grains, and olive oil, as well as a moderate consumption of fish and poultry, and a low intake of sweets, red meat and dairy products [2,3]. Being poor in saturated fat intake and rich in monounsaturated fat intake, it provides a high amount of fibre, glutathione and antioxidants, and it is characterized by a balanced ratio of n-6/n-3 essential fatty acids [4,5]. The adoption of the MD on a large scale has long been reported to be protective against the occurrence of several different health outcomes [6].

Thanks to all these healthy aspects, the MD has been associated with a lower risk of cardiovascular mortality [7–9] and coronary diseases [10], obesity, type 2 diabetes, mellitus and metabolic syndrome in adults [11,12].

In pregnancy, a higher adherence to the MD has been associated with a lower risk of neural tube defects [13], preterm birth [14,15] and fetal growth restriction [16].

Moreover, it seems to influence the fetus' susceptibility to gain weight later in life, as it has been associated with lower offspring waist circumference at preschool age [17] and lower offspring cardiometabolic risk [18].

How an adherence to the MD during pregnancy could have positive effects in offspring, not only during fetal life, but also later in life, is still unclear, but the induction of epigenetic modifications represents a possible explanation [19].

Despite this almost indisputable scientific evidence, some ambiguous effects highlighted in specific studies are considered depending on the definition of the MD standards and the indexes of the adhesion to the same standard used [20], so a few concerns arise when we refer to the definition of the MD, in view of the different opinions in the scientific literature [21] on how it has to be technically defined. Moreover, citizens and consumers who need to be persuaded to adopt it often have confused ideas about the foods that are part of this diet, [22]. In effect, since the MD has become an increasingly popular topic of interest worldwide, several myths and misconceptions are now associated with its nutritional pattern, and this may be a further obstacle to its correct diffusion, since the main challenges for its desirable transferability in non Mediterranean areas largely derive from these misrepresentations.

In consideration of the scientific evidence, it seems increasingly appropriate to maintain the Mediterranean paradigm by way of an overall food composition, suggesting the possibility of implementing a Mediterranean-type dietary pattern within the context of a non-Mediterranean population. Even if the paucity of data does not give a clear picture of the health effects of the MD in non-Mediterranean countries [23], the transferability of the MD pattern to non-Mediterranean settings is desirable, and has been studied and deemed possible. However, it requires a multitude of changes in dietary habits, practical resources, and knowledge to accomplish these changes [24]. New strategies to increase the adherence to its principles among citizens are considered necessary above all due to the fact that some recent studies support the role of the MD in preventing obesity development in children [25–27], a thorny issue which is worth examining briefly.

Methods: This narrative review was performed with a multidisciplinary approach to identify publications about the regulatory instruments used to increase adherence to the Mediterranean Diet and stop the spread of obesity. A multidisciplinary and multilevel approach is chosen due to the nature of the topic itself: obesity is a multifactorial, multifaceted problem. Given that poor diets are a component of a more complex array of factors and owing to the complexity of the obesity epidemic, prevention strategies and policies across multiple levels and disciplines are needed in order to have a measurable effect. In order to set up population strategies prevention, combination and collaboration between different disciplines and competences has become essential to tackle this multifactorial problem. The search strategy was conducted in the following database: PubMed, Embase, and selected gray literautre sources. Reports, working papers, government documents, white papers and evaluation materials and research produced by organizations outside of the traditional commercial or academic publishing and distribution channels have been consulted for research and duly indicated in the bibliography.

Relevant keywords relating to the Mediterranean Diet in combination with public policy terms and text words ("Public Policy", "Mediterranean Diet," or "diet" or "dietary pattern" "Mediterranean," or "adherence" or "score") were used in combination with words relating to health status ("health" or "mortality" or "morbidity," or "cardiovascular diseases" or "obesity" and "childhood obesity"). The search strategy had no language restrictions. The date range was from the inception of the respective database until March 2019, when multiple articles for a single study were present, we used the latest publication and supplemented it, if necessary, with data from the most complete or updated publication.

2. Obesity as a Global Disease

According to the NCD Risk Factor Collaboration (Non Communicable Diseases Study Group's research) [28], the rising trends in children's and adolescents' BMI have plateaued in many high-income countries, although at high levels, but have accelerated in some parts of Asia, with these trends no longer correlated with those of adults. Mean BMI and prevalence of obesity increased worldwide in children and adolescents from 1975 to 2016, with the rate of change in mean BMI moderately correlated with that of adults until around 2000, but only weakly correlated afterwards.

The NCD Study Group research highlights that the number of children and adolescents aged 5–19 years in the world who are moderately or severely underweight remains larger than those who are obese, showing the continued need for policies that enhance food security in low-income countries and households, especially in south Asia. The experiences of East Asia and Latin America and the Caribbean show that the transition from underweight to overweight and obesity can be rapid and can overwhelm the national capacity needed to engender a healthy transition. Furthermore, populations have changed their habits in an unhealthy nutritional shift: an increase in nutrient-poor, energy-dense foods can lead to stunted growth along with weight gain in children, adolescents, and adults, resulting in higher BMI and worse health outcomes throughout an individual's lifespan.

In particular, obese children and adolescents are at increased risk for a large number of medical disorders, including hypertension, insulin resistance, dyslipidaemia, fatty liver disease and obstructive sleep apnoea disorder [29].

Moreover, obesity may lead not only to physical but also to psychological and social complications, such as low self-esteem, depression and stigma [30,31]. Childhood obesity is also difficult to reverse and it increases the likelihood of obesity in adulthood and the development of health problems, mainly cardiovascular diseases such as coronary heart disease, which is the leading cause of adult mortality and morbidity [32].

Therefore, it is important to prevent the onset of obesity in childhood in order to reduce the onset of obesity-related complications later in life.

With the exception of rare genetic disorders like *Prader-Willi* syndrome and some endocrine diseases like thyroid dysfunction, obesity is due to an imbalance between calorie intake and calories utilized that results in an excess of body adiposity. A sedentary lifestyle, lack of physical activity and poor dietary habits, together with genetic predisposition, all contribute to this phenomenon [33].

However, the rapid increase in BMI worldwide cannot be entirely explained by genetics; environmental factors also play an important role in childhood obesity. This is why family and school environments are so relevant to this topic. The most frequent unhealthy food choices seen in schoolchildren and adolescents include: skipping breakfast, eating at fast-food restaurants and consuming a high amount of sweets and junk food, which are calorie dense, while parents are still at work. All these behavior patterns increase the risk of childhood obesity and its comorbidities. In order to realize how much eating habits have changed in various parts of the world and how widespread the threat of obesity is, it's worth taking a look at several recent studies on the point. In 2010, more than one third of children in the United States were classified as overweight or obese [34], but even at that time obesity and its related diseases were not limited to Western countries. In effect, mostly in the past two decades, urbanization in many Asian countries, where the prevalence of obesity was historically very low, has led to a sedentary lifestyle and overnutrition, setting the stage for the epidemic of obesity and conditions like non-alcoholic fatty liver disease [35]. In the last decade the spread of obesity has been increasing at an alarming rate, especially in China, Japan, and India [36]. In particular, China presents a unique model for weight change, as the country has experienced a shift from a history of undernutrition to a very rapid increase in obesity [37].

Some studies point out that China's food consumption patterns and eating, along with the country's cooking behaviors changed dramatically between 1991 and 2011: prior to the last decade there was essentially no snacking in China except for hot water or green tea, while currently the changes in cooking and eating styles include a decrease in the proportion of food steamed, baked, or boiled and a parallel increase in snacking and eating away from home. In addition to this, most recently the intake of foods high in added sugar has increased, together with a major growth in consumption of processed foods and beverages, while the profusion of supermarkets and convenience stores are dramatically changing the nature of China's food supply, showing how dietary shifts are greatly affected by a wild Western urbanization [38,39].

The shifts in diet are also profound in the Latin America and the Caribbean region, which faces a major diet-related health problem accompanied by enormous economic and social costs [40].

Not even Africa has escaped this problem: the prevalence of overweight and obesity among children under five years of age was 5% in 2017, and in absolute numbers there has been an increase of almost 50% since 2000, from 6.6 million to 9.7 million in 2017 [41,42].

Overweight and obesity are a major public health issue in Australia, where their rates have risen over recent decades, with nearly 2 in 3 adults, and 1 in 4 children considered overweight or obese in 2014–2015. In addition, if compared with non-Indigenous Australians, Indigenous adults are more likely to be overweight or obese, and Indigenous children and adolescents are more likely to be obese. Unlike the previous examples, those who live outside of major urban areas are more likely to be overweight or obese than others [43].

It therefore appears evident that inadequate eating habits now constitute a multilevel problem threatening healthcare sustainability worldwide. In most of the aforementioned studies it is noted that consumer choices turn irremediably towards Western diets, abandoning autochthonous and typical diets. And this indisputable fact entails serious problems for healthcare sustainability [44].

3. The Choice: Mediterranean Diet Versus Western Diets

Insufficient levels of adherence to the MD are specifically considered to be a major factor in the concerning spread of the obesity epidemic in Southern Europe [45], where a Western type Diet that is high in saturated fats and refined carbohydrates, poor in quality and high in calorie intake is now spreading rapidly. This creates an astounding paradox, well highlighted during the European Congress on Obesity held in Vienna in May 2018, regarding the fact that within the very geographical area in which the MD was developed, there has been an extreme and undeniable shift in the population's nutritional choices towards another diet that is full of saturated fats, sugars and processed meats [46]. According to the World Health Organization (WHO) [47], the abandonment of the MD is making children in the Mediterranean area fatter and generally less healthy than their Swedish counterparts, who from a young age become accustomed to a MD made up of more fish and vegetables.

Some recent studies report that adherence to the MD significantly began to decrease between 1961–65, whereas from 2004–2011 there was a stabilization of the trends in adherence values and even an increase among 16 countries [48]. After all, since 1961 there had been quite dramatic changes in the European Union (EU) diet: at the level of macronutrients, convergence was the most notable tendency, with Mediterranean countries increasing their intake of free sugars, saturated fats and cholesterol, while the highest-intake Northern European countries moderated their consumption of these nutrients [49].

In effect, a significant role in the Sixties was certainly played by the growing industrialization of the food market, taking into consideration that in many countries of Southern Europe these years coincided with those of the well-being generated by the consolidation of the post-war economic boom, which led to new nutritional options based on a greater quantity of processed foods and expanded availability of red meats and sugar, to the detriment of vegetables and cereals. Housewives became workers and the time to prepare meals was dramatically reduced, while ready-made meals became a common usage. The subsequent globalization and urbanization have in a few decades greatly worsened the effects of these factors [50].

Nowadays, the Westernization of the diet is particularly evident, especially among the younger generations [51]. This process, which is generally referred as the *modernization* of a society, implies a number of unhealthy lifestyle habits, not just limited to modification of food preferences toward western foods, but also relative to other common activities (electronic devices, computer and television use), which facilitated a radical shift in a population's habits, leading to an overall imbalance between energy intake and expenditure [52,53].

In other words, the essence of the matter is that the general adoption of sedentary lifestyle and westernized dietary patterns generated the global rise of obesity and diabetes worldwide over the last few decades [54–58]. Large swathes of populations choose Western diets on a daily basis [59], both in Western and Southern Europe [60–63] and in developing countries [64], which is not a optimal choice for healthy living [65,66].

In effect, the rising prevalence of childhood obesity is a particularly concerning aspect of the phenomenon [67], the underlying causes of which are complex and interconnecting, involving social, cultural, familial, physiological, genetic, metabolic, and behavioral factors. The only safe and effective treatment is a real long-term change in lifestyle, as obesity is the result of unhealthy behaviors that may be difficult to change.

Table 1 reports the main dietary foods of the Mediterranean and Western Diets. The greatest difference between the Mediterranean and the Western Diets is the sources and proportion of dietary fat [2].

Table 1. Comparison of dietary foods between Mediterranean and Western Diets.

Foods	Mediterranean Diet	Western Diets
Vegetables	Every main meal (≥2 servings)	Rarely
Fruits	Every main meal (1–2 servings)	Rarely
Bread/pasta/rice/couscous/other cereals	Every main meal (1–2 servings, preferably whole grain)	Rarely whole grain cereals, often refined grains
Olive Oil	Every main meal (3–4 servings, expecially extra virgin)	Rarely olive oil, often replaced by margarine and butter
Nuts/seeds/olives	Every day (1–2 servings)	Occasionally
Dairy Foods	Every day in moderate portions (2 servings, preferably low fat)	Often high fat dairy foods
Herbs/spices/garlic/onions	Every day (less added salt)	Less often
Legumes	Weekly (≥2 servings)	Less often
Potatoes	Weekly (≤3 servings)	Less often
Eggs	Weekly (2–4 servings)	Less often
Fish/seafood	Weekly (≥2 servings)	Less often
White meat	Weekly (2 servings)	Less often
Red meat	Weekly (<2 servings)	Often
Processed meat	Weekly (≤1 serving)	Often
Sweets	Weekly (≤2 servings)	Often

In view of all this, the choice between Mediterranean and Western Diets is mainly determined by a set of socio-economic, demographic and conjunctural factors. But that is not all: obesity is a complex, multifactorial, multilevel disease that not only has a significant impact on physical health but also on psychosocial well-being and therefore on quality of life. Obese people experience substantial impairments in quality of life as a consequence of their weight, and these can impact significantly on their mental health, which in turn can further impact on their physical health [68].

Clearly, important changes in the social determinants, whatever they may be, are unlikely in the absence of social, fiscal or legislative change, which remains a decisive tool for change: a brief examination of impact of such tool therefore seems appropriate.

4. Public Policy Measures to Tackle the Phaenomenon

Every government needs to urgently adopt policies that make a healthy diet easily accessible and affordable for all, in order to reach healthcare sustainability [69,70]. It is a fight in which time is an enemy, due to the extraordinary growth rates of the epidemic [71].

Law and regulation are now definitely considered essential tools in tackling childhood obesity [72–74], but unfortunately the legal interventions focused on public health are still at an early stage and the impact they may have on the obesity epidemic is not yet completely perceptible. After more than a decade of research on the topic [75,76], what is most evident is that the effectiveness of the attempt to change citizens' behavior is subject to the quality of the public health policy choices, which should be structured in such a way as to protect citizens' health, especially for the most disadvantaged groups. This fact calls into question the responsibility of public health policies in the planning of actions to combat obesity, from the perspective of the economic sustainability of healthcare.

In this context, the Mediterranean-style diet is not considered a specific diet, but rather a collection of eating habits [77]. Primarily it is characterized by a substantially reduced consumption of meat, especially red and processed meat, and as not being based on a lot of sophisticated and very expensively marketed products, but centered on a very simple and humble set of foods that have to be appropriately chosen, washed and prepared with care and time, it represents a dietary plan that can be followed everywhere.

In terms of sustainability, cost-effectiveness analyses and sensitivity analyses have all shown that the MD remained highly cost effective under all scenarios [78], but the choice to adhere to its prescriptions is, however, substantially affected by the reduction of family time due to the increase in female work force participation [79]. What remains debateable today is whether the cost linked to a healthy diet that promotes the use of fish, vegetables and cereals, in place of often less expensive processed foods and ready meals, plays a significant role in citizens' less healthy food choices [80].

Cross-sectional results [81] show how a low income is strictly associated with a poor adherence to the MD and a higher prevalence of obesity, while in the wider framework, inequalities in health are closely entwined in a worrying way with socio-economic inequality [82], especially among children. The relevance of socio-economic factors in determining such differences is evident: the structural determinants and conditions of daily life cause much of the health inequity between and within countries [83]. The creation of supportive environments for health is a basic action principle of health promotion, and equality is a connected core value.

A setting approach determines in fact an opportunity to link these two, highlighting the interplay between individual, environmental and social determinants of health [84].

This means that the environmental approach, focused on public health practice, necessarily goes through special policy actions, operating upon the intersection between Behavior, Environment, Health, and Public Policy [85].

However, current prevention programs have had little success to date and have proven ineffective in reversing the constantly rising rates of childhood obesity, so much so that the epidemic is growing rapidly even where once it did not exist, as previously discussed. If behavioral and environmental factors are so relevant, these disappointing observations reveal the urgent need to better understand the complex mechanisms involved in social conditions that lead to obesity, in order to propose better disease prevention and care.

5. The Three Pillars and the Public Health Choices

Although environmental factors are important, there is considerable evidence that genes also have a significant role in the pathogenesis of obesity [86], but very little can be done from this point of view with public policy. For this reason we hereby set about discussing only the interventions that can be undertaken through models such as regulation. Moreover, we must consider that there are currently three main treatment methods for obesity, which are easily identifiable in three different pillars represented by pharmacotherapy, bariatric surgery, and lifestyle modifications. The first two are treatments to be carried out on an individual basis and, due to the fact that they are extremely expensive and particularly invasive, they are commonly debated [87]. Furthermore, they are not to be taken into consideration for subjects of a developmental age, even if for some minors, bariatric surgery may be the only option to save their lives or avoid severe disease. For others, bariatric surgery may be considered morally wrong when more beneficent alternatives exist [88].

The cornerstone of lifestyle modifications includes changes to dietary and exercise habits that only public policy can effectively induce. While the first two pillars can obtain excellent results, they achieve nothing from a social point of view other than increasing social and health inequality. It is not exactly a correct use of public health policy to rely on such invasive and non-reversible surgeries, instead of intensifying a social commitment towards a substantial improvement of the conditions of disadvantaged groups [89] who are forced to live in environments that cannot prevent the onset of the disease. Moreover, the first two pillars can only help when obesity has been diagnosed, unlike the third pillar, which can also effectively be used to prevent the onset.

In this context, prevention is more necessary than ever in order to halt the increase of social and health inequality: only preventing obesity can decrease the number of years lived with diseases and tackle the spreading of the continuous rise of the epidemic. A clear policy implication is the need for careful monitoring and following-up of public health intervention, with a focus on effects—those intended or otherwise—in different socioeconomic groups [90].

One major issue is the scarcity of strong evidence on how to prevent obesity: prevention surely requires a complex, multilevel, environmental, socioeconomic, and lifespan approach, acting on changeable causal factors, such as diet or physical activity [91].

Despite a few isolated areas of improvement, no country has yet reversed its obesity epidemic [92]. However, since incontrovertibly strong scientific and experiential data from research carried out over the last two decades highlights the relevance of environmental factors in the development of obesity and how its effects can modify citizens' lifestyle, important steps have already been made in the development of systems for the monitoring of socio-economic inequality in health. In some European member states, considerable efforts have been made over the last two decades to use existing data sources to monitor socio-economic differences in health indicators [93]. Given the direct connection, this could provide a good basis for identifying areas of epidemiological onset, in order to dispense directed and appropriate interventions.

In fact, the practice has shown that imposing regulations regardless of the epidemiological knowledge of the onset of the disease has very limited effects.

6. Facts and Patterns of the Onset of the Epidemic: the Relevance of Environmental Factors

New habits then [94] can lead to obesity in certain environments, and epidemiological studies [95] reveal that obesity occurs and develops systematically here and there, but mostly in low-income urban and suburban areas [96]. As a consequence, the recognition of obesogenic environments, the importance of which have been acknowledged for some time [97], can be verified through defined parameters. This means that we can avoid dispersed intervention in order to promote specific actions for the change of microenvironments with appropriate control and surveillance [98].

Getting people to change is not easy [99] and the role of public action remains that of modeling interventions in relation to the epidemiological evidence, in conformity with the aspects of health character and the administrative and accounting procedures of the territory, respecting the different needs of each specific area. The correct use of social accounting in the Local Health Units could play a very important role in the interception and monitoring of disadvantaged areas, thus enhancing the sustainability that these instruments can achieve for stakeholders.

Therefore, it is necessary to change the choices that affect the lifestyle of citizens in an effective manner. Some positive results to this aim seem to have been obtained through the specific public policies of *social marketing* [100] and *nudges* [101], despite the heated debates that the latter caused over time [102,103]. These policies have helpfully directed the dietary behavior of consumers according to various aims [104]. They have achieved this through a correction of certain characteristics of the environments in which citizens live and by concentrating on the reasons behind their unhealthy dietary choices. Even though some recent analyses demonstrate that nudge techniques can be an effective public health strategy for combatting obesity [105], these instruments can certainly not be considered a cure-all, but should be included in a framework of directed measures, in consideration of the multidisciplinary nature of the problem [106]: they can help to put in place a systematic action aimed at getting to know the benefits of the MD as well.

The nudge action can be structured in different degrees of effectiveness, in accordance with the aims to be pursued: providing information, communicating and informing citizens; enabling people to make good choices; educating them; leading them to the right choice through changing the default option; making the default option the healthier choice; using incentives to guide people to opt for the healthiest choice; using disincentives to discourage them from making harmful decisions; regulating, containing or definitively eliminating the prospects of choice. It can be applied in limited areas, concurrently with other measures aimed at improving the environment, contributing to positively affect the quality of citizens' choices. Since it is a question of modifying environments, the effort must be multilevel and multi-competency and cannot be limited to isolated actions. In view of all of this, it is now clear that a single measure to tackle obesity will have a largely insignificant result, if it is implemented without an orderly vision of the epidemiological characteristics of the disease that it is put in place to control.

The public law research on this topic is well advanced, and since the Nineties, some European governments, aware of the effects of the spread of obesity, have not hesitated to implement new proposals, like excises on unhealthy foods and traffic light food labeling. Of course, even if the law is considered to be a decisive tool for addressing childhood obesity and NCD in general [107], it seems appropriate to verify the effectiveness of some of these measures in light of the studies that have dealt with them.

This paper therefore is proposed to proceed to a general examination of the currently known policies to tackling obesity, trying to highlight the criticalities that each regulatory intervention entails, as well as the potentially achievable advantages.

The most widespread public policies adopted to reduce childhood obesity are schematically indicated in Figure 1.

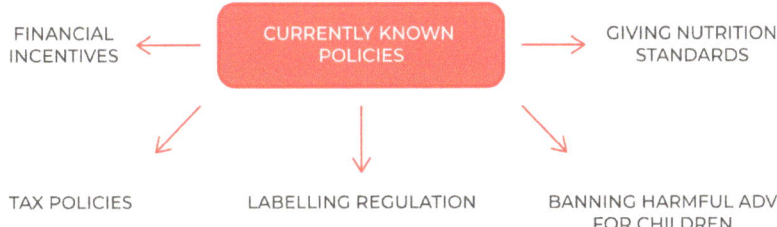

Figure 1. Currently known policies to tackle childhood obesity.

7. Fiscal Strategies for A Healthier Lifestyle: Do They Work?

Excise taxes on junk food often generate strong debates when they are proposed in order to modify the nutritional choices of citizens. However, we cannot disregard a very brief examination of the effects of their application in a thorough assessment of what may be the most effective measures to spread the adoption of the MD as much as possible.

Very sugary drinks have no place in the MD and are unanimously considered to be harmful foods, but it is very difficult to eliminate them from the diets of adults and children. To reduce their consumption, governments have imposed excise duties on these products since 1920 [108], principally with the aim of generating revenue [109], but nowadays this sort of taxation is considered more as a social instrument to stop the increasing obesity rate. Therefore, they are currently in place in a number of countries [110], while elsewhere [111] they have had a short lifespan and only marginal results.

The real objective of an excise of this kind should be the adoption of healthy regimes and the consequent reduction of obesity, but despite all the heated discussions generated, it is still not clear if they really can help to reach this goal.

For example, there is empirical evidence that connects taxation with a considerable decrease in sales [112], and yet there is still no clear evidence that taxation can lead to a real improvement in a population's health. What is more, even if we were to have high quality data on the population's health, which currently we do not, it would be very difficult to establish whether the improvement was due to a single specific political measure [113].

The results of some studies investigating the extension of a value-added tax to certain categories of food products have shown that it is indeed possible to obtain small health benefits, but unexpected results are also possible; for example, they have shown that taxing saturated fats leads to an increase in salt intake and greater overall mortality [114].

On the other hand, a connection between fizzy drinks and a large number of diseases has long been established: these diseases include cardiac and cerebrovascular disease [115] and reduction of bone strength [116].

Not only it has been hypothesized that fizzy drinks can contribute to causing erectile dysfunction, but it is also been highlighted that monosaccharide fructose is the most harmful sugar component in terms of weight gain and metabolic disturbances, while high-fructose corn syrup is gradually replacing sucrose as the main sweetener in soft drinks and has been accused of being potentially responsible for the current high prevalence of obesity. There is also considerable evidence that fructose, rather than glucose, can be the more damaging sugar component in terms of cardiovascular risk [117].

However, it should be noted that no one would think of reducing the intake of fructose from fresh fruit.

Even if it is well known today that soft drinks have detrimental metabolic effects and that their consumption should be limited, they only represent a very small part of the problem, given that the consumer frequently consumes them alongside other junk food, which is full of salt, sugar and trans-fats, almost all of which is industrially produced and processed.

We are talking about food available at very low prices on the market, which we have come to associate with images of happiness and socializing due to the amount and invasive nature of obsessively repeated advertising, which for this reason, makes the food even more dangerous for minors. Another aspect of this food that is perhaps even more attractive than its price, is the fact that it is readily available almost everywhere, from large urban areas to smaller provincial towns [118], and it is ready prepared and can be eaten immediately. In today's society, where time is an increasingly rare resource, this is an aspect that cannot be overlooked.

Therefore, we must ask ourselves whether the various sugar or soda taxes can truly represent a realistic solution that is both feasible and desirable in a context where the real purpose would be to encourage citizens to adopt voluntarily a healthy regime.

The answer is not immediately clear: some studies [119] have proposed an examination of the advantages and disadvantages of implementing a tax on junk food as an intervention to halt the increase of obesity in North America. The results have confirmed that although it is probable that modest excises produce substantial revenue, it is however improbable that these excices have any real influence on the rates of obesity. It is more likely that higher excises on soft drinks would have a direct impact on the weight of populations at risk, but it is less likely that they would be politically acceptable or sustainable.

As things stand, the efficiency of these taxes seems to be irrelevant because the consumption of soft drinks is a small part of overweight people's diets and the drinks that can substitute for sugary drinks can often be even more calorific than the original soft drinks.

In fact, evidence shows that consumption often merely shifts from one unhealthy product to another: a reduction in soda consumption is shown to be completely offset by increases in the consumption of other high-calorie drinks [120], leaving the calorie count unchanged and meaning the action was undertaken in vain. Only replacing sugar-sweetened beverages with natural water is associated with a reduction in total calories and weight loss [121,122].

Moreover, if the aim of imposing taxation on soft sugary drinks lies in wanting to reduce the rate of obesity, then the increase in revenue should go towards financing projects and programs that would work towards this goal. This sort of taxation would then be worth considering more carefully.

Usually governments, for political convenience, don't have the ability to direct the increase in revenue derived from these taxes to social aims and the consumers have little control over the final use of these funds. Indeed, the effectiveness of healthcare programs and subsidiaries allocated *ad hoc* are probably only a determining factor of the fiscal success in the fight against obesity if proposed in a well-devised, multidisciplinary framework.

What's more, the analyses and contributions of some researchers [123] demonstrate that selective taxation distorts the market, reducing the consumer's freedom of choice; and tends to have a regressive impact [83], impoverishing the less-advantaged social groups, confirming that the excises on sugary drinks usually only weigh upon the less advantaged classes.

Instead, these taxes need to be inserted into a wider plan, one that possibly includes incentives for healthy foods, gently pushing people to improve their choices. For example, some studies show that about a quarter of consumers claim to not eat enough fresh fruit, but that they would eat more fruit if it cost a little less; around a fifth of citizens would do the same with vegetables.

The same studies show that, in reality, in some environments, the actual diet rarely coincides with the healthiest one, but this does not reduce the weight of public-healthism as an ethical and practical nutritional reference point, as it has the ability to generate a sense of mass guilt, even in areas where it cannot have an effect on healthy eating in practice [124]. Certainly, cost is an important factor when we talk about nutritional choices and the impact of the price of fruit and vegetables—the most important part of the MD—on the pocket of the consumer, should certainly be re-evaluated in the context of fiscal planning based on citizens' lifestyle. This is also the line of the WHO, which recommends the use of financial incentives in a complete and coherent political context [125].

It is true that: "The cost of basic food commodities, such as corn and soy, is very low owing to economic strategies for food production including direct and indirect subsidies or tax advantages implemented as part of the farm bill. These crops are highly profitable because they are the raw ingredients of most processed foods and beverages. Corn and soy are also the primary feed for livestock; thus, the prices of beef and poultry are also very low by historic and international standards. By contrast, production of fruits and vegetables, which receives little governmental support, remains expensive" [95].

These circumstances make it difficult to achieve a healthy remodeling of behaviors and habits of individuals and families. A few cents more will not be enough to address the consumer in the right direction [126], as a buying choice is motivated by many other impulses. Indeed, recent scientific evidence shows that the cerebral neurochemistry, when in a state of sugar withdrawal, conditions behavior, pushing the consumer to satisfy their need in any way possible, in a worrying parallel to other addictions [127]. Moreover, high consumption levels of soft drinks containing sugar have long been associated with mental health problems among adolescents, even after adjustments have been made in research for possible confounders [128], this is why a small price difference is not relevant in effectively influencing behavior towards better choices, and even if it was a price problem, as already discussed above, the subject's preference would simply turn towards other drinks, which are often no less calorific and just as harmful.

Labeling systems seem to be equally insufficient in the positive conditioning of citizens' choices. For a while different studies [129] have shown that the information directed at changing eating habits, communicated only through labeling, has provided limited results in the conditioning of citizens' behavior and can even lead to excesses of consumption.

It is quite clear then, just how difficult it is to change nutritional choices on a large scale for wide sectors of the population with the only help of fiscal strategies. In reality, the areas that the legal instrument would need to touch upon are numerous and influenced by different causal factors. It is therefore necessary to swiftly examine the other aspects that political action must consider in order to halt and control the multifaceted and multilevel problem of obesity, particularly considering other actors that could participate in attempts to stop the spread of the epidemic.

8. The Role of the Food and Drink Industry

When buying processed foods, people are not able to clearly evaluate the food's levels of saturated and trans fats, sugar and salt. Instead, they usually rely on brand reputation to determine their choice. In general, labels do not help with clear evaluation, as everyone reading them has different backgrounds. To be effective, they require the consumer to already have a high level of nutritional education and then also a willingness to devote the time to reading and reacting to labeling information while shopping.

It is said that the food industry uses too many ingredients that are deemed unhealthy because they contribute to the taste and the manufacturing process, and are relatively inexpensive: some Food and Beverage Corporations (hereinafter FBC) and manufacturers have often been held responsible for facilitating the explosion of obesity around the world [130,131].

In effect, governments' relationships with industrial enterprises are an equally significant factor in the fight to prevent the spread of obesity, especially in terms of agreements for improving the ingredients in products and remodeling commercial communications.

In England the food industry has failed to hit its target of cutting sugar by 5% over the past year, with experts describing the results as hugely disappointing and suggesting the government may be forced to introduce a tax, as with sugary drinks [132]. A voluntary approach has been tried and tested with sugar and has been found to be lacking, as progress has been slow and too reliant on a handful of responsible manufacturers.

Obviously, it is very difficult to convince manufacturers to change their products to make them less harmful. It is made even more difficult in advanced countries by the presence of laws that protect the rights of profit margins, just as there are laws to protect the rights of the citizens' health, with the same constitutional level of protection generating conflict.

It is well known that food and beverage manufacturers often ignore the rise in obesity rates, since their purpose—which they must report to their shareholders—remains that of tending to profit and seeking to increase sales as much as possible. Many unhealthy products represent a major source of profitability for some companies, so the spectre of government regulation is particularly threatening [133,134].

The conflict of interests is clear [135]. Many multinational corporations insist that they will help reduce obesity rates, but it must be noted that they do not promise to solve them, which leaves room for them to promote plans to improve nutrition, while simultaneously continuing to promote unhealthy products. It may be useful to remember the case of salt in Britain: in 2003 the food industry was invited to take voluntary measures to reduce salt in processed food products, including bread, hamburgers, pasta and biscuits. In 2018, Public Health England (PHE), published the first comprehensive report on the voluntary salt reductions that had been achieved by food producers and retailers [136]. Only slightly more than half of the goals had been reached. In fact, seven product categories did not meet any of the average targets set for them, these included ready-made meals, soups and meat alternatives, making them some of the largest contributors to salt intake with a huge variability in salt content. Many of the main contributors to salt are more frequently consumed by children, such as ham, fried potatoes, pizza, bread, breakfast cereals, beans, cakes, pastries, fruit pies and sauces. These foods are also more likely to be consumed by those in lower socio-economic groups. This report confirms that voluntary targets need comprehensive monitoring and guidance to be effective and, most crucially, that the food industry cannot, and must not, be made solely responsible for lowering our salt intakes. And this does not only apply to salt.

Depending on the choices of public policy, the government can opt for the targets to be made mandatory, with penalties if the targets are not met, or alternatively to choose to intensify communication and education for the most disadvantaged groups of consumers to make them aware of the risks of consumption.

In any case, it is easy to understand how the adaptation of a normative model for the current needs of reducing childhood obesity cannot be achieved whilst the obesity epidemic is growing so exponentially that it is unthinkable that it can be slowed only by preventing citizens from eating harmful foods by the use of regulation.

On the other hand, the same goal will not be achieved either by demanding producers to make their products healthier as quickly as possible. The spread of obesity is simply too rapid.

It is necessary, above all, to improve citizens' daily nutritional options promoting knowledge. Encouraging appropriate choices that can lead to a greater adherence of the MD is just as important, as evidenced by the majority of the population, who already eat well due to simple cultural choices, avoiding eating sweets, fats and processed meats for every meal or drinking water instead of fizzy drinks. It is therefore necessary to ensure that citizens' purchases respond to more rational and informed impulses, especially with regard to minors.

On this topic, it is widely assumed too that children are more susceptible than adults to persuasion by clever advertising and are more influenced by peer pressure. Junk food advertising is widely connected with poor nutrition, which has led to the policy response of banning junk food advertising for children [137].

To this end, limiting advertising for harmful foods could help, above all for the more impressionable bands of society such as minors, but this measure should also be accompanied by social marketing and appropriate education. Food marketing intentionally targets children who are too young to distinguish advertising from truth and induces them to eat high-calorie, low nutrient, but often highly profitable, junk food. Manufacturers and FBC are so successful in this marketing that business-as-usual cannot be allowed to continue without appropriate limits being imposed on them.

Such legislation, however, should be introduced in a wider framework of actions to combat childhood obesity [138]. This is an action that many European countries have already undertaken, given that it is now definitively established that the effects of these forms of advertising are extremely harmful [139]. A study drawn up by the WHO [140] indicates that existing policies and regulations are markedly insufficient when it comes to addressing the continuing challenges in this sensitive area. This is because they often tend to use too narrow definitions and criteria, meaning that standards are applied only to certain types of media, rather than to those with the largest audience of children. Furthermore, the complex challenges faced by cross-border marketing are hardly ever dealt with. The multiple causes of these situations are underpinned by both strong control and opposition from parts of the private sector, and the weakness of some self-regulation schemes.

9. The Nature of the Obstacles to the Adoption of the MD: Addressing Research

Generally, people prefer to eat everyday foods that correspond to predetermined patterns within their food culture, so that each food can satisfy an already known standard. The parameters of these standards are compatible with their lifestyle: not too expensive, with the nutrition they deem they need, prepared in the time they have and fitting to social norms with expected costs. Because trying a new food represents a risk of waste, simplifying seems to be the best option.

Attempts to steer consumers toward cheaper yet nutrient dense foods have encountered resistance and the main barriers to adoption are generally affordability, a lack of compatibility with taste preferences, and the belief that diet recommendations are often too time-consuming [141].

In this sense, the MD provides a socially acceptable framework for the inclusion of a set of fresh vegetables and dried fruit in a nutrient-rich everyday diet. Many of the products included in MD are themselves economical—except for some types of fish which can be replaced with cheaper ones—but consumers generally resist eating these less-familiar foods on a daily basis, particularly if they believe that doing so means abandoning their cultural heritage, or that those foods are associated with a different culture or a different social class.

As for this problem, there is evidence of a social gradient in diet quality: some studies demonstrate that generally, MD products are more likely to be consumed by groups of higher socio-economic status, while the consumption of refined grains, processed meats and added fats have been associated with a lower socio-economic status [142]. This fact can represent the real challenge, because the determinants of food choice are both complex and multifactorial, but food price is one of the most relevant determinants [143]. The lowest-cost diets, both energy rich and shelf stable, are also the least healthy, as composed by dry packaged and processed foods, likely to contain refined grains, added sugars, and added fats.

In many industrialized countries, there are socio-economic gradients in diet, so that those who are better off consume healthier diets than those less well-to-do. Almost everywhere the available evidence reveals that income affects food intake both directly and indirectly through the dispositions associated with particular social class locations [144]. Economic differences often generate cultural thresholds that constitute the most consistent problem: understanding how to overcome them and structuring adequate public policies is particularly important for resolving the problems faced by those that are most vulnerable to the choice of insecure food.

The multiple challenges involved in improving diet quality include helping people recognize the lower cost foods within their own cultural heritage, increasing the convenience and accessibility of lower cost, lower energy dense foods, and finally, doing so without sacrificing taste or enjoyment.

The MD represents a real intangible cultural heritage that flourished in a specific socio-cultural context, the dictates of which have become the biomedical model of a cultural representation [145], leading to a greater awareness of the importance of the social and cultural context in which a food model develops. This not only includes the choice of food in itself, but also corresponds particularly to the idea of conviviality, preparation and the pleasure of shared meals. The environment in which the MD was once consumed saw populations that were physically active enjoy a diet that basically rested on local plant foods. The challenges to promoting the Mediterranean Diet within and outside the Mediterranean region have been much researched and a significant point of evaluation has been how accurately the cultural ideals recognized by United Nations Educational, Scientific and Cultural Organization (UNESCO) [146] really represent the region and how culturally acceptable these ideals are to populations outside of the Mediterranean [147].

In particular, the act of eating together is seen to promote cultural identity and ensures social continuity. This special aspect of the MD represents an opportunity for social exchange, sharing time together, creating a special connection and promoting a space for community values and hospitality. A complete cultural process, expressed through the safeguarding of culinary techniques and the transmission of social values, is at the core of the life-style regime, along with the acknowledgment of pleasure as a fundamental part of a sustainable eating pattern. This point differentiates the MD from most dietary models focusing on the role of diet to meet biological needs rather than the role that foods can play as a vehicle for cultural processes and social interactions. Achieving the balance between pleasurable eating and health can obviously be more troublesome in the current environment, where media is a dominant presence and consumers are faced with an overabundance of calorific and processed food. In effect, economic growth and the globalization of food production are the reasons behind the desertion of the MD in countries where it once flourished [148].

It is clear that in the current obesogenic environment, reconstructing the same socio-environmental model is the most difficult challenge and the feeble voice of nutrition is almost lost amidst all the competing interests from the food industry and the perennially incumbent media. Living in cultural environments continually exposed to an excess of harmful foods makes it difficult opt out to healthy choices, while such choices remain almost non-existent or ineffective because they are dispersive, which means the clear identification of a correct nutritional modality is necessary. This is the reason why the structuring of an adequate and systematic health communication that takes these elements into account to be effective in contrasting childhood obesity and the sustainability of health systems now seems essential. Clearly indicating what is not suitable for long-term human nutrition and allowing consumers to explore their shared cultural food heritage through proper culinary education might represent a first step to restructuring, explicitly showing the benefits of joining the MD. Adapting traditional food preparation techniques to the modern world would also help to promote the adoption of this healthy lifestyle.

Gradually replacing harmful processed foods with high caloric density is a process that can be assimilated with proper communication, correct information and extensive education. If consumers are required to maintain a dietary pattern, they need to be clear on what that this pattern is.

Figure 2 shows a communication framework of actions aimed at enhancing the adoption of the MD.

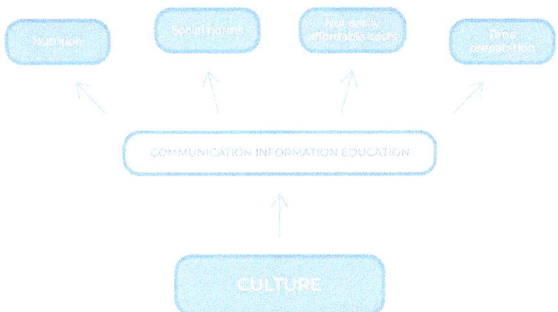

Figure 2. A communication framework of actions.

As previously mentioned, there are clear links between low socio-economic status, poor health and obesity, and it is a priority that health messages be made accessible to all sectors of society. The precise balance between good nutrition, affordability, culture and acceptable social norms is an area that deserves further study [149] as it is directly connected to the problem of the consumer's empowerment. Further research is also needed to gain clarity as to what pleasurable eating means to different bands of consumers [150] and whether the practice of eating convivially is accessible and relevant to general populations. If research needs to go beyond examining the validity of the nutritional components of the MD, more than anything else it has to explore the legitimacy of its cultural ideals.

10. Individual Choices and Actions to be Implemented

In view of the above, it is clear that the magic recipe to reduce obesity has not yet been discovered. Diet, exercise and behavior modifications will remain the cornerstones of obesity treatment for the foreseeable future, with a set of well structured public measures needed to increase their diffusion, acting in multi-competence, in a system of different levels of intervention.

In this context, where prevention remains the most obvious key, obesity continues to impose an economic burden on both public and private payers and the high public-sector spending for obesity remains a major cause for concern in terms of sustainability. Countering the continuing spread of the Western diet could be considered a primary goal of prevention, in favor of greater adherence to the MD.

Figure 3 shows the consequencences of a massive adherence to the principles of the Western Diet: the consequences of less adherence to MD and the connection between rising rates of obesity and undeniable rising medical spending. Without a strong and sustained reduction in obesity prevalence through more adherence to MD, major costs will be imposed on the healthcare system for the foreseeable future.

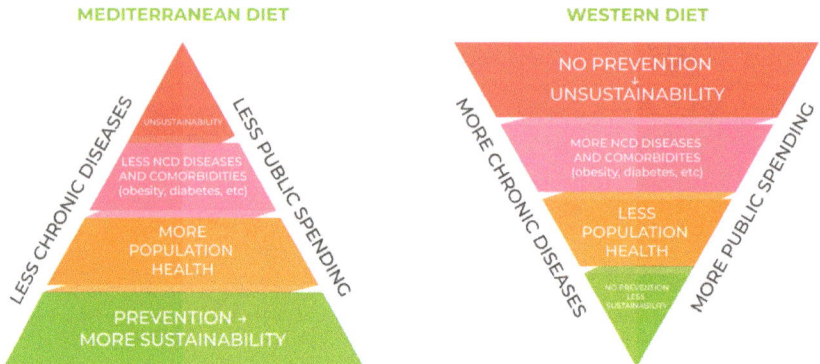

Figure 3. The consequences of the consumer's daily choice.

However, it must be kept in mind that is always up to the individual to formulate and continuously redefine the level of health and well-being that they intend to achieve. They must have the will to incorporate knowledge about what is healthy, together with the fulfillment of the consequent choices and actions to be implemented.

While on the one hand society tends to lack stable and shared orientations, it certainly opens the way to individual empowerment [151], which in turn leads to an awareness of the role of citizens in the social context: individual choices, after all, have consequences at both community and corporate level.

Even though people often modify their behavior in unpredictable ways, they can still be helped to improve their basic standards: obesity-inducing lifestyles are just an adaptation to external factors, and if our aim is to decrease obesity or improve diet quality through external measures using regulation and a selected set of practices, external conditions must be properly changed, starting with the pricing of healthy foods, the cost of sport and recreational activities, improving microenvironments and urban environments [152], and the promotion of a heuristic approach to make it easier for citizens learning about healthy eating.

Precisely in consideration of these topics, preforming *ad hoc* forms of architecture through the modification of micro-environments in order to *nudge* subjects to make advantageous choices seems to be a step forward for reducing the problem [153,154].

Cities often concentrate risks and hazards that can promote the development of obesity, diabetes and their comorbidities. In order to tackle the challenge, policy makers and urban planners must understand how their communities and families live and work in order to develop the best interventions and start to engender a shift in attitude and culture in how they look at their own health. Education and culture play a decisive role here: taste has long been recognized as a question of education, learning, and therefore, of belonging [155]. The concept of culture itself [156] has recently acquired very significant meanings for the medical and scientific fields that are full of consequences for future political choices in healthcare. In effect, health communication is becoming an important tool for determining citizens' behavior, because food is not only a necessity, but also, and above all, it represents a language, a means of communication, and therefore a privileged point of observation for the study of human and societal culture [157].

In order to be effective, the public policy approach must therefore be at the same time environmental and individual, effectively balancing its interventions [158]. It is increasingly being recognised that effective responses must go beyond interventions that only focus on a specific individual, social or environmental level and instead embrace system-based multilevel intervention approaches that address both the individual and environment.

The specific effects on different population groups should be considered in the design, modulation and monitoring of interventions, while also requiring a thorough understanding of the behavior and the target audience [159,160]. In effect, interventions should be targeted and based on relevant audience characteristics.

The scheme proposed in Figure 4. Summarily contains the instruments of action, where the indicated disciplines are to be considered among the most effective and diffused practices and models for individual/behavioral improvement of lifestyles [161,162], with the aim to create engagement even when there is resistance to change [163]. Their further analysis does not concern the subject of the present discussion.

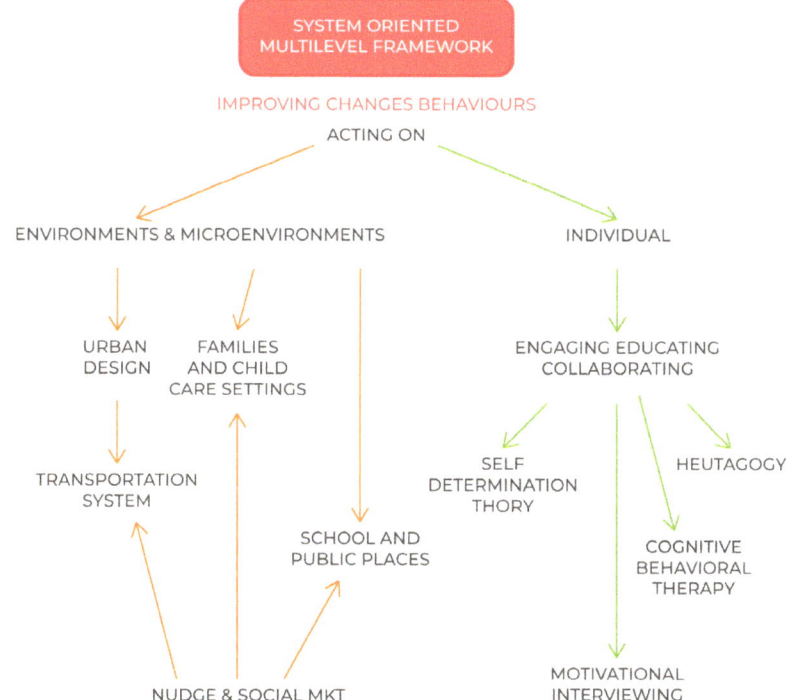

Figure 4. A system oriented multilevel framework.

11. Conclusions

In this scenario, having shown that the Mediterranean Diet (MD) prevents many diseases, the dissemination of its principles must be placed at the center of health policies.

For improvement to be effective, externality must also be pervaded by adequate and coherent communication, because in a dietary and food context, imperfect and asymmetric information is very often synonymous with poor efficacy.

In reverse, if well-conceived, carefully structured, implemented, and well-sustained public health communication programs have the capacity to elicit change among citizens by raising awareness, increasing knowledge, shaping attitudes, and changing behaviors and lifestyle [164], effectively influencing health outcomes.

Even if the evidence obviously suggests that poor diets and lifestyle cannot be changed by information policy alone, improved information is nevertheless essential for a conscious choice.

This means that policy measures should include the allocation of funds to expressly encourage a greater adherence to the MD in childhood environments through appropriate information and education. In consideration of the substantial evidence that supports its effects in chronic disease prevention and management, the Mediterranean Model could be designed while considering the needs of the period we are experiencing, of the current food supply, which is obviously different from that of the Sixties, and designing specific practical strategies to further spread and implement, considering that nutritional habits are homogenizing everywhere. In effect, the greater issue is that the importance of having the majority of a population following a healthy diet like the MD is hugely underestimated. In a general prevention context, speaking abstractly about generic dietary patterns is not what's needed. Instead, one model needs to be unequivocally promoted, that which has been identified as having proved to be the most effective amongst many others in terms of the prevention of obesity-related diseases.

The aim is to translate the MD traditional principles, identifying the key food-based components, in order to be able to adapt them also to populations with different nutritional traditions, or in multicultural settings, as already successfully experimented [165]. In other words, the MD Model should represent the translation of the key elements of the traditional MD to populations outside the Mediterranean Region in order to increase the likelihood of acceptability and sustainability.

Encouraging people to adopt MD habits would not only be beneficial from a public health perspective, but above all it would be a concrete measure of intervention in terms of economic sustainability.

Author Contributions: The contributions refer to the different areas of competence: Law, Regulation and Human Sciences: S.D.; Figure 2, Figure 3, Figure 4: S.D.; Pediatrics: C.B. and M.L.; Everything has been shared among the Authors. All authors read, revised, and approved the final manuscript.

Funding: This research received no external funding.

Conflicts of Interest: The authors declare no conflict of interest.

References

1. Romagnolo, D.F.; Selmin, O.I. Mediterranean Diet and Prevention of Chronic Diseases. *Nutr. Today* **2017**, *52*, 208–222. [CrossRef] [PubMed]
2. Bach-Faig, A.; Berry, E.M.; Lairon, D.; Reguant, J.; Trichopoulou, A.; Dernini, S.; Medina, F.X.; Battino, M.; Belahsen, R.; Miranda, G.; et al. Mediterranean Diet Foundation Expert Group. Mediterranean diet pyramid today. Science and cultural updates. *Public Health Nutr.* **2011**, *14*, 2274–2284. [CrossRef]
3. Willett, W.C.; Sacks, F.; Trichopoulou, A.; Drescher, G.; Ferro-Luzzi, A.; Helsing, E.; Trichopoulos, D. Mediterranean diet pyramid: A cultural model for healthy eating. *Am. J. Clin. Nutr.* **1995**, *61*, 1402S–1406S. [CrossRef]
4. Simopoulos, A.P. The Importance of the Omega-6/Omega-3 Fatty Acid Ratio in Cardiovascular Disease and Other Chronic Diseases. *Exp. Biol. Med.* **2008**, *233*, 674–688. [CrossRef]
5. Marventano, S.; Kolacz, P.; Castellano, S.; Galvano, F.; Buscemi, S.; Mistretta, A.; Grosso, G. A review of recent evidence in human studies of n-3 and n-6 PUFA intake on cardiovascular diseases, cancer, and depressive disorders: Does the ratio really matter? *Int. J. Food Sci. Nutr.* **2015**. [CrossRef] [PubMed]
6. Sofi, F.; Abbate, R.; Gensini, G.F.; Casini, A. Accruing evidence on benefits of adherence to the Mediterranean diet on health: An updated systematic review and meta-analysis. *Am. J. Clin. Nutr.* **2010**, *92*, 1189–1196. [CrossRef] [PubMed]
7. Rees, K.; Hartley, L.; Clarke, A.; Thorogood, M.; Stranges, S. Mediterranean' dietary pattern for the primary prevention of cardiovascular disease. *Cochrane Database Syst. Rev.* **2012**, *2012*. [CrossRef]
8. Rosato, V.; Temple, N.J.; La Vecchia, C.; Castellan, G.; Tavani, A.; Guercio, V. Mediterranean diet and cardiovascular disease: A systematic review and meta-analysis of observational studies. *Eur. J. Nutr.* **2019**. [CrossRef]
9. Estruch, R.; Ros, E. Primary Prevention of Cardiovascular Disease with a Mediterranean Diet Supplemented with Extra-Virgin Olive Oil or Nuts. *N. Engl. J. Med.* **2018**, *378*, e34. [CrossRef]

10. Dontas, A.S.; Zerefos, N.S.; Panagiotakos, D.B.; Valis, D.A. Mediterranean diet and prevention of coronary heart disease in the elderly. *Clin. Interv. Aging* **2007**, *2*, 109–115. [CrossRef]
11. Huo, R.; Du, T.; Xu, Y.; Xu, W.; Chen, X.; Sun, K.; Yu, X. Effects of Mediterranean-style diet on glycemic control, weight loss and cardiovascular risk factors among type 2 diabetes individuals: A meta-analysis. *Eur. J. Clin. Nutr.* **2015**, *69*, 1200–1208. [CrossRef] [PubMed]
12. Kastorini, C.M.; Milionis, H.J.; Esposito, K.; Giugliano, D.; Goudevenos, J.A.; Panagiotakos, D.B. The effect of Mediterranean diet on metabolic syndrome and its components: A meta-analysis of 50 studies and 534,906 individuals. *J. Am. Coll. Cardiol.* **2011**, *57*, 1299–1313. [CrossRef] [PubMed]
13. Fischer, M.; Stronati, M.; Lanari, M. Mediterranean diet, folic acid, and neural tube defects. *Ital. J. Pediatr.* **2017**, *43*, 74. [CrossRef] [PubMed]
14. Mikkelsen, T.B.; Osterdal, M.L.; Knudsen, V.K.; Haugen, M.; Meltzer, H.M.; Bakketeig, L.; Olsen, S.F. Association between a Mediterranean-type diet and risk of preterm birth among Danish women: A prospective cohort study. *Acta Obs. Gynecol. Scand.* **2008**, *87*, 325–330. [CrossRef] [PubMed]
15. Smith, L.K.; Draper, E.S.; Evans, T.A.; Field, D.J.; Johnson, S.J.; Manktelow, B.N.; Seaton, S.E.; Marlow, N.; Petrou, S.; Boyle, E.M. Associations between late and moderately preterm birth and smoking, alcohol, drug use and diet: A population-based case-cohort study. *Arch. Dis. Child. Fetal Neonatal Ed.* **2015**, *100*, F486–F491. [CrossRef] [PubMed]
16. Martínez-Galiano, J.M.; Olmedo-Requena, R.; Barrios-Rodríguez, R.; Amezcua-Prieto, C.; Bueno-Cavanillas, A.; Salcedo-Bellido, I.; Jimenez-Moleon, J.J.; Delgado-Rodríguez, M. Effect of Adherence to a Mediterranean Diet and Olive Oil Intake during Pregnancy on Risk of Small for Gestational Age Infants. *Nutrients* **2018**, *10*, 1234. [CrossRef]
17. Fernandez-Barres, S.; Romaguera, D.; Valvi, D.; Martinez, D.; Vioque, J.; Navarrete-Munoz, E.M.; Amiano, P.; Gonzalez-Palacios, S.; Guxens, M.; Pereda, E.; et al. Mediterranean dietary pattern in pregnant women and offspring risk of overweight and abdominal obesity in early childhood: The INMA birth cohort study. *Pediatr. Obes.* **2016**, *11*, 491–499. [CrossRef]
18. Chatzi, L.; Rifas-Shiman, S.L.; Georgiou, V.; Joung, K.E.; Koinaki, S.; Chalkiadaki, G.; Margioris, A.; Sarri, K.; Vassilaki, M.; Vafeiadi, M.; et al. Adherence to the Mediterranean diet during pregnancy and offspring adiposity and cardiometabolic traits in childhood. *Pediatr. Obes.* **2017**, *12* (Suppl. 1), 47–56. [CrossRef]
19. Gonzalez-Nahm, S.; Mendez, M.; Robinson, W.; Murphy, S.K.; Hoyo, C.; Hogan, V.; Rowley, D. Low maternal adherence to a Mediterranean diet is associated with increase in methylation at the MEG3-IG differentially methylated region in female infants. *Environ. Epigenetics* **2017**, *3*, dvx007. [CrossRef]
20. D'Alessandro, A.; De Pergola, G. The Mediterranean Diet: Its definition and evaluation of a priori dietary indexes in primary cardiovascular prevention. *Int. J. Food Sci. Nutr.* **2018**. [CrossRef]
21. Davis, C.; Bryan, J.; Hodgson, J.; Murphy, K. Definition of the Mediterranean Diet; a literature review. *Nutrients* **2015**, *7*, 9139–9153. [CrossRef]
22. Altomare, R.; Cacciabaudo, F.; Damiano, G.; Palumbo, V.D.; Gioviale, M.C.; Bellavia, M.; Tomasello, G.; Monte, A.I. The Mediterranean Diet: A History of Health. *Iran. J. Public Health* **2013**, *42*, 449–457. [PubMed]
23. Mocciaro, G.; Ziauddeen, N.; Godos, J.; Marranzano, M.; Chan, M.Y.; Ray, S. Does a Mediterranean-type dietary pattern exert a cardio-protective effect outside the Mediterranean region? A review of current evidence. *Int. J. Food Sci. Nutr.* **2017**. [CrossRef] [PubMed]
24. Martínez-González, M.; Hershey, M.; Zazpe, I.; Trichopoulou, A. Transferability of the Mediterranean Diet to Non-Mediterranean Countries. What Is and What Is Not the Mediterranean Diet. *Nutrients* **2017**, *9*, 1226. [CrossRef] [PubMed]
25. Romaguera, D.; Norat, T.; Vergnaud, A.C.; Mouw, T.; May, A.M.; Agudo, A.; Buckland, G.; Slimani, N.; Rinaldi, S.; Couto, E.; et al. Mediterranean dietary patterns and prospective weight change in participants of the EPIC-PANACEA project. *Am. J. Clin. Nutr.* **2010**, *92*, 912–921. [CrossRef]
26. Bonaccio, M.; Iacoviello, L.; De Gaetano, G. The Mediterranean diet: The reasons for a success. *Thromb. Res.* **2012**, *129*, 401–404. [CrossRef] [PubMed]
27. Tognon, G.; Hebestreit, A.; Lanfer, A.; Moreno, L.A.; Pala, V.; Siani, A.; Tornaritis, M.; De Henauw, S.; Veidebaum, T.; Molnar, D.; et al. Mediterranean diet, overweight and body composition in children from eight European countries: Cross-sectional and prospective results from the IDEFICS study. *Nutr. Metab. Cardiovasc. Dis.* **2014**, *24*, 205–213. [CrossRef] [PubMed]

28. NCD Risk Factor Collaboration (NCD-RisC). Available online: www.thelancet.com (accessed on 10 May 2019).
29. Braet, C.; Mervielde, I.; Vandereycken, W. Psychological aspects of childhood obesity: A controlled study in a clinical and nonclinical sample. *J. Pediatr. Psychol.* **1997**, *22*, 59–71. [CrossRef] [PubMed]
30. Kelsey, M.M.; Zaepfel, A.; Bjornstad, P.; Nadeau, K.J. Age-related consequences of childhood obesity. *Gerontology* **2014**, *60*, 222–228. [CrossRef] [PubMed]
31. Hartlev, M. Stigmatisation as a public health tool against obesity—A health and human rights perspective. *Eur. J. Health Law* **2014**, *21*, 365–386. [CrossRef] [PubMed]
32. Karnik, S.; Kanekar, A. Childhood obesity: A global public health crisis. *Int. J. Prev. Med.* **2012**, *3*, 1–7. [PubMed]
33. Tsakiraki, M.; Grammatikopoulou, M.G. Nutrition transition and health status of Cretan women: Evidence from two generations. *Public Health Nutr.* **2011**, *14*, 793–800. [CrossRef] [PubMed]
34. Ogden, C.L.; Carroll, M.D.; Kit, B.K.; Flegal, K.M. Prevalence of obesity and trends in body mass index among US children and adolescents, 1999–2010. *JAMA* **2012**, *307*, 483–490. [CrossRef] [PubMed]
35. Fan, J.G.; Kim, S.U.; Wong, V.W. New trends on obesity and NAFLD in Asia. *J. Hepatol.* **2017**, *67*, 862–873. [CrossRef] [PubMed]
36. Chakraborty, C.; Das, S. Dynamics of diabetes and obesity: An alarming situation in the developing countries in Asia. *Mini Rev. Med. Chem.* **2016**, *16*, 1258–1268. [CrossRef] [PubMed]
37. Gordon-Larsen, P.; Wang, H.; Popkin, B.M. Overweight Dynamics in Chinese Children and Adults. *Obes. Rev.* **2014**, *15*, 37–48. [CrossRef] [PubMed]
38. Liu, X.; Wu, W.; Mao, Z.; Huo, W.; Tu, R.; Qian, X.; Zhang, X.; Tian, Z.; Zhang, H.; Jiang, J.; et al. Prevalence and influencing factors of overweight and obesity in a Chinese rural population: The Henan Rural Cohort Study. *Sci Rep.* **2018**, *8*, 13101. [CrossRef]
39. Zhai, F.; Du, S.; Wang, Z.; Zhang, J.; Du, W.; Popki, B. Dynamics of the Chinese Diet and the Role of Urbanicity, 1991–2011. *Obes. Rev.* **2014**, *15*. [CrossRef]
40. Popkin, B.M.; Reardon, T. Obesity and the food system transformation in Latin America. *Obes. Rev.* **2018**, *19*, 1028–1064. [CrossRef]
41. UNICEF-WHO-The World Bank Group. *Joint Child Malnutrition Estimates—Levels and Trends*, 2018 ed.; World Health Organization: Geneva, Switzerland, 2018; Available online: Http://www.who.int/nutgrowthdb/estimates2017/en/ (accessed on 17 May 2018).
42. Klingberg, S.; Draper, C.E.; Micklesfield, L.K.; Benjamin-Neelon, S.E.; Van Sluijs, E.M.F. Childhood Obesity Prevention in Africa: A Systematic Review of Intervention Effectiveness and Implementation. *Int. J. Environ. Res. Public Health* **2019**, *16*, 1212. [CrossRef]
43. Australian Government, Australian Institute of Health and Welfare. A Picture of Overweight and Obesity in Australia. Available online: https://www.aihw.gov.au/getmedia/172fba28-785e-4a08-ab37-2da3bbae40b8/aihw-phe-216.pdf.aspx?inline=true (accessed on 12 May 2019).
44. Finkelstein, E.A.; Trogdon, J.G.; Cohen, J.W.; Dietz, W. Annual Medical Spending Attributable to Obesity: Payer-and Service-Specific Estimates. *Health Aff.* **2009**, *28*, w822–w831. [CrossRef] [PubMed]
45. Esposito, K.; Kastorini, C.M.; Panagiotakos, D.B.; Giugliano, D. Mediterranean diet and weight loss: Meta-analysis of randomized controlled trials. *Metab. Syndr. Relat. Disord.* **2011**, *9*, 1–12. [CrossRef] [PubMed]
46. Laccetti, R.; Pota, A.; Stranges, S.; Falconi, C.; Memoli, B.; Bardaro, L.; Guida, B. Evidence on the prevalence and geographic distribution of major cardiovascular risk factors in Italy. *Public Health Nutr.* **2012**, *30*, 305–315. [CrossRef] [PubMed]
47. Childhood Obesity Surveillance Initiative (COSI) Factsheet. Highlights 2015–2017. 2018. Available online: http://www.euro.who.int/en/health-topics/disease-prevention/nutrition/activities/who-european-childhood-obesity-surveillance-initiative-cosi/cosi-publications/childhood-obesity-surveillance-initiative-cosi-factsheet.-highlights-2015-17-2018 (accessed on 20 March 2019).
48. Vilarnau, C.; Stracker, D.M.; Funtikov, A.; da Silva, R.; Estruch, R.; Bach-Faig, A. Worldwide adherence to Mediterranean Diet between 1960 and 2011. *Eur. J. Clin. Nutr.* **2018**. [CrossRef] [PubMed]
49. Schmidhuber, J.; Traill, W.B. The changing structure of diets in the European Union in relation to healthy eating guidelines. *Public Health Nutr.* **2006**, *9*, 584–595. [CrossRef] [PubMed]

50. Moreno, L.A.; Sarria, A.; Popkin, B.M. The nutrition transition in Spain: A European Mediterranean country. *Eur. J. Clin. Nutr.* **2002**, *56*, 992–1003. [CrossRef]
51. Grosso, G.; Galvano, F. Mediterranean diet adherence in children and adolescents in southern European countries. *NFS J.* **2016**, *3*, 13–19. [CrossRef]
52. Caballero, B. *The Nutrition Transition: Global Trends in Diet and Disease*; Lippincott Williams & Wilkins: Philadelphia, PA, USA, 2005; pp. 1717–1722.
53. Kearneys, J. Food Consumptions trends and drivers. *Philos. Trans. R. Soc. B Biol. Sci.* **2010**, *365*, 2793–2807. [CrossRef]
54. Oggioni, C.; Lara, J.; Wells, J.C.; Soroka, K.; Siervo, M. Shifts in population dietary patterns and physical inactivity as determinants of global trends in the prevalence of diabetes: An ecological analysis. *Nutr. Metab. Cardiovasc. Dis.* **2014**, *24*, 1105–1111. [CrossRef]
55. Thow, A.M. Trade liberalization and the nutrition transition: Mapping the pathways for public health nutritionists. *Public Health Nutr.* **2009**, *12*, 2150–2158. [CrossRef]
56. Ogden, C.L.; Kuczmarski, R.J.; Flegal, K.M.; Mei, Z.; Guo, S.; Wei, R.; Grummer-Strawn, L.M.; Curtin, L.R.; Roche, A.F.; Johnson, C.L. Centers for Disease Control and Prevention 2000 growth charts for the United States: Improvements to the 1977 National Center for Health Statistics version. *Pediatrics* **2002**, *109*, 45–60. [CrossRef] [PubMed]
57. Lobstein, T.; Baur, L.; Uauy, R. Obesity in children and young people: A crisis in public health. *Obes. Rev.* **2004**, *5* (Suppl. 1), 4–104. [CrossRef]
58. Magarey, A.M.; Daniels, L.A.; Boulton, T.J. Prevalence of overweight and obesity in Australian children and adolescents: Reassessment of 1985 and 1995 data against new standard international definitions. *Med. J. Aust.* **2001**, *174*, 561–564. [PubMed]
59. Popkin, B.M. Global nutrition dynamics: The world is shifting rapidly toward a diet linked with noncommunicable diseases. *Am. J. Clin. Nutr.* **2006**, *84*, 289–298. [CrossRef] [PubMed]
60. Finucane, M.M.; Stevens, G.A.; Cowan, M.J.; Danaei, G.; Lin, J.K.; Paciorek, C.J.; Singh, G.M.; Gutierrez, H.R.; Lu, Y.; Bahalim, A.N.; et al. National, regional, and global trends in body-mass index since 1980: Systematic analysis of health examination surveys and epidemiological studies with 960 country-years and 9.1 million participants. *Lancet* **2011**, *377*, 557–567. [CrossRef]
61. Bleich, S.N.; Cutler, D.; Murray, C.; Adams, A. Why Is the Developed World Obese? *Annu. Rev. Public Health* **2008**, *29*, 273–295. [CrossRef] [PubMed]
62. Bagarani, M.; Forleo, M.; Zampino, S. Household Food Expenditure Behaviours and Socioeconomic Welfare in Italy: A Microeconometric Analysis. In Proceedings of the European Association of Agricultural Economists (EAAE) > 113th Seminar, Chania, Crete, Greece, 3–6 September 2009; Available online: https://tind-customer-agecon.s3.amazonaws.com/1f27feaf-1359-44e9-afee-e9b4da06f434?response-content-disposition=inline%3B%20filename%2A%3DUTF-8%27%27Bagarani.pdf&response-content-type=application%2Fpdf&AWSAccessKeyId=AKIAXL7W7Q3XHXDVDQYS&Expires=1559637196&Signature=Y9Kt8nHvnsmR0HPkafRGIzBQNuY%3D (accessed on 4 May 2019).
63. Baourakis, G.; Mattas, K.; Zopounidis, C.; Van Dijk, G. *A Resilient European Food Industry in a Challenging World*; Nova Science Publishers: Hauppauge, NY, USA, 2010; ISBN1 978-1611220322. ISBN2 1611220327.
64. Conforti, P. *Looking Ahead in World Food and Agriculture. Perspectives to 2050*; Food and Agriculture Organization of the United Nations, Economic and Social Development Department, Agricultural Development Economics Division: Rome, Italy, 2011.
65. Behlasen, R. Nutrition transition and food sustainability. *Proc. Nutr. Soc.* **2014**, *73*, 385–388. [CrossRef]
66. Archero, F.; Ricotti, R.; Solito, A.; Carrera, D.; Civello, F.; Di Bella, R.; Bellone, S.; Prodam, F. Adherence to the Mediterranean Diet among School Children and Adolescents Living in Northern Italy and Unhealthy Food Behaviors Associated to Overweight. *Nutrients* **2018**, *10*, 1322. [CrossRef]
67. Ritchie, L.D.; Ivey, S.L.; Woodward-Lopez, G.; Crawford, P.B. Alarming trends in pediatric overweight in the United States. *Soc. Prev. Med.* **2003**, *48*, 168–177.
68. McPherson, K.; Marsh, T.; Brown, M. Foresight, Tackling Obesities: Future Choices—Modelling Future Trends in Obesity and the Impact on Health. 2007. Available online: http://citeseerx.ist.psu.edu/viewdoc/download?doi=10.1.1.629.2896&rep=rep1&type=pdf (accessed on 10 May 2019).
69. Rappange, D.R.; Brouver, W.B.F.; Hoogenveen, R.T.; Van Baal, P.H.M. Healthcare Costs and Obesity Prevention, Drug Costs and Other Sector-Specific Consequences. *Pharmacoeconomics* **2009**, *27*. [CrossRef]

70. Kelly, T.; Yang, W.; Chen, C.S.; Reynolds, K.; He, J. Global burden of obesity in 2005 and projections to 2030. *Int. J. Obes.* **2008**, *32*, 1431–1437. [CrossRef] [PubMed]
71. WHO. Key Facts. 2018. Available online: https://www.who.int/news-room/fact-sheets/detail/obesity-and-overweight (accessed on 27 March 2019).
72. Swinburn, B.A. Obesity prevention: The role of policies, laws and regulations. *Aust. New Zealand Health Policy* **2008**, *5*, 12. [CrossRef] [PubMed]
73. Gortmaker, S.L.; Swinburn, B.A.; Levy, D.; Carter, R.; Mabry, P.L.; Finegood, D.T.; Moodie, M.L. Changing the future of obesity: Science, policy, and action. *Lancet* **2011**, *378*, 838–847. [CrossRef]
74. Trust for America's Health. R.W. Johnson Foundation. Available online: https://stateofobesity.org/wp-content/uploads/2018/09/stateofobesity2018.pdf (accessed on 30 September 2018).
75. Dietz, W.H.; Benken, D.E.; Hunter, A.S. Public health law and the prevention and control of obesity. *Milbank Q.* **2009**, *87*, 215–227. [CrossRef] [PubMed]
76. Mensah, G.A.; Goodman, R.A.; Zaza, S.; Moulton, A.D.; Kocher, P.L.; Dietz, W.H.; Pechacek, T.F.; Marks, J.S. Law as a tool for preventing chronic diseases: Expanding the range of effective public health strategies. *Prev. Chronic Dis.* **2004**, *1*, A13. [PubMed]
77. Martinez-Gonzalez, M.A.; Bes-Rastrollo Serra-Majem, L.; Lairon, D.; Estruch, R.; Trichopoulou, A. Mediterranean food pattern and the primary prevention of chronic disease: Recent development. *Nutr. Rev.* **2009**, *67*, S111–S116. [CrossRef]
78. Saulle, R.; Semyonov, L.; La Torre, G. Cost and Cost-Effectiveness of the Mediterranean Diet: Results of a Systematic Review. *Nutrients* **2013**, *5*, 4566–4586. [CrossRef] [PubMed]
79. Traill, W.B.; University of Reading. Poor Diets in Europe: Causes and Implications for Policy. Available online: http://ilo.unimol.it/sidea/images/upload/convegno_2009/plenarie/relazione%20plenaria_traill.pdf (accessed on 3 March 2019).
80. Lopez, C.N.; Martinez-Gonzalez, M.A.; Sanchez-Villegas, A.; Alonso, A.; Pimenta, A.M.; Bes-Rastrollo, M. Costs of Mediterranean and western dietary patterns in a Spanish cohort and their relationship with prospective weight change. *J. Epidemiol. Community Health* **2009**, *63*, 920–927. [CrossRef]
81. Bonaccio, M.; Bonanni, A.E.; Di Castelnuovo, A.; De Lucia, F.; Donati, M.B.; De Gaetano, G.; Iacoviello, L.; Moli-sani Project Investigators. Low income is associated with poor adherence to a Mediterranean diet and a higher prevalence of obesity: Cross-sectional results from the Molisani study. *BMJ. Open* **2012**, *2*. [CrossRef]
82. Tiffin, R.; Salois, M. Inequalities in diet and nutrition. *Proc. Nutr. Soc.* **2012**, *71*, 105–111. [CrossRef]
83. Marmot, M.; Friel, S.; Bell, R.; Houweling, T.A.; Taylor, S. Closing the gap in a generation: Health equity through action on the social determinants of health. *Lancet* **2008**, *372*, 1661–1669. [CrossRef]
84. Shareck, M.; Frolich, K.L.; Poland, B. Reducing social inequalities in health through settings-related interventions—A conceptual framework. *Glob. Health Promot.* **2013**, *20*, 39–52. [CrossRef] [PubMed]
85. Brownell, K.D. Weight Bias: Nature, Consequences, and Remedies. In *Eating Disorders and Obesity*, 3rd ed.; A Comprehensive Handbook; Guilford Publications: New York, NY, USA, 2005.
86. Choquet, H.; Meyre, D. Genomic insights into early-onset obesity. *Genome Med.* **2010**, *2*, 36. [CrossRef] [PubMed]
87. Kass, D.; Haslam, D. Is bariatric Surgery the Right Approach to Obesity? 2015. Available online: https://www.pharmaceutical-journal.com/opinion/comment/is-bariatric-surgery-the-right-approach-to-obesity/20067632.article?firstPass=false (accessed on 17 December 2018).
88. Hofmann, B. Bariatric surgery for obese children and adolescents: A review of the moral challenges. *BMC Med Ethics* **2013**. [CrossRef] [PubMed]
89. Anderson, P.M.; Butcher, K.F.; Whitmore Schanzenbach, D. *Childhood Disadvantage and Obesity: Is Nurture Trumping Nature?* NBER Working Paper No. 13479, Issued in October 2007, NBER Program(s): Children, Labor Studies; National Bureau of Economic Research 1050 Massachusetts Avenue: Cambridge, MA, USA, 2007.
90. Allebeck, P. The prevention paradox or the inequality paradox? *Eur. J. Public Health* **2008**, *18*, 215. [CrossRef] [PubMed]
91. Chiolero, A. Why causality, and not prediction, should guide obesity prevention policy. *Lancet Public Health* **2018**. [CrossRef]

92. Roberto, C.A.; Swinburn, B.; Hawkes, C.; Huang, T.T.; Costa, S.A.; Ashe, M.; Zwicker, L.; Cawley, J.H.; Brownell, K.D. Patchy Progress in Obesity Prevention, Emerging Examples, Entrenched Barriers and New Thinking. Available online: https://www.thelancet.com/journals/lancet/article/PIIS0140-6736(14)61744-X/fulltext (accessed on 19 January 2019).
93. EU Working Group on Socio-Economic Inequalities in Health. Monitoring Socio-Economic Inequalities in Health in the European Union: Guidelines and Illustrations. 2001. Available online: http://ec.europa.eu/health/ph_projects/1998/monitoring/fp_monitoring_1998_frep_06_a_en.pdf (accessed on 22 January 2019).
94. McAllister, E.J.; Dhurandhar, N.V.; Keith, S.W.; Aronne, L.J.; Barger, J.; Baskin, M.; Benca, R.M.; Biggio, J.; Boggiano, M.M.; Eisenmann, J.C.; et al. Ten putative contributors to the obesity epidemic. *Crit. Rev. Food Sci. Nutr.* **2009**, *49*, 868–913. [CrossRef] [PubMed]
95. Malik, V.S.; Willett, W.C.; Hu, F.B. Global obesity: Trends, risk factors and policy implications. *Nat. Rev. Endocrinol.* **2013**, *9*, 13–27. [CrossRef]
96. Samouda, H.; Ruiz-Castell, M.; Bocquet, V.; Kuemmerle, A.; Chioti, A.; Dadoun, F.; Kandala, N.; Stranges, S. Geografical variation of overweight, obesity and related risk factors, Findings from the European Health Examination Survey in Luxembourg 2013–2015. *PLoS ONE* **2018**. [CrossRef]
97. Brownell, K.D. Behavioral, psychological, and environmental predictors of obesity and success at weight reduction. *Int. J. Obes.* **1984**, *8*, 543–550.
98. WHO. Available online: http://www.euro.who.int/__data/assets/pdf_file/0004/258781/COSI-report-round-1-and-2_final-for-web.pdf?ua=1 (accessed on 2 March 2019).
99. Haber, B. The Mediterranean diet: A view from history. *Ame. J. Clin. Nutr.* **1997**, *66*, 1053S–1057S. [CrossRef] [PubMed]
100. Evans, W.D.; Christoffel, K.K.; Necheles, J.W.; Becker, A.B. Social Marketing as a Childhood Obesity Prevention Strategy. *Obesity* **2010**. [CrossRef] [PubMed]
101. Lycett, K.; Miller, A.; Knox, A.; Dunn, S.; Kerr, J.A.; Sung, V.; Wake, M. 'Nudge' interventions for improving children's dietary behaviours in the home: A systematic review. *Obes. Med.* **2017**. [CrossRef]
102. Oliver, A. Is nudge an effective public health strategy to tackle obesity? Yes. *BMJ* **2011**, *342*, d2168. [CrossRef] [PubMed]
103. Rayner, G.; Lang, T. Is nudge an effective public health strategy to tackle obesity? No. *BMJ* **2011**, *342*, d2177. [CrossRef] [PubMed]
104. Bianchi, F.; Garnett, E.; Dorsell, C.; Aveyard, P.; Jebb, S.A. Restructuring physical micro-environments to reduce the demand for meat: a systematic review and qualitative comparative analysis. *Lancet Planet. Health* **2018**, *2*, e384–e397. [CrossRef]
105. Arno, A.; Thomas, S. Restructuring physical micro environmentsto reduce the demand for meat:a systematic review and qualitative and comparative analysis The efficacy of nudge theories strategies in influencing adult dietary behaviours, a systematic review and meta analysis. *BMC Public Health* **2016**, *16*, 676–697. [CrossRef]
106. Smith, M.; Topprakkiran, N. Behavioural Insight, Nudge and the Choice in Obesity Policy. Available online: https://rsa.tandfonline.com/doi/full/10.1080/01442872.2018.1554806?scroll=top&needAccess=true#.XBPuja2h3q3 (accessed on 9 March 2019).
107. WHO. Key Considerations for the Use of Law to Prevent Noncommunicable Diseases in the WHO European Region Report of an Intensive Legal Training and Capacity-Building Workshop on Law and Noncommunicable Diseases. 2016. Available online: http://www.euro.who.int/__data/assets/pdf_file/0009/333954/Moscow-report.pdf?ua=1 (accessed on 28 January 2019).
108. Holcombe, R.G. Selective Excise Taxation from an Interest-Group Perspective. In *Taxing Choice: The Predatory Politics of Fiscal Discrimination*; William, F., Shughart, I.I., Eds.; Rutgers—The State University of New Jersey: New Brunswick, NJ, USA, 1998; pp. 81–100.
109. Fletcher, J.M.; Frisvold, D.; Tefft, N. Can Soft Drink Taxes Reduce Population Weight? Available online: http://www.economics.emory.edu/Working_Papers/wp/2008wp/Frisvold_08_08_paper.pdf (accessed on 28 January 2019).
110. Kerry. *Global Map of the Sugar Tax*, 2018. Available online: https://kerrydotcomcdn.azureedge.net/cdprod/Media/infographics/kerry-sugar-tax-infographic (accessed on 28 January 2019).
111. Bødker, M.; Pisinger, C.; Toft, U.; Jørgensen, T. The Danish fat tax—Effects on consumption patterns and risk of ischaemic heart disease. *Prev. Med.* **2015**, *77*, 200–203. [CrossRef]

112. Silver, L.D.; Ng, S.W.; Ryan-Ibarra, S.; Taillie, L.S.; Induni, M.; Miles, D.R.; Poti, J.M.; Popkin, B.M. Changes in prices, sales, consumer spending, and beverage consumption one yearafter a tax on sugar-sweetened beverages in Berkeley, California, US: A before-and-after study. *PLoS Med.* **2017**. [CrossRef]
113. Thelancet.com/diabetes-endocrinology Vol 5 April. Available online: https://www.thelancet.com/pdfs/journals/landia/PIIS2213-8587(17)30070-0.pdf (accessed on 26 January 2019).
114. Mytton, O.; Gray, A.; Rayner, M.; Rutter, H. Could targeted food taxes improve health? *J. Epidemiol. Community Health* **2007**, *61*, 689–694. [CrossRef]
115. Brown, C.M.; Dulloo, A.G.; Montani, J.P. Sugar drinks in the pathogenesis of obesity and cardiovascular diseases. *Int. J. Obes. (Lond.)* **2008**, *32* (Suppl. 6), S28–S34. [CrossRef]
116. Choi, H.K.; Willett, W.; Curhan, G. Fructose-rich beverages and risk of gout in women. *JAMA* **2010**, *304*, 2270–2278. [CrossRef] [PubMed]
117. Adamowicz, J.; DrewaIs, T. Is there a link between soft drinks and erectile dysfunction? *Cent. Eur. J. Urol.* **2011**, *64*, 140–143. [CrossRef] [PubMed]
118. Satterthwaite, D.; McGranahan, G.; Tacoli, C. Urbanization and its implications for food and farming, review. *R. Soc. Philos. Trans. B* **2010**, *365*, 2809–2820. [CrossRef] [PubMed]
119. Franck, C.; Grandi, S.M.; Eisenberg, M.J. Taxing junk food to counter obesity. *Am. J. Public Health* **2013**, *103*, 1949–1953. [CrossRef] [PubMed]
120. Fletcher, J.M.; Frisvold, D.E.; Tefft, N. The effects of soft drink taxes on child andadolescent consumption and weight outcomes. *J. Public Econ.* **2010**, *94*, 967–974. [CrossRef]
121. Chen, L.; Appel, L.J.; Loria, C.; Lin, P.H.; Champagne, C.M.; Elmer, P.J.; Ard, J.D.; Mitchell, D.; Batch, B.C.; Svetkey, L.P.; et al. Reduction in consumption of sugar-sweetened beverages is associated with weight loss: The PREMIER trial. *Am. J. Clinnutr.* **2009**, *89*, 1299–1306. [CrossRef] [PubMed]
122. Wang, Y.C.; Ludwig, D.S.; Sonneville, K.; Gortmaker, S.L. Impact of change in sweetened caloric beverage consumption on energy intake among children and adolescents. *Arch. Pediatr. Adolesc. Med.* **2009**, *163*, 336–343. [CrossRef]
123. Williams, R.; Christ, K. Mercatus on Policy, Taxing Sin: Are Excise Taxes Efficient? N°52. Available online: https://www.mercatus.org/system/files/RSP_MOP52_Taxing_Sins_web.pdf (accessed on 2 January 2019).
124. Studio Censis Coldiretti. Primo Rapporto Sulle Abitudini Alimentari Degli Italiani Sintesi dei Principali Risultati. Available online: https://www.coldiretti.it/archivio/censis-il-primo-rapporto-sulle-abitudini-alimentari-degli-italiani-alcuni-flash-19-05-2010 (accessed on 24 January 2019).
125. WHO. Fiscal Policies for Diet and the Prevention of NCD. 2016. Available online: http://apps.who.int/iris/bitstream/handle/10665/250131/9789241511247-eng.pdf;jsessionid=3A372C03CFB2A8FC33E4A03A37CFF073?sequence=1,pag.23 (accessed on 24 January 2019).
126. Garde, A.; Bartlett, O.; Ward, K. Fizzy Drinks Tax Alone Won't Solve Childhood Obesity Nightmare. Available online: https://theconversation.com/fizzy-drinks-tax-alone-wont-solve-childhood-obesity-nightmare-56523 (accessed on 24 January 2019).
127. Di Nicolantonio, J.J.; O'Keefe, J.H.; Wilson, W.L. Sugar addiction: Is it real? A narrative review. *Br. J. Sports Med.* **2018**, *52*, 910–913. [CrossRef]
128. Lien, L.; Lien, N.; Heyerdahl, S.; Thoresen, M.; Bjertness, E. Consumption of Soft Drinks and Hyperactivity, Mental Distress, and Conduct Problems Among Adolescents in Oslo, Norway. *Am. J. Public Health* **2006**, *96*, 1815–1820. [CrossRef]
129. Wansick, B.; Chandon, P. Can "Low-Fat" Nutrition Labels Lead to Obesity? *J. Mark. Res.* **2006**, *43*, 605–617. [CrossRef]
130. Scholsser, E. *Fast-Food Nation*; Allen Lane The Penguin Press: London, UK, 2001.
131. Schlosser, E. Still a Fast Food Nation: Eric Schlosser Reflects on 10 Years Later. *Retrieved* **2012**, *2*, 2017.
132. Public Health England. Sugar Reduction and Wider Reformulation Programme: Report on Progress towards the First 5% Reduction and Next Steps. Available online: https://assets.publishing.service.gov.uk/government/uploads/system/uploads/attachment_data/file/709008/Sugar_reduction_progress_report.pdf (accessed on 29 March 2019).
133. Nestle, M. *Food Politics: How the Food Industry Manipulates What We Eat to the Detriment of Our Health*; University of California Press: Berkeley, CA, USA, 2002.
134. Critser, G. *Fat Land: How Americans Became the Fattest People in the World*; Houghton Mifflin: New York, NY, USA, 2002.

135. Garde, A.; Jeffery, B.; Rigby, N. Implementing the WHO Recommendations whilst Avoiding Real, Perceived or Potential Conflicts of Interest. *Eur. J. Risk Regul.* **2017**, *8*, 237–250. [CrossRef]
136. Public Health England. Salt Targets 2017: Progress Report a Report on the Food Industry's Progress towards Meeting the 2017 Salt Targets. 2018. Available online: https://assets.publishing.service.gov.uk/government/uploads/system/uploads/attachment_data/file/765571/Salt_targets_2017_progress_report.pdf (accessed on 3 February 2019).
137. Garde, A.; Davies, S.; Landon, J. The UK Rules on Unhealthy Food Marketing to Children. *Eur. J. Risk Regul.* **2017**, *8*, 270–280. [CrossRef]
138. Nestle, M. Food Marketing and Childhood Obesity—A Matter of Policy. *N. Engl. J. Med.* **2006**, *354*, 2527–2529. [CrossRef] [PubMed]
139. Cezar, A. The Effects of Television Food Advertising on Childhood Obesity. *Nev. J. Public Health* **2008**, *5*, 2.
140. WHO. Evaluating Implementation of the WHO Set of Recommendations on the Marketing of Foods and Non-Alcoholic Beverages to Children, Progress, Challenges and Guidance for Next Steps in the WHO European Region. Available online: http://www.euro.who.int/__data/assets/pdf_file/0003/384015/food-marketing-kids-eng.pdf (accessed on 20 February 2019).
141. Fuhrer, R.; Shipley, M.J.; Chastang, J.F.; Schmaus, A.; Niedhammer, I.; Stansfeld, S.A.; Goldberg, M.; Marmot, M.G. Socioeconomic position, health, and possible explanations: A tale of two cohorts. *Am. J. Public Health* **2002**, *92*, 1290–1294. [CrossRef] [PubMed]
142. Darmon, N.; Drewnowski, A. Does social class predict diet quality? *Am. J. Clin. Nutr.* **2008**, *87*, 1107–1117. [CrossRef] [PubMed]
143. Schroder, H.; Marrugat, J.; Covas, M.I. High monetary costs of dietary patterns associated with lower body mass index: A population-based study. *Int. J. Obes.* **2006**, *30*, 1574–1579. [CrossRef] [PubMed]
144. Power, E.M. SUPPLEMENT 3: Understanding the Forces That Influence Our Eating Habits: What We Know and Need to Know (JULY/AUGUST 2005). *Can. J. Public Health* **2005**, *96*, S37–S42. Available online: https://www.jstor.org/stable/41994471 (accessed on 20 February 2019).
145. Phull, S. The Mediterranean Diet: Socio-cultural Relevance for Contemporary Health Promotion. *Open Public Health J.* **2015**, *8*, 35–40. [CrossRef]
146. UNESCO. Representative List of the Intangible Cultural Heritage of Humanity. 2013. Available online: Http://www.unesco.org/culture/ich/RL/ (accessed on 29 April 2014).
147. Keys, A. Mediterranean diet and public health: Personal reflections. *Am. J. Clin. Nutr.* **1995**, *61* (Suppl. 6), 1321S–1323S. [CrossRef] [PubMed]
148. León-Munoz, L.M.; Guallar-Castillón, P.; Graciani, A.; López-García, E.; Mesas, A.E.; Aguilera, M.T.; Banegas, J.R.; Rodríguez-Artalejo, F. Adherence to The Mediterranean Diet pattern has declined in Spanish adults. *J. Nutr.* **2012**, *142*, 1843–1850. [CrossRef] [PubMed]
149. Drewnowski, A.; Eichelsdoerfer, P. Mediterr. Diet: Does It Have Cost More? *Public Health Nutr.* **2009**, *12*, 1621–1628. [CrossRef] [PubMed]
150. OECD. Measuring Leisure in OECD Countries. In *Society at a Glance 2009*; OECD Social Indicators; OECD: Paris, France, 2009; pp. 19–49.
151. Laverack, G. *Public Health, Power, Empowerment and Professional Practice*; Palgrave McMillan: Basingstoke, UK, 2009.
152. Handy, S.L.; Boarnet, M.G.; Ewing, R.; Killingsworth, R.E. How the built environment affects physical activity: Views from urban planning. *Am. J. Prev. Med.* **2002**, *23*, 64–73. [CrossRef]
153. Thorndike, A.N.; Sonnenberg, L.; Riis, J.; Barraclough, S.; Levy, D.E. A 2-Phase Labeling and Choice Architecture Intervention to Improve Healthy Food and Beverage Choices. *Am. J. Public Health* **2012**, *102*, 527–533. [CrossRef] [PubMed]
154. Wansink, B.; Just, D.R.; Payne Collin, R. Mindless Eating and Healthy Heuristics for the Irrational. *Am. Econ. Rev.* **2009**, *99*, 165–169. [CrossRef]
155. Bourdieu, P.; Saint-Martin, M. Anatomie dugoût. *Actes Rech. Sci. Soc.* **1976**, *2*, 18–43.
156. Napier, A.D.; Ancarno, C.; Butler, B.; Calabrese, J.; Chater, A.; Chatterjee, H.; Guesnet, F.; Horne, R.; Jacyna, S.; Jadhav, S.; et al. Culture and health. *Lancet* **2014**, *384*, 1607–1639. [CrossRef]
157. Marrone, G. *Semiotica del Gusto. Linguaggi Della Cucina, del Cibo, Della Tavola*; Mimesis Insegne: Sesto San Giovanni, Milano, Italy, 2016.

158. World Health Organization (WHO). *Behaviour Change Strategies and Health: The Role of Health Systems*; EUR/RC58/Tbilisi, Georgia; WHO: Geneva, Switzerland, 2008.
159. Sassi, F.; Cecchini, M.; Lauer, J.; Chisholm, D. Improving lifestyles, tackling obesity: The health and economic impact of prevention strategies. In *OECD Health Working Papers*; OECD Publishing: Paris, France, 2009.
160. Ward, D.S.; Welker, E.; Choate, A.; Henderson, K.E.; Lott, M.; Tovar, A.; Wilson, A.; Sallis, J.F. Strength of obesity prevention interventions in early care and education settings: A systematic review. *Prev. Med.* **2017**, *95*, S37–S52. [CrossRef]
161. Abraham, C.; Kok, G.; Schaalma, H.; Luszczynska, A. *Health Promotion. The International Association of Applied Psychology Handbook of Applied Psychology*; Martin, P., Cheung, F., Kyrios, M., Littlefield, L., Knowles, L., Overmier, M., Eds.; Wiley-Blackwell: Oxford, UK, 2010.
162. Nixon, C.A.; Moore, H.J.; Douthwaite, W.; Gibson, E.L.; Vogele, C.; Kreichauf, S.; Wildgruber, A.; Manios, Y.; Summerbell, C. Identifying effective behavioural models and behaviour change strategies underpinning preschool-and school-based obesity prevention interventions aimed at 4–6-year-olds: A systematic review. *Obes. Rev.* **2012**. [CrossRef]
163. Britt, E.; Hudson, S.M.; Blampied, N.M. Motivational interviewing in health settings: A review. *Patient Educ. Couns.* **2004**, *53*, 147–155. [CrossRef]
164. Bernhardt, J.M. Communication at the Core of Effective Public Health. *Am. J. Public Health* **2004**, *94*, 2051–2053. [CrossRef] [PubMed]
165. George, E.; Kucianski, T.; Mayr, H.; Moschonis, G.; Tierney, A.; Itsiopoulos, C. A Mediterranean diet model in Australia: Strategies for Translating the Traditional Mediterranean Die tinto a Multicultural Setting. *Nutrients* **2018**, *10*, 465. [CrossRef] [PubMed]

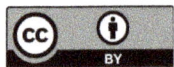

© 2019 by the authors. Licensee MDPI, Basel, Switzerland. This article is an open access article distributed under the terms and conditions of the Creative Commons Attribution (CC BY) license (http://creativecommons.org/licenses/by/4.0/).

MDPI
St. Alban-Anlage 66
4052 Basel
Switzerland
Tel. +41 61 683 77 34
Fax +41 61 302 89 18
www.mdpi.com

Nutrients Editorial Office
E-mail: nutrients@mdpi.com
www.mdpi.com/journal/nutrients

www.ingramcontent.com/pod-product-compliance
Lightning Source LLC
LaVergne TN
LVHW071940080526
838202LV00064B/6642